THIRD EDITION

THOS. FLINT, Jr., M.D.

Associate Physician, Kaiser Foundation Rehabilitation
Center and Senior Consultant, Emergency Department
and Division of Industrial Relations, Kaiser Foundation
Hospital, Vallejo, California

Formerly Director, Division of Industrial Relations, Permanente
Medical Group, Oakland and Richmond, California; Chief,
Emergency Department, Permanente Medical Group, Kaiser Foundation
Hospital, Richmond, California

EMERGENCY
TREATMENT
AND
MANAGEMENT

W. B. Saunders Company   Philadelphia and London   1964

Emergency Treatment and Management

Foreword

The third edition of this well-known work continues to exemplify the best traditions in the communication of practical modern emergency care established in the first and second editions. Its information is contemporary, comprehensive, concise and clear.

Emergencies are ubiquitous and omnipresent; they frequently occur under the most unlikely and inopportune conditions. When disaster strikes, the physician who is called upon to cope with the situation does not have the opportunity for a leisurely trip to a medical library or for perusal and evaluation of lengthy emergency treatises with dissertations on various and variable methods of treatment.

Under the trying conditions often associated with severe acute illness and injury, a book of the caliber of Doctor Flint's carried in the medical bag or automobile glove compartment and immediately available will help the physician to initiate rapid and effective action.

I am sure that the new readers around the world who refer to this book will have the same enthusiasm for the third edition as do those of us who are familiar with Doctor Flint's prior writings.

SEDGWICK MEAD, M.D., *Medical Director*
Kaiser Foundation Rehabilitation Center
Vallejo, California

Preface to the Third Edition

In recent years improvement in over-all medical care, the hallmark as well as the goal of a concerned and skilled profession, has proceeded at an accelerated pace. Management and treatment of emergency conditions has not been an exception. Important modifications in the handling of urgent medical and surgical situations have been developed, tested thoroughly, and established. For instance, closed cardiac massage has almost completely supplanted the open chest method in the treatment of cardiac arrest, and direct expired-air respiration is now accepted as the method of choice for emergency resuscitation in acute respiratory failure. New and wider uses of many potentially dangerous substances, together with the development of completely new toxic agents, have necessitated revision of portions of the section on Poisoning and the addition of new material. Changing medicolegal concepts have required interpretation and incorporation in several sections—among them Death Cases, Abandonment and Malpractice.

Throughout this third edition, related conditions have been grouped together under general topic headings whenever possible. This rearrangement, together with further simplification of the cross reference system, has been designed to facilitate and expedite locating of a specific subject—essential in an emergency text.

Although I appreciate that in different areas variations exist in legal provisions covering such subjects as privileged communications, statutes of limitation, treatment of minors, validity of treatment and autopsy permits, and causes for malpractice actions, I have found that the authorization and permit forms suggested in the text (especially in Topic 70) have wide application. Unless otherwise stated, recommendations as a rule are based on, and are in compliance with, California statutes; therefore, under other jurisdictions some modifications of details rather than principles may be necessary.

Whenever a proprietary name of a drug, compound, or preparation is mentioned in the text, it is used only as a representative of a generic class and not as an endorsement or recommendation of the specifically named proprietary preparation. In accordance with the present-day trends, all dosages are given in the metric system. As in the previous editions, the dosages given are for adults unless otherwise specified and should be modified for infants, children, and elderly or debilitated persons.

For obvious reasons it is impractical for me to thank individually all the persons who by their writings, suggestions, and critical reviews have contributed directly and indirectly to this book as well as to previous editions. However, for two important reasons I am most grateful to Dr. Sedgwick Mead, Medical Director of the Kaiser Foundation Rehabilitation Center at Vallejo —first, for his contributions to the section on Neurologic Disorders, and second, for his encouragement and tolerance during the lengthy period in which the manuscript has been in the process of preparation. To Dr. Harvey D. Cain I would like to express my deep appreciation and sincere thanks, not only for his interest and assistance in the preparation of major portions of the sections on Medical Bag Contents, Fluid Replacement, Gastrointestinal Emergencies, Phenothiazine Toxicity, and Vascular Emergencies but also for his detailed analysis and constructive criticism of the remainder of the text. Suggestions by Dr. Beatrice Lei, Dr. Marianne Leppman, and Dr. Donovan McCune, of the Pediatrics Departments of the Kaiser Hospitals at Richmond, Oakland, and Vallejo respectively have been of great assistance to me in the revision of the section on Pediatric Emergencies. Finally, I am indebted to Mrs. Florence Kerr for accurate and painstaking typing and checking of the manuscript.

Thos. Flint, Jr., M.D.
Vallejo, California

Preface to the First Edition

Many excellent texts are available covering first aid procedures, and surgical and medical care in acute conditions. The following pages, however, have a much more limited objective —the presentation of the treatment and management of the patient by the Emergency Physician from first examination until disposition for definitive treatment can be arranged. To borrow a phrase from current labor relations, I have endeavored to outline *in a rapidly available form* "portal-to-portal" care in emergency situations.

The term "Emergency Physician" has been used throughout this book to designate the physician in charge of the patient in the emergency room, department or private office. In large hospitals this physician may be on a full-time basis; in smaller units he may have numerous other duties, or be on part-time emergency call. Too often he is an intern, resident, or general practitioner of very limited experience in the management and treatment of acute conditions. To all these physicians whose contribution to the welfare of the patient is often overshadowed by a spectacular surgical procedure or a brilliant medical diagnosis, I am dedicating this book, with the hope that the information herein contained may be of some assistance to them in fulfilling their very great, and often unrecognized, responsibilities.

"Emergency Care" is used in this book in the sense of the examination, treatment and disposition of a person who has developed or sustained an unforeseen condition which is believed to call for prompt action. Examination may disclose no urgent or pressing need for treatment, and reassurance of the patient or his family may be all that is necessary. On the other hand, prompt and proper handling of the case may result in saving a life, preventing a long illness, or preserving maximum function.

In the first section are grouped some important generally applicable miscellaneous medical procedures. Administrative, medicolegal, and clerical principles and procedures which I have found to be of value in the operation of an efficient emergency service are covered in the third section. Since, by the nature of the cases which he is called upon to handle, the physician treating emergencies is especially vulnerable to legal action, the medicolegal aspects have been outlined in considerable detail. The underlying legal principles used as the basis for the medicolegal points involved are widely accepted although minor variations may occur in some localities.

In order to facilitate rapid reference all conditions covered in the second section are listed alphabetically, and cross-references are indicated. Although in some instances the most important diagnostic points have been given, I have made no attempt to cover this aspect fully. The methods of treatment suggested are *not necessarily the only proper therapeutic methods*, but they are based upon several years of experience in the handling of a large volume of emergency cases as well as upon accepted methods of emergency care. The drugs mentioned are those available in any well equipped emergency room or office. The dosages given are for adults unless otherwise specified and should, of course, be modified for infants, children or elderly persons. Whenever the use of Plazmoid is recommended, dextran, PVP (polyvinylpyrrolidone), serum albumin, or any of the other accepted plasma volume expanders can be substituted. If facilities for typing and cross matching are available the use of whole blood transfusions is even more desirable.

No attempt has been made to specify or suggest therapeutic measures after immediate emergency care with the exception of supportive therapy during ambulance transportation and occasional instructions to be carried out at home before receiving hospital or office treatment.

It will be noted that repetition and duplication occur rather frequently, particularly in the section covering *Poisoning, Acute*

[Topic 49]. I believe that *for the purpose of quick reference* this repetition will be found to be of value.

The political and social unrest so prevalent throughout the world suggests the possibility that many physicians not familiar with emergency measures may be called upon to treat large numbers of serious civilian casualties. This possibility—remote though it may be—in my opinion justifies the presentation of this summary at this time.

I should like to express my thanks to Dr. E. M. MacKay for his encouragement, constructive criticism and guidance in the preparation of this book. I am also grateful to Dr. Glenn Lubeck for his suggestions on *Cardiac Emergencies* and to Dr. Arthur Michels for the section on *Shock*. The interpretation and clarification of the medicolegal problems by Mr. James French and Mr. C. H. Brandon have been invaluable. Finally, I wish to thank Miss Bernice Turkovich for her very great assistance in the preparation of the manuscript.

THOS. FLINT, JR., M.D.

Contents

EMERGENCY TREATMENT OF SPECIFIC CONDITIONS

ADMINISTRATIVE, CLERICAL AND MEDICOLEGAL PRINCIPLES AND PROCEDURES

GENERAL MEDICAL
PRINCIPLES AND PROCEDURES

1. ABUSE OF EMERGENCY FACILITIES

1–1. Public utilization of emergency facilities as convenient 24-hour-a-day, drop-in clinics for nonurgent care has become more and more alarming during the last few years. Analyses of emergency department case loads indicate that in many localities the ratio between nonurgent and urgent cases is as high as ten to one. As a result, facilities designed, equipped and staffed for handling emergency conditions have been swamped with nonurgent patients at times when care of true emergencies [Topic 20 (Urgency Evaluation)] suddenly and unexpectedly has become imperative. In several instances in my own personal experience, this unfortunate blocking of emergency facilities has been the direct cause of detrimental delay in treatment of persons with legitimate urgent emergency conditions.
1–2. Another disturbing result of the constantly increasing public abuse of emergency facilities has been replacement of physicians who are trained and experienced—and interested— in traumatology, toxicology and urgent medical care by others whose chief knowledge and interest is in the more leisurely and less dramatic (and often more lucrative) cases usually seen in offices and nonemergency clinics. This shift in the type of professional staffing is relatively unimportant in large university-type teaching hospitals where consultants in all specialties are available on short notice around the clock, but in smaller, less elaborately staffed facilities, the inevitable result is less efficient and less proficient management of urgent cases.

2. ADDICTION

The two most common and least recognized examples of addiction in everyday life are the use of coffee and tobacco. Both fulfill the requirements for true addiction (increased tolerance and withdrawal symptoms), but social condemnation for habitual use of either has never become widespread, although it does occur in certain religious, sociologic and professional groups. The possible results of rigid government control (tried unsuccessfully and eventually repealed for alcohol and now in effect for barbiturates and narcotics) is an interesting topic for surmise. Widespread and indiscriminate use of "mood modifiers" (stimulants and tranquilizers) has introduced other problems which currently are requiring consideration.

Public attention at the present time is focused upon three main causes for addiction.

2–1. **Alcohol**

Acute dehydration and malnutrition may make hospitalization for fluid replacement necessary (Topic 7). *Delirium Tremens* (Topic 36–3) and *Alcoholic Neuritis* (Topic 47–4) as well as degenerative mental changes may require institutional care. For the toxic picture and treatment of acute alcoholism see Topic 49–227 (*Ethyl Alcohol*).

2–2. **Barbiturates**

Chronic barbiturate addiction rarely requires emergency care unless an overdose has been taken, but hospitalization is often indicated for definitive therapy since too rapid withdrawal may result in convulsions, irreversible mental changes and even death. For signs, symptoms and treatment of acute poisoning see Topic 49–76.

2–3. **Narcotics**

Whenever addiction to any of the substances covered by the Narcotics Act is known or suspected, certain restrictions apply (see 2–5, below). Most of the substances covered by the Act are included in the following list:

Alpha and beta eucaine (Topic 49–52)
Alphaprodine (Nisentil) (Topic 9–2)
Apomorphine (Topic 49–61)
Cocaine and its salts, preparations, compounds and derivatives (Topic 49–152)
Codeine and its salts, preparations, compounds and derivatives (Topic 49–153)
Dihydrocodeinone (Hycodan) (Topic 9–2)
Dihydromorphinone (Dilaudid) (Topic 49–194)
Hemp and its extracts and compounds (Topic 49–332)
Heroin (diacetylmorphine) (Topic 49–268)
Laudanum (tincture of opium) (Topic 49–370)
Levorphan (Levodromoran)
Lophorphora (mescal, peyote) (Topic 49–261 and 347)
Marihuana (*Cannabis sativa*) (Topic 49–332)
Meperidine (Demerol) (Topic 9–2)
Metapon (methyl dihydromorphinone)
Methadone (Adanon, Dolophine, Methadon)

Morphine and its salts, preparations, compounds and derivatives
(Topic 49–370)

Opium and its salts, preparations, compounds and derivatives (Topic
49–420)

Pantopon (pantopium hydrochloride) (Topic 49–420)

Paregoric (camphorated tincture of opium) (Topic 49–439)

Racemorphan (Dromoran, methylmorphinan)

2–4. **Signs and symptoms of addiction to opiate-type drugs**

A. In spite of widespread publicity to the contrary, a
habitual user of opium derivatives or synthetics of
similar action who is taking his regular dose at
accustomed intervals will rarely show any outward
evidences of his dependence on the drug. Mental
impairment of any type almost never occurs;
neither does physical or social degeneration, provided the addict is economically able to support his
very expensive habit without interruption and provided degenerative mental or physical processes
were not already present when habitual use became
established.

B. Scars—old, recently healed, healing and fresh—from
subcutaneous, intramuscular or intravenous injections.

C. Pinpoint or small pupils which react sluggishly to light.
Pupillary signs demonstrable by the usual tests may
be completely absent in persons accustomed to large
doses at frequent intervals. The nalorphine hydrochloride (Nalline) test (Topic 18–3) is of great
diagnostic value in this type of case.

2–5. **Restrictions on treatment of narcotic addiction**

In many states and countries all over the world, ambulatory
treatment of narcotic addiction is unlawful. As a result, in these
areas addicts can be treated only if they are under complete
control—usually in government certified institutions. Therefore,
only palliative symptomatic care (sedation, hydration, supportive therapy, etc.) can be given while arranging for disposition of the patient with the proper, certified agencies.

Whenever possible, patients should be encouraged to arrange
voluntarily for treatment in a controlled environment by physicians especially trained in this very difficult therapy.

The usual exceptions to these restrictions are:

A. An acute condition which in itself requires use of a
narcotic drug.

B. If the patient has been booked and is in custody of a law enforcement officer.

C. If the patient has an incurable or terminal condition. In this instance the patient must be registered with the proper enforcement agency. The following form is usually required:

MAIL TO:
BUREAU OF NARCOTIC ENFORCEMENT

NAME OF PATIENT	AGE
ADDRESS	
STREET	CITY
QUANTITY AND KIND OF NARCOTIC	
DAILY DOSAGE	
DIAGNOSIS OF INJURY OR AILMENT	
HAS PATIENT PREVIOUSLY USED NARCOTICS?	ADDICTED?
	YES OR NO YES OR NO
PHYSICIAN'S SIGNATURE	
ADDRESS	
STREET	CITY
DATE OF REPORT	FED. REG. NO.

3. COMA

Common causes of coma (complete loss of consciousness— no response to painful stimuli) are listed below. For clinical approach to management of coma of undetermined origin see Topic 47–1 (*Neurologic Disorders*).

3–1. **Acute infectious diseases**

Especially in children, acute infectious diseases may cause deep coma. Treatment depends upon the causative condition (see Topic 32, *Contagious and Communicable Diseases*, Topic 48, *Pediatric Emergencies*, and Topic 63, *Virus Infections*).

3–2. **Cardiac decompensation.** See Topic 29 (*Cardiac Emergencies*).

3–3. **Diabetes mellitus**

    A. Two conditions directly related to diabetes may require emergency care, hyperglycemia (diabetic coma) and hyperinsulinism (insulin shock). Each may be fatal if not recognized promptly and treated adequately, and each responds spectacularly to proper therapy.

    Laboratory determinations of blood sugar levels and carbon dioxide combining power are sometimes essential for differential diagnosis but, unfortunately, they are seldom available in emergency situations. Therefore, the attending physician may be forced to base his diagnosis on any history which he may be able to obtain from members of the family, friends or persons who observed the onset of the condition, and on careful clinical examination and observation (Topic 47–1). If there is any doubt concerning the differential diagnosis, a small amount of dextrose given intravenously is a valuable diagnostic test. If the coma is hyperglycemic, no harm will result; on the other hand, additional insulin may be fatal to a person already in insulin shock.

B. Differential Diagnosis

	Hyperglycemia (Diabetic Coma)	Hyperinsulinism (Insulin Shock or Reaction)
History	Known diabetes; progressively increasing thirst, air hunger, sleepiness; nausea and vomiting	Rapid onset following dose of insulin; may not have eaten usual meal before or after dose; may have taken excessive dose of insulin
Diet	Too much food	Not enough food
Nausea and vomiting	Often present	Seldom present

	Hyperglycemia (*Diabetic Coma*)	*Hyperinsulinism* (*Insulin Shock or Reaction*)
Fever	May be present	Seldom present
Facies	Looks toxic	Looks pale and weak
Eyeballs	Soft	Normal
Skin	Dry	Moist
Respiration	Rapid; air hunger	Normal
Abdominal pain	Common; may simulate an acute surgical abdomen	Absent
Mental state	Gradual development of coma	Sudden onset of delirium followed by deep coma; bizarre neurologic pictures may develop rapidly
Infection	May bring on symptoms	No effect
Insulin	May have omitted usual dose	Always has taken dose; sometimes excessive amount
Urine	Sugar and diacetic acid present	Sugar may be present, diacetic acid absent in first specimen; second specimen, both absent
Blood sugar (normal, 80–120 mg. %)	Above normal level	Below normal level
CO_2 combining power (normal, 45–70 volumes %)	20 volumes % or less	Normal
Response to treatment	Slow	Rapid (may be delayed if protamine zinc or NPH insulin overdosage)

C. Treatment of Diabetic Coma

1. WHEN THE PATIENT IS FIRST SEEN—*not* in a hospital:
   a. Draw 20 ml. of blood for serum sugar, plasma acetone, potassium, BUN, HCO_3, and pH, and for typing and crossmatching when facilities are available. This blood specimen must be sent with the patient to the hospital.
   b. Start intravenous infusion of 500 ml. of ⅙ molar sodium lactate solution.
   c. Give 100 units of regular insulin intravenously at

once through the infusion tubing if Kussmaul's respiration and a 4 plus acetone and sugar are present.

d. Treat shock (Topic 15–7). Keep the patient warm but not hot—room temperature is satisfactory.

e. Transport the patient immediately to an adequately equipped hospital.

2. WHEN THE PATIENT REACHES THE HOSPITAL:

a. Complete the blood tests specified above.

b. Obtain a hematocrit, white blood count and differential.

c. Obtain a urine specimen without catheterization if possible; otherwise, insertion of an indwelling catheter (Topic 17–3) is mandatory.

d. Start hourly urine volume, sugar and acetone determinations.

e. Obtain an electrocardiogram.

f. If febrile, culture according to the source of infection.

g. Wash the stomach; continue suction through a nasogastric tube until the patient becomes responsive and cooperative.

h. Start an intravenous infusion of 750 ml. of ⅙ molar sodium lactate plus 250 ml. of normal saline with the following modifications:

(1) When the urine output is adequate and the ECG does not show evidence of an increased potassium level, add 1 to 4 gm. of potassium chloride, depending on the need.

(2) Do not add dextrose until the serum glucose level is under 250 ml. %.

(3) Adjust the rate of infusion according to the degree of dehydration. Five to 7 liters of fluid plus electrolytes (Topic 7) may be required in the first 24 hours. If indicated, give 500 ml. of whole blood or plasma simultaneously with the molar lactate–normal saline infusion.

i. Inject 200 units of regular insulin intravenously every 2 hours until the blood sugar level is less than 300 mg. %, then decrease the regular insulin to 40 units or less subcutaneously.

Continue close observation and recording of vital signs every hour until stabilized.

D. Treatment of Insulin Shock or Reaction
1. Give 30 ml. of 50% dextrose in water intravenously.
2. Inject 0.5 to 1.0 mg. of glucagon hydrochloride (glucagon) intramuscularly or intravenously.
3. When the patient is conscious enough to swallow, give orange juice or sweet soft drinks by mouth. Glucose solution can also be given through the nasogastric tube.
4. Watch carefully for relapses which may occur in the presence of long acting hypoglycemic agents if therapy is not continued.

3–4. **Eclampsia.** See Topic 50–9 and 10 (*Pre-eclamptic Toxemia*).

3–5. **Electrical shock**
   A. Severe cases are usually caused by contact with low voltage circuits and are characterized by ventricular fibrillation and respiratory paralysis. Once the former is established, resuscitative measures (Topic 13) are rarely successful; however, closed chest cardiac massage (Topic 17–2,A) and expired air respiration (Topic 17–1) should be tried, with external defibrillation (Topic 17–2,A,9) when and if equipment is available. WHEN IN DOUBT, DEFIBRILLATE!
   B. If there is perceptible heart action:
   1. Start mouth-to-mouth respiration (Topic 17–1,A) and continue until mechanical methods such as a close-fitting face mask or intranasal catheter and rebreathing bag can be substituted. Closed chest cardiac massage (Topic 17–2,A) may be required as an adjunct to weak or irregular heart action. Resuscitation should be continued FOR AT LEAST 4 HOURS before declaring the patient dead. The attending physician should remember that the presumptive signs of death (Topic 4–2) often do not apply following an electrical shock and that normal breathing and heart action have been re-established as long as 8 hours after contact with the current.

    2. Keep the patient comfortably warm (but not hot) during resuscitative measures.

    3. Do not give stimulant (analeptic) drugs; they are of no value until the breathing center has recovered and spontaneous respiration has been established.

3–6. Emphysema

Comatose patients with pulmonary emphysema are frequently (and mistakenly) considered as being beyond aid. However, recognition of the condition and immediate institution of the following measures may result in restoring persons with this condition to useful activity:

    1. Tracheotomy (Topic 17–11,B,2) to lessen airway resistance, using a large diameter tube.

    2. Cleansing of the airway by suction to remove mucus plugs from the large bronchi.

    3. Intermittent positive pressure breathing by use of a Bird, Bennett or other mechanical respirator. Depression of the respiratory center by intravenous morphine sulfate may be necessary to allow the apparatus to function efficiently. Moisture should be supplied by a saline spray. Detergents should never be used.

    4. Restoration of normal fluid balance (Topic 7).

    5. Administration of broad spectrum antibiotics.

3–7. Epilepsy. See also Topic 33 (*Convulsive Seizures*).

Prevention of injury (especially tongue biting) and, in severe cases, sedation by intravenous administration of a rapidly acting barbiturate, is all that can be done in emergencies of this type. Cerebral stimulants to shorten the unconscious periods are definitely contraindicated; they may result in severe prolonged headaches and extreme exhaustion. Restraint may be necessary during the convulsive episode. Complete recovery is the rule and hospitalization is rarely necessary. The need for carefully supervised long-term therapy should be stressed.

3–8. Episodic or recurrent unconsciousness. See Topic 51–8.

3–9. Excessive heat. See Topic 57–4 (*Heat Stroke*) and Topic 57–8 (*Sunstroke*).

3–10. Hepatic coma

Treatment

    1. Treatment of shock (Topic 15–7) and hemorrhage (Topic 8).

    2. Reduction of body protein breakdown by intravenous

infusion of 800 calories of dextrose in hypertonic solution per day.

3. Reduction of intestinal ammonia caused by bacterial decomposition. Give 1.0 gm. of neomycin orally every 6 hours.

4. Sedation with chloral hydrate or paraldehyde as needed.

5. Balancing of fluid input and output if hepatorenal symptoms are present, with avoidance of saline. Protein intake should be sharply limited.

6. Administration of vitamin K oxide.

7. Cautious treatment of anemia.

3–11. **Intracranial pathology.** See Topic 43 and Topic 60–2.

3–12. **Myxedema.** See Topic 35–5,A,1.

3–13. **Poisons**

The poisons listed in this section are those which are characterized by rapid action, with coma usually the main or presenting symptom.

   A. Alcohol. See Topic 49–227 (*Ethyl Alcohol*).

   B. Barbiturates. See Topic 49–76.

   C. Carbon Monoxide. See Topic 49–119.

   D. Chloral Hydrate. See Topic 49–128.

   E. Morphine and Related Opiates. See Topic 9 (*Narcotics*); and Topic 49–370 (*Morphine*).

3–14. **Shock following trauma, severe burns or hemorrhage.** See Topic 15.

3–15. **Uremia**

If uremic convulsions or coma have developed, symptomatic treatment is all that can be done. Sedatives, hypnotics and narcotics may be given as required while hospitalization is being arranged.

3–16. **Rare causes of coma**

   A. Syphilis of the central nervous system.

   B. Malaria.

   C. Tuberculosis, acute miliary, meningeal form.

   D. Encephalitis.

   E. Brain tumors.

   These conditions require only supportive and symptomatic care before and during transfer for hospitalization.

3–17. **Coma of undetermined etiology.** See Topic 47–1.

4. DEATH CASES

4–1. Absence of accepted criteria for determining time of death

Modern methods of resuscitation (Topic 17–1 and 2) have been spectacularly successful—so much so that the point at which death ends human existence has become difficult to determine. Although respiratory and higher nervous system centers have been destroyed by prolonged anoxia, viability of what has been termed "a human heart-lung preparation" may be continued for lengthy periods by various means. It seems probable that at some time in the future some type of civil action—for instance, an important will contest—will result in establishment of generally accepted basic medicolegal criteria for "life," "existence" and "death."

4–2. Presumptive signs of death

A. No response to painful stimuli.

B. No pulse or heart beat by palpation or auscultation.

C. No breath sounds on auscultation; no fogging of a freshly polished mirror held close to the nostrils or mouth.

D. Complete absence of corneal and deep tendon reflexes.

E. Absence of evidence of blood pressure by sphygmomanometer.

F. A flat base line on all electrocardiographic (ECG) leads.

G. Doughy resistance to passive motion suggestive of developing rigor mortis.

H. Dependent lividity and cyanosis.

I. Decreased body temperature in relation to environment.

These presumptive signs are usually considered to be adequate for determination of death when they occur following severe trauma or in the terminal stages of chronic illnesses such as malignancy with metastases or uremia in a patient with whom the attending physician is thoroughly familiar. They are NOT adequate for determination of death when catastrophic emergency conditions such as acute poisoning (Topic 49), myocardial infarction (Topic 29–5) or electrical shock (Topic

3–5) have occurred, or if the attending physician is not familiar with the patient's underlying condition and with the events leading up to, and climaxed by, the apparent terminal state.

4–3. **Conclusive signs of death**

    A. Complete partition of parts of the body incompatible with life (examples: complete decapitation, separation of the trunk into two or more completely detached parts with no one portion containing adequate vital organs, etc.).

    B. Generalized body putrefaction.

    C. Fully established rigor mortis.

    D. Flat lines without evidence of rhythm in all leads of an electroencephalographic (EEG) tracing, not modified by loud noises. When there have been no EEG changes present for one hour, the attending physician is fully justified in certifying to the death of the patient and in terminating resuscitative measures, even if agonal cardiac ventricular activity is still demonstrable by electrocardiogram. The time at which cardiac circulatory support was discontinued should be entered on the clinical record and indicated on the death certificate (Topic 66–6,B) as the time of death. The clinical record should give an accurate account of findings and therapy and, if possible, should be countersigned by another physician.

4–4. **Dead on arrival (DOA) cases**

These should be registered in the usual manner (Topic 67), using "John Doe" or "Jane Doe" if unidentified. Any available information regarding details of the illness or accident, cause of death, etc., together with external signs of trauma and other objective findings, should be entered in detail on the emergency record.

Any physician called upon to examine a suspected DOA has the very great responsibility of determining to the best of his ability if life is, in fact, extinct. If there is any suspicion in his mind that life might still be present, immediate and vigorous resuscitative and supportive measures should be begun (Topic 13). Careful recheck examinations should be done at frequent intervals until there is ABSOLUTELY no doubt in the mind of the attending physician that life is no longer present.

CASES IN WHICH A SPARK OF LIFE IS SUSPECTED, AND WHICH RECEIVE ANY TREATMENT, SHOULD NOT BE CLASSIFIED AS "DOA."

All DOA cases must be reported at once to the coroner's office and the remains, together with any personal belongings, turned over to the coroner or his representative.

4–5. **Coroner's or medical examiner's cases**

    A. The circumstances under which a death case comes under the jurisdiction of the coroner (in some areas called the medical examiner) vary in minor details in different localities, but, in general, responsibility is transferred from the attending physician to the coroner or medical examiner in the locality or political subdivision in which the death occurs in the instances listed below. When a coroner or medical examiner assumes responsibility, his authority is supreme and completely supersedes the usual rights of the surviving spouse or next of kin (4–6,B, below).

      1. All DOAs (4–4, above).

      2. All deaths without previous medical care.

      3. All suicides (Topic 16).

      4. All violent deaths.

      5. All deaths resulting directly or indirectly from an accident at any time in the past.

      6. All cases in which there are reasonable grounds for suspecting that death may have resulted from criminal acts of another person or persons.

      7. When the deceased had not been seen by his attending physician for 7 or more days before death.

      8. When the patient had been hospitalized for 24 hours or less.

      9. All instances in which the attending physician is unable or unwilling to sign the death certificate (Topic 66–6,B).

    B. The attending physician CANNOT sign the death certificate (Topic 66–6,B) or arrange for or perform an autopsy (4–6, below) in coroner's cases unless specifically designated to do so by the coroner or his representative. The decision regarding the need for an autopsy, and its extent, is made solely by the coroner.

4–6. **Autopsies (postmortem examinations)**

  A. Coroner's Cases. The request for autopsy must be signed
      by a representative of the coroner's office. The
      signature of any other person is of no value.

  B. Non-coroner's Cases

    1. REQUEST AND PERMIT FOR AUTOPSY. Any type of
       postmortem examination, with or without re-
       moval of tissue, requires completion BEFORE
       THE EXAMINATION IS BEGUN of a properly
       signed and witnessed autopsy permit (Topic
       70–3). Any type of postmortem examination
       without such permission constitutes actionable
       assault. There are no universal specifications in
       regard to the persons who may authorize post-
       mortem examinations but, in general, priority is
       usually considered to be as follows:

      a. The surviving spouse.
      b. Surviving children over 21 years of age.
      c. Surviving parents of the deceased.
      d. Surviving adult siblings of the deceased.
      e. Other surviving adult kin in order of closest blood
         relationship.

Although the signature of only one of several persons of the
same degree of blood relationship is required by law, it is always desirable to obtain as many as practical without delaying
the autopsy.

    2. Any limitations or restrictions on the extent and scope
       of the postmortem examination, or unusual spe-
       cial instructions, must be specified on the "Au-
       topsy Permit" form (Topic 70–3) and must be
       scrupulously observed by the autopsy surgeon or
       pathologist. Any examination or removal of tis-
       sues in excess of, or in addition to, those spe-
       cifically authorized is prima facie evidence of
       law violation even if, in the opinion of the au-
       topsy surgeon, such additional examination is
       absolutely necessary to determine the cause of
       death.

       Examples: "No brain examination"
                 "Enucleation of both eyes for donation to
                 _____ Hospital for
                 scientific purposes."

"Bone for donation to _____
Hospital Bone Bank."

3. No specific authorization [except if coroner's cases (4–5, above)] is required for postmortem examinations on industrial cases (Topic 76).

4–7. Disposal of remains

A. If the decedent leaves written instructions in a will or other document, his remains should be disposed of in accordance with his instructions even if other provisions of the will are subject to dispute.

B. If the decedent leaves no will or written instructions, the decision regarding disposition follows the same priority as outlined under Autopsy Permits (4–6,B, above and Topic 70–3).

C. *Stillbirths* (for definition see Topic 66–4).

When the parents do not wish custody of a dead fetus, a permit "to preserve or dispose" (Topic 70–10), should be properly signed and witnessed.

4–8. Religious rites

Considerable variation exists among religious groups regarding procedural rites before, at or after death. Accepted procedures, in some of which the attending physician may of necessity be forced to participate, are outlined under sections A, B and C, on page 18.

A. Premature or Other Infants in Critical Condition: Stillbirths, Abortions

General Instructions	Roman Catholic	Jewish	Protestant
	Excluding Anglo-Catholic, Eastern Orthodox and Polish National Catholic	The Conservative, Orthodox and Reform branches specify minor differences in certain rites.	Presbyterian, Episcopalian, Lutheran, Moravian, etc.
Notify the closest representative of the patient's church group, but if death is imminent, do not await his arrival.	Call a priest (addressed as "Father").	Call a rabbi (addressed as "Rabbi").	Call a minister (addressed generally as "Mister" or "Doctor," never as "Reverend"; Lutheran, "Pastor"; high church Episcopal, "Father").
BAPTISM "I baptize you in the name of the Father and of the Son and of the Holy Spirit, Amen."	Required for infants in danger of death and for all products of conception, no matter how early. Water must flow on the skin. If born with membranes intact, immerse in water and break membranes. If in utero, hypodermic injection of sterile water through membranes. (Must be done by a physician.)	No. Jewish males are circumcised on the 8th day after birth—no religious rites of any type for females.	Required for all viable infants and stillbirths, not for early products of conception. (Exceptions —Baptists and Disciples of Christ not baptized.) Water must touch skin— excess poured off— cloths, cotton, etc., used to wipe skin or head must be burned at once.
Name Necessary?	No. Give full details to priest on his arrival.	No.	Yes. If no given name, specify "Baby Boy Doe." Give full details to minister on his arrival.

B. Persons on Critical List for Any Reason

	Roman Catholic	Jewish	Protestant
Physician's responsibility	Call a priest to administer the required sacraments of Penance, Holy Communion and Extreme Unction. Arrange complete privacy for confession.	Call a rabbi—preferably of the branch (Conservative, Orthodox, Reformed) to which the patient belongs.	Call a minister—preferably of the patient's own denomination. In certain instances, Holy Communion, Penance and Extreme Unction may be required. Arrange for privacy.

C. Death Cases

	Roman Catholic	Jewish	Protestant
Last rites	Call a priest. If last rites have not been given before death, Extreme Unction can be administered conditionally for several hours afterward, provided the body has not been shrouded or covered.	No last rites. Notify a rabbi or a responsible member of the Jewish community so that arrangements for disposition of remains, burial, etc., can be made.	No last rites after death.
Permission for autopsy?	No objection on religious grounds.	Because of religious objections, permission will have to be obtained through a rabbi.	No moral or religious objection to autopsy.

5. DRUG DOSAGE IN CHILDREN

The following dosage table is satisfactory for emergency use except in those instances where a specific dose/age, dose/weight, or dose/skin surface ratio is specified in the text.

Age	Comparison with Adult Dose	Age	Comparison with Adult Dose
1 month	$\frac{1}{20}$	3 years	$\frac{1}{5}$
3 months	$\frac{1}{15}$	4 years	$\frac{1}{4}$
6 months	$\frac{1}{10}$	5–6 years	$\frac{1}{3}$
9 months	$\frac{1}{9}$	7–8 years	$\frac{1}{2}$
1 year	$\frac{1}{7}$	9–12 years	$\frac{5}{8}$
2 years	$\frac{1}{6}$	13–15 years	$\frac{3}{4}$

Infants are especially susceptible to the action of narcotics; therefore, from the age of 6 months to 2 years doses should be reduced below this schedule by at least one half.

DO NOT GIVE ANY NARCOTICS OF ANY KIND UNDER ANY CIRCUMSTANCES TO ANY INFANT UNDER SIX MONTHS OF AGE.

6. EMERGENCY MEDICAL BAG CONTENTS

The contents of an emergency bag will, of course, vary to some extent according to the owner's type of practice and individual preferences, and with the proximity of a well-equipped emergency room. Some physicians may wish to add to or delete some items from the lists suggested below. However, a bag containing the basic items specified under Equipment (Diagnostic) (6–1, below), Medications (6–2, below), and Therapeutic Supplies (6–3, below) will give the emergency physician enough equipment and supplies to give practical, efficient and satisfactory emergency care for almost all urgent conditions (Topic 20). A strongly constructed bag 17 inches long, 9 inches wide, and 11 inches deep, with covered side compartments in the top, will accommodate all of the basic equipment suggested in 6–1, 2 and 3 (below), with a total over-all weight of between 20 and 25 pounds.

The basic emergency bag contents suggested below are listed alphabetically, not in order of importance. Each article should, if possible, be packaged separately, labeled clearly for rapid identification, and kept in one specific place in the bag. Medications (especially solutions) should be in separate individual doses and not in stock bottles. Parenteral medications should, when practical, be carried in single-dose sterile vials.

REPLACEMENT OF EACH ITEM as soon as possible after use IS IMPERATIVE! Expiration dates should be checked monthly.

6–1. Equipment (diagnostic)

ITEM	QUANTITY	DESCRIPTION AND USE
1.	1 set	Batteries and bulb (spare) to fit electrical diagnostic equipment. A battery-containing universal handle to fit laryngoscope, ophthalmoscope, otoscope and flashlight is highly recommended to save space and weight. A nickel-cadmium battery unit, rechargeable for short use in 5 minutes, is even better and obviates carrying spare batteries.
2.	4	Finger cots, assorted sizes, for digital examination and protection of small finger dressings and for use as "flutter" valves in tension pneumothorax, etc.
3.	2	Fluorescein ophthalmic solution (1%); one dose packages.
4.	2 pairs	Gloves, sterile, disposable.
5.	3	Laryngoscope with 3 blades (infant, medium, large) to fit universal handle (Item 1, above).
6.	1	Ophthalmoscope–otoscope combination to fit universal handle (Item 1, above).
7.	1	Phenylephrine hydrochloride (Neo-Synephrine), 10% solution, 5 ml. dropper vial (for funduscopic examination).
8.	1	Rectal lubricant (K-Y Jelly) 2 oz. in airtight container.
9.	1	Reflex hammer, preferably containing a camel's hair brush and sharp stylet in the handle.
10.	1	Sphygmomanometer, aneroid, with self-adherent cuff (can also be used as a tourniquet).
11.	1	Spinal puncture needle with stylet (22 gauge).
12.	1	Stethoscope, preferably of the folding type with flexible tubes.
13.	2	Thermometers (oral and rectal) in break-resistant case.
14.	1	Thoracentesis needle, 18 gauge, short bevel, 3" long, hypodermic (for pericardial aspiration and treatment of tension pneumothorax).
15.	4	Tongue blades, individually packaged.

6-2. Medications

ITEM	QUANTITY	NAME	HOW GIVEN	DESCRIPTION AND AMOUNT
16.	2	Aminophylline	I.V.	Ampules, 0.5 gm.
17.	3	Amobarbital sodium (Amytal Sodium)	I.M. or I.V.	Ampules, 250 mg.
18.	4	Atropine sulfate	Oral, I.M. or I.V.	H.T., 0.4 mg.
19.	2	Caffeine sodiobenzoate	I.M. I.V.	Ampules, 0.5 gm.
20.	4	Codeine sulfate	Oral I.M.	H.T., 30 mg.
21.	1	Dextrose in water (50%)	I.V.	Ampule, 50 ml.
22.	4	Digoxin (Lanoxin)	I.V.	Ampules, 2 ml. (0.25 mg./ml.)
23.	10	Digoxin (Lanoxin)	I.M. Oral	Tablets, 0.25 mg.
24.	1	Digoxin (Lanoxin)	Oral	Bottle, 60 ml. (0.05 mg./ml.) Pediatric elixir
25.	1	Diphenylhydantoin	I.M. I.V.	Ampule, 250 mg.
26.	2	Diphenylhydramine (Benadryl)	I.M. I.V.	Ampules, 1 ml. (50 mg./ml.)
27.	4	Epinephrine hydrochloride (Adrenalin Hydrochloride)	I.M. I.V.	Ampules, 1 ml. of 1:1000 solution
28.	1	Hydrocortisone succinate (Solu-Cortef)	I.V.	Mix-O-Vial, 100 mg.
29.	1	Ipecac, syrup of	Oral	Bottle, 30 ml.
30.	2	Isoproterenol hydrochloride (Isuprel)	I.V.	Ampules, 5 ml. (1 mg.)
31.	1	Mephenteramine (Wyamine)	I.M. I.V.	Vial, 10 ml. (30 mg./ml.)
32.	1	Meralluride (Mercuhydrin)	I.M. I.V.	Vial, 10 ml.

ITEM	QUANTITY	NAME	HOW GIVEN	DESCRIPTION AND AMOUNT
33.	2	Methylergonovine maleate (Methergine)	I.M.	Ampules, 1 ml. (0.2 mg./ml.)
34.	6	Morphine sulfate	I.V. Oral	H.T., 15 mg.
35.	4	Nitroglycerin	Sublingual	Tablets, 0.3 mg.
36.	2	Penicillin G potassium (Crystapen)	I.V.	Vials, sterile powder, 1.5 million units
37.	1	Phenobarbital sodium	I.M.	Vial, 130 mg.
38.	10	Phenoxymethyl penicillin (V-Cillin)	Oral	Tablets, 250 mg.
39.	2	Pontocaine ½%	Local	One dose packages for anesthesia of eye
40.	1	Procainamide hydrochloride (Pronestyl)	I.M.	Vial, 10 ml. (10 mg./ml.)
41.	1	Procaine hydrochloride	H. I.M.	Vial, 20 ml. of 1% solution for local anesthesia
42.	1	Prochlorperazine (Compazine)	I.M. I.V.	Vial, 10 ml. (5 mg./ml.)
43.	10	Secobarbital (Seconal)	Oral	Capsules, 100 mg.
44.	1	Sodium bicarbonate	I.V.	Vial, 50 ml. (3.75 gm.)
45.	2	Tetracycline	I.M.	Vials, 100 mg.
46.	10	Tetracycline phosphate complex (Sumycin)	Oral	Capsules, 250 mg. and suspension (60 ml.)
47.	4	Water (sterile)		Ampules, 10 ml.

6–3. Therapeutic supplies

ITEM	QUANTITY	DESCRIPTION
48.	1 roll	Adhesive tape—3".
49.	1	Alcohol 70%, 120 ml. in plastic nonbreakable bottle with screw top.
50.	6	Applicators, cotton-tipped, sterile, individually packaged.
51.	1 pair	Bandage scissors.
52.	1 box	Bandages, sterile, assorted sizes (Band-Aids)
53.	2	Eye patches.
54.	1	File, small, for opening ampules and vials.
55.	2	Gauze roller bandages, sterile, 1".
56.	2	Gauze roller bandages, sterile, 2".
57.	8	Gauze pads, sterile, 2" x 2", individually packaged.
58.	4	Gauze pads, sterile, 4" x 4", individually packaged.
59.	8	Hypodermic needles, sterile, individually packaged and labeled.
		2 26 gauge, ⅞" long
		2 24 gauge, 1½" long
		3 22 gauge, 2" long
		1 18 gauge, 3" long
60.	8	Hypodermic syringes, glass, Luer type, sterile, individually packaged and labeled.
		2 syringe, 1 ml. (tuberculin)
		4 syringe, 2 ml.
		1 syringe, 5 ml.
		1 syringe, 10 ml.
		(Disposable plastic syringes can be substituted for glass type but are not so satisfactory for intravenous injections.)
61.	3	Laryngeal intubation tubes (assorted sizes) including one No. 16 rubber catheter.
62.	1 doz.	Matches, friction type, in waterproof container.
63.	1	Pad—prescription.
64.	1	Pad—notes.
65.	1	Pocket knife, large pointed blade.
66.	2	"Resusitubes" (plastic), small and large, for expired air ventilation.
67.	6	Safety pins, assorted sizes, nonsterile, in plastic box. (Can be bent to form small self-retaining retractors.)
68.	1 roll	Scotch tape, ¾" width.
70.	1	Tincture of benzoin, 30 ml. bottle.
69.	1	Tincture of merthiolate, 30 ml. bottle.

6–4. **Additional equipment**
(Optional—can be carried in the car trunk separately from the basic bag.)

A. Intravenous Starter Set
1. 1 Dextrose, 5% in saline, 500 ml.
2. 1 Dextrose, 5% in water, 500 ml.
3. 1 Plasma, dried, 1 unit.
4. 1 Sodium lactate, 1/6 molar solution, 500 ml.
5. 2 Needles, blunt bevel, 20 gauge, 2" long.
6. 2 Disposable tubing sets.

B. Lavage and Catheterization Setup

ITEM	QUANTITY	DESCRIPTION
1.	4	Adaptors (plastic or metal, *not* glass) to fit funnel, catheters, gastric lavage tubes and rubber tubing.
2.	2	Adaptors (plastic or metal), Y-tube.
3.	4	Catheters (sterile), individually packaged, 3 male (small, medium and large); one female (plastic, nonbreakable) with adaptor to fit plastic funnel, bulb syringe and rubber tubing.
4.	1	Funnel (plastic) with adaptors to fit lavage tubes, catheters and rubber tubing.
5.	3	Gastric lavage tubes (Ewald type), small, medium and large.
6.	1	Syringe, rubber bulb type, large, with rubber tubing.

C. Obstetric—Gynecologic
1. 1 clamp, large (Kocher), sterile.
2. Forceps, sterile.
3. 2 silver nitrate solution (1%), individual dose package. (For prophylactic use on newborns).
4. 2 umbilical cord ties (sterile).
5. 1 vaginal speculum, medium size.

D. Orthopedic

ITEM	QUANTITY	DESCRIPTION
1.	1	Aluminum, sheet, malleable, 14" x 5", for small splints.
2.	1 pair	Electrician's pliers, 6", alligator—nose tips.
3.	1 pair	Mechanic's pliers with side-cutting jaws.
4.	1 pair	Metal scissors, heavy enough to cut sheet aluminum (Item 1).
5.	3	Finger splints, metal.
6.	8	Plaster of paris rolls + 2 rolls padding (sheet wadding).
		2 1" rolls
		3 2" rolls
		3 3" rolls
7.	1 roll	Stockinette, bias-cut.

E. Poison Kit. Certain physicians will wish to carry with them a separate bag for treatment of poisoning of all types. This kit should contain the following items, some of which are duplicated in the basic emergency bag described in 6–1, 2 and 3, above:

Acetic acid, 5%
Ammonia water, 0.2%
Amyl nitrite pearls
Amytal Sodium (parenteral)
Apomorphine (parenteral)
Atropine sulfate (parenteral)
Caffeine and sodiobenzoate
  (parenteral)
Calcium gluconate, 10%
  (parenteral)
Dimercaprol (BAL)
Edathamil calcium disodium
  (EDTA)
Hydrocortisone succinat. or
  phosphate (parenteral)
Ipecac syrup
Magnesium hydroxide (milk of
  magnesia)
Metaraminol bitartrate
  (Aramine) (parenteral)
Methylene blue, 1% aqueous
  (parenteral)

Nalorphine or levallorphan
Paraldehyde
Phenobarbital sodium (parenteral)
Phenylephrine hydrochloride (Neo-
  Synephrine) (parenteral)
Potassium chloride (tablets and
  parenteral)
Potassium permanganate
Procainamide (parenteral)
Sodium bicarbonate, 5%
Sodium formaldehyde
  sulfoxylate, 5%
Sodium thiosulfate, 25%
  (parenteral)
Starch
"Universal antidote"
  (Topic 49–10)
Vitamin K_1 oxide (AquaMephyton)
Water (distilled, sterile) for
  dilution and injection

F. Specimen Collection Setup

QUANTITY	DESCRIPTION
1	Clinitest packet containing dropper, test tube, individually wrapped Clinitest and Acetest tablets.
2	Culture tubes, 5 ml., plastic screw top, small blank label attached.
1 box	Labels, gummed, small.
2	Microscope slides, in container.
2	Tubes, sterile, 10 ml., screw tops, blank label attached, for blood samples.
2	Bottles, sterile, large mouth, screw top, 120 ml., for specimens of urine, vomitus, stool, etc.

G. Surgical Setup

QUANTITY	DESCRIPTION
4	Clamps (hemostats), sterile, individually packaged: 2 small (mosquito or Kelly); 2 large (Carmalt or Kocher).
1	Eye scalpel, bistoury point, sterile, separately wrapped.
1	Eye spud, small.
3	Forceps (sterile), individually packaged and labeled.
	1 thumb forceps, plain tip
	1 thumb forceps, rat-tooth tip
	1 splinter forceps, small

QUANTITY	DESCRIPTION
1	Probe, flexible wire, ball tip.
1	Razor, safety, with package of blades.
1	Scalpel handle (Bard-Parker No. 3) with 3 individually packaged sterile blades, assorted shapes, to fit handle.
1 pair	Scissors, Mayo type (1 sharp, 1 rounded point).
1	Ring cutter in case.
3	Suture sets in individual tubes,
	1 5–0 Dermalon with affixed needle
	1 3–0 Dermalon with affixed needle
	1 2–0 Plain catgut with affixed needle

H. Oxygen Tank (small) with attached face mask and rebreathing bag.

I. Electrocardiograph, portable.

J. Miscellaneous

Emergency textbook.

Flashlight.

Road and street map.

Restraint straps (4), 1″ webbing, airplane-type quick release buckles.

Rubber tubing (2 rolls) ¼″ to ⅜″ bore, 18 to 31 inches long for use as tourniquets, etc.

6–5. Precautions

A. The basic emergency bag, as well as optional kits, should be kept out of public view as much as possible, preferably locked in the luggage compartment. If carried on the seat or floor of the car, they should be covered. All equipment will be safer if the car does not carry M.D. identification.

B. When a physician receives an emergency night call, a spotlight, either transportable or mounted on the car, and a good map of any unfamiliar localities are invaluable.

C. If calls for emergency treatment are received from persons who are not known to the physician, or if the circumstances of the call are unusual, it may be prudent for the physician to request a police escort, particularly if the area to be visited has a high crime rate.

7. *FLUID REPLACEMENT IN EMERGENCIES*

Proper replacement of fluid is an often overlooked and neglected aspect of the care of emergency cases that in certain situations may be lifesaving. The following principles of replacement therapy may require modification because of limited facilities for laboratory determination but, in many instances, clinical examination will allow institution of therapy which can be continued during transfer to a hospital where accurate confirmatory laboratory tests can be obtained. In all instances an ACCURATE record of intake, both parenteral and oral, and of output must be sent with the patient.

7–1. Basic elements in electrolyte balance

Element	Chemical Symbol	Atomic Weight	Valence	Range of Concentration in Extracellular Fluid (mEq./L.)
Sodium	Na	23	1	135–148
Potassium	K	39	1	4.4–5.6
CO$_2$ combining power	..	..	1	25.0–30.0
Chloride	Cl	35	1	99–108
Calcium	Ca	40	2	4.5–5.5

7–2. Calculations for repair of electrolyte imbalance are usually expressed in milliequivalents per liter, abbreviated to mEq./L.

$$mEq./L. = \frac{mg./100\ ml. \times 10}{atomic\ weight} \times valence = \frac{vol.\ \% \times 10}{22.4}$$

7–3. Basic requirements (fluids and electrolytes) per day
A. The amount of fluids and electrolytes required every 24 hours depends upon the patient's age, weight and skin surface (usually indicated in square meters [M^2]). Approximate relationships between the weight in kilograms and the skin surface area (S.A.) in square meters (M^2) are as follows:

Weight in Kilograms	S. A. (M²)	Weight in Kilograms	S. A. (M²)	Weight in Kilograms	S. A. (M²)	Weight in Kilograms	S. A. (M²)
1.0	0.10	11.0	0.52	21.0	0.85	31.0	1.13
1.5	0.12	12.0	0.55	22.0	0.87	32.0	1.15
2.0	0.15	13.0	0.58	23.0	0.90	33.0	1.18
2.5	0.18	14.0	0.61	24.0	0.93	34.0	1.20
3.0	0.20	15.0	0.64	25.0	0.95	35.0	1.25
4.0	0.25	16.0	0.71	26.0	1.00	36.0	1.25
5.0	0.29	17.0	0.74	27.0	1.03	37.0	1.27
6.0	0.33	18.0	0.76	28.0	1.06	38.0	1.30
7.0	0.38	19.0	0.79	29.0	1.08	39.0	1.32
8.0	0.42	20.0	0.82	30.0	1.11	40.0	1.34
9.0	0.45						
10.0	0.49			S.A. of average (70 kg.) adult = 1.72 M²			

B. Water (H₂O) Requirements per day

Average physical condition	1500 ml./M²
Moderately dehydrated	2400 ml./M²
Severely dehydrated	3000 ml./M²
Hyperventilating	500 ml./M² additional
Hyperpyrexic	1500 ml./M² + 4.5% for each centigrade degree above normal (8% for each degree Fahrenheit)

C. Potassium Ion Requirements per day 40 mEq./M²

D. Sodium Chloride (NaCl) Requirements per day by age

Age	NaCl	
	Gm.	mEq.
Newborn	0.25	4
1–3 months	0.35	6
3–6 months	0.5	8
6–12 months	0.75	12
1–2 years	1.0	17
2–4 years	2.0	34
4–7 years	3.0	51
7–12 years	4.0	68
12–18 years	5.0	85
18 years up	6.0–7.0	100–120

7–4. Output

Physiologic elimination of fluids and electrolytes from the body must be given full consideration in estimating replacement therapy. So must pathologic processes (excessive perspiration, hyperpyrexia, rapid respiration, vomiting, diarrhea and bleeding).

Types and Approximate Average Amounts of Output (mEq./L).

Type	Na	K	Cl	HCO₃	Av. Output per Day (Adults)
Bile	140	10	100	30	500
Bowel	120	10	105	25	3000
Gastric	35	12	125	..	2500
Pancreatic	140	10	75	75	700
Perspiration	85	5	85	..	....
Saliva	10	25	10	10	1000
Urine	100	50	100	..	1000

7–5. Conversion factors (mEq. per gm.)
  Na = 43 mEq.
  NaCl = 17 mEq. of Na and Cl.
  K = 26 mEq.
  KCl = 15 mEq. of K and Cl.
  Cl = 29 mEq.

7–6. Replacement solutions (mEq. to volume indicated)

	Volume or Amount	Na	K	Cl	Lactate
Ammonium chloride (0.9% solution)	per liter	....	....	167	...
Butler's solution	per liter	57	25	50	25
Multiple electrolyte solution (MES)	per liter	40	35	40	20
Normal saline	per liter	154	....	154	...
Plasma	per 250 ml.	35	1.2	25	...
Sodium bicarbonate (3.75 gm.)	per 50 ml.	44.6	....	...	...
Sodium lactate (⅙ molar solution)	per liter	166	....	...	166
Potassium penicillin	per million units	....	1.7	...	...
Sodium penicillin	per million units	1.6	....	...	...

7–7. Fluid requirements of a burned adult in the first 24 hours (Modified from standard procedure in Brooke Army Hospital)

 A. Dextrose in Water (fixed amount)   2000 ml.
 B. Electrolyte Solutions
   Formula: (Body weight in kilograms) × (% of
    body surface burned) × 1.5 ml.
   Example: 70 kg. adult with 40 % S.A. burn
    70 × 40 × 1.5 =   4200 ml.
 C. Colloid Solutions (blood, plasma, plasma volume ex-
   panders)
   Formula: (Body weight in kilograms) × (% of
    body surface burned) × 0.5 ml.
   Example: 70 × 40 × 0.5 =   <u>1400 ml.</u>
      Total in example <u>7600 ml.</u>
   One half of the total (3800 ml.) should be given
   in the first 8 hours; then one quarter (1900 ml.)
   in the next two 8-hour periods, modified by clinical
   judgement.

7–8. Oral solution for mass casualty use

Drinking large amounts of a solution containing one level
teaspoonful of table salt and one-half teaspoonful of baking
soda dissolved in a quart of water may be lifesaving.

8. HEMORRHAGE

8–1. Control of bleeding of varying degrees of severity as
soon as possible is one of the chief functions of the physician
in an emergency (Topic 20). If the hemorrhage is from a portion of the body which is accessible, one or more of the following measures may be adequate:

 A. Direct pressure over the bleeding area or vessel.
 B. Proper application of a tourniquet (above systolic blood
   pressure) to an extremity. Too loose an application
   often causes an increase in, or continuation of,
   bleeding. If dangerous hemorrhage has been controlled, the tourniquet should NOT be loosened
   until facilities are available for surgical control.
 C. Clamping and tieing, or insertion of mattress sutures
   incorporating the bleeding vessels, followed by

closure of the skin with interrupted nonabsorbable sutures.

D. Packing with sterile gauze.

E. Application of hemostatics to areas of excoriation or avulsion.

8–2.   **General measures**

A. Absolute rest in a position of comfort.

B. Treatment of shock (Topic 15–7). Replacement of blood volume (Topic 7) as soon as possible is essential.

C. Morphine sulfate, 10 to 15 mg., intravenously to control pain, restlessness and apprehension unless intracranial damage (Topic 43 and Topic 60–2) or intrathoracic injuries (Topic 31) are causative factors, or extreme respiratory depression is present.

D. Plasma volume expanders intravenously (Topic 7).

E. Hospitalization as soon as the patient's condition has stabilized if blood loss has been excessive, extensive surgical repair is needed, or damage to a major blood vessel (especially an artery) is evident or suspected (Topic 60–1).

8–3.   **Hemorrhage from special sites**

A. *Adenoid Fossa.* Severe hemorrhage following adenoidectomy can usually be controlled by proper insertion of a posterior nasal pack (Topic 17–6,B). Enough blood may be lost to require transfusion.

B. *Arteries (Major).* See Topic 60–1.

C. *Ears.* Following trauma to the head, bleeding from an ear is pathognomonic of skull fracture (Topic 43–12), provided there are no lacerations of the external auditory canal.

Treatment. Hospitalize AT ONCE for head injury care. No attempt should be made to cleanse the canal. A sterile pad may be applied over the ear, but nothing should be inserted into the external auditory canal.

D. *Epidural.* See Topic 43–20 and Topic 48–22.

E. *Epistaxis.* See Topic 46–3.

F. *Esophageal.* See Topic 39–4.

G. *Extradural.* See Topic 43–20 and Topic 48–22.

H. *Eyes.* See Topic 37–32.

I. *Gastrointestinal Tract.* See 8–3,X, below, and Topic 31–4, –6 and –24.

J. *Head.* See Topic 43–19 and Topic 48–28 (*Head Injuries in Children*).

K. *Intra-abdominal.* See Topic 22 and Topic 55–1.

L. *Intra-alveolar.* See 8–3,P, below, and Topic 31–3 (*Chest Injuries*).

M. *Intracranial*
   1. NONTRAUMATIC. See Topic 60–2.
   2. TRAUMATIC. See Topic 43–19 and Topic 48–28 (*Head Injuries in Children*).

N. *Intrapericardial.* See Topic 29–4.

O. *Liver.* See Topic 55–1.

P. *Lungs.* See also Topic 31–3.

   Gross hemorrhage from the lungs from any cause requires immediate hospitalization. Morphine sulfate or dihydromorphinone hydrochloride (Dilaudid) may be given subcutaneously or intravenously to allay the characteristic acute apprehension. Treatment of shock (Topic 15–7) may be necessary before and during transportation to a hospital. Bleeding following therapeutic pneumothorax can sometimes be controlled by diluting 1 ml. of surgical Pituitrin to 10 ml. with normal salt solution and administering it intravenously very slowly— no faster than 1 ml. per minute.

Q. *Major Blood Vessels.* See 8–2, above, Topic 20 and Topic 60–1.

R. *Mediastinal.* See Topic 31.

S. *Neck.* Knife slashings and glass cuts (accidental, suicidal or homicidal) may cause hemorrhage from the large superficial neck vessels and must be controlled immediately to prevent exsanguination. Digital pressure or pinching of the bleeding vessels or clamping with hemostats may be necessary. No attempt should be made to tie off the vessels in severe cases; blood loss should be countered by intravenous volume expanders (Topic 7) and the patient transferred by ambulance to a hospital with the clamps in place, accompanied, if possible, by a physician, nurse or other trained attendant. If the patient is in profound shock, metaraminol bi-

tartrate (Aramine) or arterenol bitartrate (Levophed) intravenously in 1000 ml. of 5% dextrose
in normal salt solution may be necessary to support the circulation until whole blood can be administered. Morphine sulfate, 10 to 15 mg., or
dihydromorphinone hydrochloride (Dilaudid), 2 to
4 mg., should be given, preferably intravenously,
before transportation to allay the typical extreme
anxiety and apprehension and to control restlessness and pain.

T. Nose. See Topic 46–3.

U. Rectum. See Topic 39–6.

V. Scalp. See Topic 43–22.

W. Spleen. See Topic 55–30.

X. Stomach. Vomiting of blood-stained or coffee-ground
material and passage of tarry stools are specific
indications for thorough clinical and laboratory investigation. Immediate hospitalization is necessary
only if gross hemorrhage with severe shock has
occurred or if anemia is profound.

Y. Subdural. See Topic 43–21 and Topic 48–28 (*Head
Injuries in Children*).

Z. Throat. In the absence of evidence of local injury to
the nose (Topic 46) or throat, bleeding from the
posterior wall of the nasopharynx following severe
trauma should be considered as indicative of a
basal skull fracture and treated as outlined under
Topic 43–16. For posttonsillectomy bleeding, see
8–4,J,4, (below).

AA. Umbilical Stump
1. Mild cases can be controlled by direct pressure.
2. Severe cases require hospitalization after control of
hemorrhage by clamping or ligatures.

BB. Urethra. See Topic 40–9.

CC. Vagina. See Topic 41–4, –6 and –7. In certain cases
examinations for rape or criminal assault (Topic
11) must be performed.

DD. Varicosities. See Topic 60–11.

8–4.   Hemorrhage from specific conditions

A. Abortions. See Topic 50–1.

B. Aneurysms. See Topic 60–2,C and D.

C. Anticoagulant Therapy

1. If caused by Dicumarol, give aqueous solution of vitamin K_1 (AquaMephyton), 5 to 15 mg., intravenously; repeat as necessary.

2. If caused by heparin, inject 50 mg. of protamine sulfate slowly, intravenously, and repeat every 15 minutes until the desired effect has been obtained. Neutralization of the effects of long-acting depot heparin may require several injections of protamine sulfate.

D. Blood Dyscrasias.
Leukemia, hemophilia, purpura, sickle cell anemia and other blood dyscrasias can cause severe intractable bleeding. Hospitalization for thorough study and transfusions and other therapy is always indicated.

E. Corticosteroid Therapy.
Gross hemorrhage from softening of scars may occur, usually in the gastrointestinal tract. Immediate hospitalization after treatment of shock (Topic 15–7) is indicated.

F. Ectopic Pregnancy.
See Topic 50–3.

G. Hepatic Disease.
Hospitalization for control of hemorrhage—usually from esophageal varices (Topic 39–4)—and treatment of the underlying cause is essential.

H. Menorrhagia.
See Topic 41–6.

I. Metrorrhagia.
See Topic 41–7.

J. Postoperative

1. MILD BLEEDING OR OOZING usually can be controlled by:

   a. Application of pressure locally or over "pressure points."

   b. Absolute rest.

   c. Sedation by rapid-acting barbiturates.

   d. Control of restlessness and anxiety by small doses of morphine sulfate subcutaneously or intravenously.

   e. Packing, clamping, tieing or suturing after exposure of the bleeding vessel.

2. SEVERE HEMORRHAGE may require heroic measures.

   a. Control of the hemorrhage by whatever means are available may mean the difference between life and death to the patient. If necessary, the following measures should be used promptly and without waiting for preparation of a sterile operating field:

(1) Digital pressure or pinching of the hemorrhaging vessel.

(2) Application of a tourniquet (8–1, above) if on an extremity.

(3) Packing with gauze.

(4) Clamping.

(5) Ligation.

b. Shock therapy. (Topic 15–7).

c. Transportation by ambulance for hospitalization as soon as the patient's condition will permit— preferably to the hospital where the surgery was done. Intravenous supportive therapy should be continued in the ambulance.

Every possible effort should be made to get in touch with the surgeon who performed the original operation. If this is not possible, a resumé outlining all emergency treatment given should be sent with the patient. In all cases, the hospital to which the patient is being sent should be notified in advance so that there will be no delay in treatment on the patient's arrival.

3. POSTEXTRACTION HEMORRHAGE can result in loss of a large amount of blood.

TREATMENT

a. Have the patient bite firmly on a small pad of gauze.

b. Pack the area with sterile cotton moistened with epinephrine hydrochloride (Adrenalin) (1: 1000 solution).

c. Inject sodium estrone sulfate (Premarin Intravenous), 20 mg., intravenously. Repeat in 1 hour if necessary.

d. Place a small piece of oxidized cellulose (Gelfoam or Oxycel) in the bleeding socket and hold firmly in place with a pad of gauze held between the teeth.

e. Give acetylsalicylic acid (aspirin), with or without codeine sulfate, for pain.

     f. If severe bleeding persists, suture the gums over the bleeding socket.

     g. If possible, refer the patient back to the dentist who performed the extraction.

     h. Instruct the patient not to eat solid foods of any kind until he has received further dental care.

  4. POSTTONSILLECTOMY BLEEDING may be delayed, profuse and difficult to control. Hospitalization for suturing under general anesthesia often is required. To prevent his swallowing blood, the patient should sit up during transportation unless signs of severe shock (Topic 15) are present. Morphine sulfate or dihydromorphinone hydrochloride (Dilaudid) subcutaneously to allay anxiety and to quiet the patient may be necessary.

K. Postpartum Bleeding. See Topic 41–10.

L. Spontaneous Hemorrhage. Although trauma is the most common cause of severe hemorrhage, spontaneous onset of bleeding of various degrees of severity may be caused by:

  1. Congenital structural blood vessel weakness.

  2. Degenerative disease processes involving the blood vessel walls.

  3. Erosion of a blood vessel by pressure from an adjacent space-consuming tumor.

  4. Drugs or other agents which interfere with normal coagulation of the blood or cause softening of previously formed scars.

  5. Familial or acquired blood dyscrasias.

The known or suspected presence of any of these factors requires hospitalization [after shock therapy (Topic 15–7)] for thorough investigation and treatment of the underlying condition.

9. NARCOTICS (OPIUM DERIVATIVES AND SYNTHETICS) IN EMERGENCY CASES

For use and toxicity of other substances listed under the Narcotic Act (Topic 2–3), see under Topic 49 (*Poisons*) and Topic 59 (*Toxic Reactions to Average Doses of Commonly Used Drugs*).

9–1. Emergency use

Opium derivatives as well as synthetic narcotics are of great value in emergency treatment provided indiscriminate use is avoided and the following principles are kept in mind.

A. Definite Indications for Use Are Present (9–2, below).
1. Control of severe pain and acute apprehension.
2. Specific effects are desired [apomorphine to induce vomiting; nalorphine (Nalline) to counteract overdoses of opiates and synthetic narcotics; morphine to control apprehension as well as pain, etc.].

B. No Contraindications Are Present. The most important contraindications are:
1. Head injuries (Topic 43). Important changes in condition may be masked by even small doses of narcotics.
2. Respiratory depression from any cause.
3. Chest injuries (Topic 31).
4. Undiagnosed abdominal pain (Topic 22).
5. Addiction, with or without withdrawal symptoms (Topic 2–3).
6. Abnormal or allergic reactions to previous doses (Topic 24).
7. Infancy or early childhood (Topic 5).
8. Pregnancy at or near term—respiratory depression may be fatal to the child.
9. Myxedema (Topic 35–5,A,2).

C. The Minimal Effective Dosage based on the age (Topic 5) and physical condition of the patient is used.

D. The Proper Means of Administration Is Chosen. Oral administration is contraindicated if vomiting may occur; subcutaneous or intramuscular injections may be totally ineffective if the patient is in circulatory collapse, producing an accumulative toxic effect when the circulation of the blood improves.

E. The Appropriate Drug Is Used. Consideration must be given to possible side effects as well as to intensity and duration of action. Morphine sulfate and dihydromorphinone hydrochloride (Dilaudid) are by far the most useful narcotics for emergency use because of their ability to control severe pain and at the same time allay apprehension. If marked contraction of smooth muscle will be detrimental, meperidine hydrochloride (Demerol) may be substituted. Demerol, however, has very little effect on severe pain and does not control acute apprehension; therefore, it should not be used in emergencies such as fractures and myocardial infarction. Codeine sulfate (9–2, below) is satisfactory for control of pain of moderate intensity and is, for practical purposes, non-habit forming.

Dihydromorphinone hydrochloride (Dilaudid) (9–2, below) has a definite use in emergency situations in place of morphine not only because of its ability to control apprehension and severe pain but also because its name is not so well known. In certain circumstances, it may be desirable to keep from the patient (or the family) the fact that administration of a powerful narcotic has been necessary. Its actions, side effects and addictive tendencies are similar to those of morphine sulfate, although its toxicity is slightly greater.

9–2. Analgesic narcotics (opiates and synthetics) of value in emergency therapy

Narcotic Drug	Average Adult Dose	Duration of Action (Hours)	Method of Administration	Indications for Use	Contraindications to Use	Analgesic Effect (Rise in Pain Threshold)	Minimal Lethal Dose for Adults (Approximate)*
Alphaprodine hydrochloride (Nisentil)	40 mg.	1–2	S.C.	Dental emergencies; minor surgery; obstetric analgesia	Same as morphine	+++	60 to 120 mg.
Camphorated opium tincture (paragoric)	4 ml.	2–3	O	Pediatrics—in children over 2 years of age*	Same as morphine	++	60 ml.
Codeine sulfate	60 mg.	2–3	O S.C. I.M.	Control of moderate pain; headache; neuralgia; myalgia; persistent cough	Allergic reactions in some persons, but usually well tolerated	++	0.8 gm.
Dihydrocodeinone bitartrate (Hycodan)	10 mg.	1–2	O	Cough depressant; does not paralyze ciliary action	None except individual hypersensitivity	+	0.3 gm.
Dihydromorphinone hydrochloride (Dilaudid)	2 mg.	3–4	O S.C. I.M. I.V.	Control of severe pain or acute apprehension; relaxation of reflex spasm	Same as morphine; slightly more toxic	++++	0.1 gm.

Meperidine hydrochloride (Demerol)	50 mg.	1–2	O I.M. I.V.	Moderate pain; obstetric analgesia; preoperative preparation; whenever smooth muscle contraction will be harmful	Severe pain or acute apprehension; head or chest injuries; shock	++	1 gm.
Morphine sulfate	15 mg.	4–5	O S.C. I.M. I.V.	Control of any type of severe pain (except psychogenic); control of acute apprehension and anxiety; shock; preoperative preparation	Head or chest injuries; respiratory depression; unstable mental make-up; when contraction of smooth muscle is detrimental	++++	0.2 gm.

* In infants (children under 2 years of age) the minimal lethal dose varies from approximately 1/100 of the adult dose in the first 2 weeks of life to 1/20 of the adult dose at the age of 2. The values given in this table do not include the occasional cases of atopic or allergic hypersensitivity.

10.   PRESCRIPTION RESTRICTIONS

10–1. **Amounts**
Only small amounts of medications of any kind should be
prescribed for patients seen on an emergency basis—enough
to obtain the desired effect until the patient can report elsewhere for definitive care (Topic 72–11).

10–2. **Barbiturates**
Minimal amounts only should be prescribed. In many localities it is required that the prescription be in the attending
physician's handwriting and give the patient's full name and
home address.

10–3. **Narcotics**
Although regulations regarding prescription of narcotics vary
in different countries, it is usually required that the prescription be in the physician's handwriting and that his office address and narcotic registration number be given. Only the
minimal amount necessary to obtain the desired effect should
be prescribed or furnished for home use. Great care should be
used in adjusting the dose to the age in children (Topic 5) and
in elderly or debilitated persons.

For restrictions on prescription of narcotics for ambulatory
treatment of addiction see Topic 2–5.

10–4. **Somnifacients**
Antihistaminics, hypnotics, muscle relaxants, narcotics, sedatives and tranquilizers are among the commonly used drugs
which may cause drowsiness and slowing of reflexes. Therefore, persons for whom any of these drugs have been prescribed
should be cautioned against operating any type of motor driven
vehicle during the duration of the effect of the drug. The same
warning should be given to persons exposed to changes in
barometric pressure (Topic 26).

11. RAPE

Examination for possible rape or criminal assault should never be done, even when requested by law enforcement officers, without a properly witnessed written consent of the patient or, if a minor, of a parent (both parents, if possible) or legal guardian. Questioning and examination should always be done in the presence of a third person (preferably a nurse, certainly a woman) and should cover the points listed below. Negative as well as positive findings should be noted in detail in the Emergency Department record.

A. Date and time of the alleged act.

B. The patient's statement regarding previous sexual relations.

C. Physical examination as soon as possible after the alleged act.
   1. The condition of the clothing.
   2. Development of the genitalia.
   3. External signs of injury (abrasions, lacerations, contusions, edema, bleeding, etc.).
   4. Presence or absence of excessive secretion (type?).
   5. Abrasions or lacerations of the vaginal canal.
   6. Condition of the hymen.

D. Collection of specimens of secretion using a pipet, from the labiae, introitus and cervix. These specimens of secretion should be examined IMMEDIATELY as wet preparations and the presence or absence of motile or nonmotile sperm noted. Smears should be made, carefully labeled for possible later identification, and sent to a qualified laboratory for staining and examination for spermatozoa and for gonococci.

   Material for cultures should also be obtained. All smears should be preserved as permanent records for at least 2 years.

E. In some localities, examination for rape requires a blood sample (10 ml.), marked carefully for identification, to be sent to a laboratory for serology tests.

11–1. **Evidence** of rape or criminal assault must be reported at once to the proper law enforcement authorities. Even if there is no evidence of penetration or seminal emission, findings indicative of trauma to the external genitalia are usually considered as evidence of criminal assault.

12. REPORTABLE DISEASES

Public health regulations regarding certain diseases require that special forms be completed and signed by the physician who established the diagnosis. The list of reportable diseases usually includes the following:

Amebiasis
Anthrax
Brucellosis (undulant fever)
Chancroid
Chickenpox (varicella)
Coccidioidomycosis, disseminated
Conjunctivitis, acute infections of the newborn (gonorrheal ophthalmia, ophthalmia neonatorum, and babies' sore eyes in the first 21 days of life)
Dengue
Diarrhea of the newborn
Diphtheria
Dysentery, bacillary (see Shigella infections)
Encephalitis, infectious
Epilepsy
Food poisoning (other than botulism)
German measles (rubella)
Gonococcus infection
Granuloma inguinale
Hemolytic streptococcal infections
Hepatitis, infectious (including hepatitis, serum)
Influenza, epidemic
Leprosy (Hansen's disease)
Leptospirosis
Lymphogranuloma venereum (lymphogranuloma inguinale)

Malaria
Measles (rubeola)
Meningitis, meningococcal, or meningococcemia
Mumps
Paratyphoid fever, A, B and C (see Salmonella infections)
Pertussis (whooping cough)
Physically handicapped children
Plague
Pneumonia, primary infectious
Poliomyelitis, acute anterior
Psittacosis
Rabies, human or animal
Relapsing fever
Rheumatic fever, acute
Rocky Mountain spotted fever
Salmonella infections (exclusive of typhoid fever cases and carriers)
Scarlet fever
Shigella infections
Smallpox (variola)
Syphilis
Tetanus
Trachoma
Trichinosis
Tuberculosis
Tularemia
Typhoid fever, cases and carriers
Typhus fever
Yellow fever

Official cards (see below) for reporting these cases should

be completed as soon as the diagnosis is made and mailed to the local health officer.

Asiatic cholera, plague, smallpox, typhus (louse-borne epidemic type) and yellow fever must be reported immediately to the director of the state department of public health *by telephone or telegraph.*

(FACE)

(REVERSE SIDE)

Morbidity Report Form

HEART-LUNG RESUSCITATION

FIRST AID: OXYGENATE THE BRAIN IMMEDIATELY

1 or 2 operators

Airway –
IF UNCONSCIOUS
REMOVE EXCESSIVE MUCUS
TILT HEAD BACK

IF NOT BREATHING

Breathe – INFLATE LUNGS 3-5 TIMES
MAINTAIN HEAD TILT
MOUTH-TO-MOUTH, MOUTH-TO-NOSE,
mouth-to-adjunct, bag-mask

- FEEL PULSE
- IF PRESENT – CONTINUE LUNG INFLATIONS
- IF ABSENT –

Circulate – *COMPRESS HEART ONCE A SECOND.*
ALTERNATE 2-3 LUNG INFLATIONS WITH
15 STERNAL COMPRESSIONS UNTIL
SPONTANEOUS PULSE RETURNS.

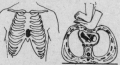

DEPRESS LEVEL OF STERNUM 1-2 INCHES IN ADULTS
USE FINGERTIPS ONLY IN INFANTS

for physicians only

START SPONTANEOUS CIRCULATION

Drugs – *EPINEPHRINE:* 1.0 mg (1.0 ml. OF 1:1000) I.V. OR 0.5 mg
REPEAT LARGER DOSE IF NECESSARY

SODIUM BICARBONATE: APPROXIMATELY 3.75 G/50 ml. (1/2 DOSE IN CHILDREN) I.V.
REPEAT EVERY 5 MINUTES IF NECESSARY

E. K. G. – • *FIBRILLATION:* EXTERNAL ELECTRIC DEFIBRILLATION. REPEAT
SHOCK EVERY 1-3 MINUTES UNTIL FIBRILLATION REVERSED

• *IF ASYSTOLE OR WEAK BEATS:* EPINEPHRINE OR
CALCIUM I.V.

A.C.: 880-1500 v 0.25 SEC.
D.C.: 150 W/SEC. 0.0025 SEC.
(CHECK MANUFACTURER'S INSTRUCTIONS).

Fluids – *I.V. PLASMA, DEXTRAN, SALINE*
Do not interrupt cardiac compressions and ventilation.
Tracheal intubation only when necessary.
AFTER RETURN OF SPONTANEOUS CIRCULATION USE VASOPRESSORS AS NEEDED,
e.g. NOREPINEPHRINE (Levophed) I.V. DRIP

SUPPORT RECOVERY   (physician - specialist)

Gauge   *EVALUATE AND TREAT CAUSE OF ARREST*

Hypothermia *START WITHIN 30 MINUTES IF NO SIGN OF CNS RECOVERY*

Intensive Care *SUPPORT VENTILATION:* TRACHEOTOMY, PROLONGED CONTROLLED
VENTILATION, GASTRIC TUBE AS NECESSARY
SUPPORT   CIRCULATION
CONTROL   CONVULSIONS
MONITOR

13.   *RESUSCITATION*

13–1.   **General principles of heart-lung resuscitation** (Fig. 1)

   A. Insurance of an adequate, unobstructed airway by digital removal of secretions, foreign bodies, etc., by gravity, by suction if available, and by supporting the angles of the jaw (Fig. 2).

   B. Oxygenation of the Brain via the lungs and blood stream by:

     1. EXPIRED AIR METHODS

       a. Mouth-to-mouth (Topic 17–1,A).

       b. Mouth-to-nose (Topic 17–1,B).

       c. Mouth-to-adjunct (Topic 17–1,C).

          These methods have the following advantages over the manual push-pull techniques (Schaefer, Sylvester, Holger, Nielsen, etc.):

       (1) Increased pulmonary ventilation.

       (2) The rescuer's hands are free to support the jaw.

       (3) Special positioning is not necessary; therefore, expired air respiration can be performed in cramped or unusual circumstances—for instance, while bringing a drowning victim to shore.

       (4) The presence of an obstruction can be recognized. If it is impossible to force air in, there is a plug in the upper respiratory tract.

     2. MANUAL METHODS

          The only one of the manual methods which is of value is the "teeter-board" method of Rickard in infants. For technique see Topic 17–1,E.

Figure 1. Three phases of cardiopulmonary resuscitation. (Modified from training poster of Pennsylvania State Department of Health, Western Pennsylvania Heart Association, and Pennsylvania Society of Anesthesiologists based on data taken from Dr. Peter Safar's editorial in the *Medical Tribune,* June 28, 1963.)

AIRWAY PATENCY

IF YOU NOTICE EXCESSIVE SECRETION,
MUCUS OR FOREIGN MATTER,
CLEAR...WITH FINGERS.

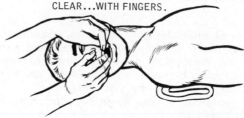

WITH SUCTION (A LARGE SYRINGE CAN BE USED
IN PLACE OF JAR).

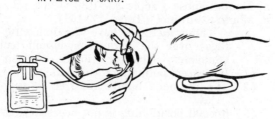

BY GRAVITY
(INFANTS AND CHILDREN).

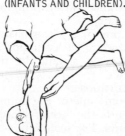

Figure 2. Two upper drawings modified from Safar, P., and McMahon,
M. C.: *Resuscitation of the Unconscious Victim—A Manual for Rescue
Breathing.* 2nd Ed. Charles C Thomas, 1961. Bottom drawing from Gordon,
A. S.: Heart-lung resuscitation. J. Occupational Medicine, 4, Jan. 1962.

    3. MECHANICAL METHODS (Topic 17–1,F)

        Administration of air and/or oxygen under intermittent positive pressure is the most efficient method of ensuring adequate ventilation and should replace expired-air and manual methods as soon as equipment is available.

C. Cardiac Compression to provide blood circulation.

    1. Closed chest (Topic 17–2,A).

    2. Open chest (Topic 17–2,B).

D. Administration of Supporting Drugs

    1. Epinephrine hydrochloride (Adrenalin) (Topic 17–2, A,8) intravenously (not intracardially).

    2. Sodium bicarbonate solution (3.75 gm. in 50 ml. of normal saline) intravenously (Topic 17–2,A,7) to combat decreased reactivity of cardiac muscle caused by metabolic acidosis.

E. Defibrillation if indicated by clinical evaluation or by ECG cardiac monitor (Topic 17–2,B,3,b). IF IN DOUBT, DEFIBRILLATE!

F. Reinforcement of Weak Respiration or Cardiac Action.

G. Administration of Supportive and Replacement Fluids (Topic 7).

H. Support of the Circulation by Vasopressors.

I. Determination and Treatment of Cause of Cardiac Arrest (Topic 29–2,A).

J. Intensive Follow-up Care. This may require tracheotomy (Topic 17–11), prolonged mechanical respiratory assistance, insertion of a nasogastric tube, hypothermia, or use of a pacemaker.

13–2. **Drowning** (See also Topic 48–18)

A. Mouth-to-mouth respiration while bringing the drowning person to shore may be lifesaving.

B. Insurance of a patent airway.

C. Heart-lung resuscitation (13–1, above).

D. Hospitalization after spontaneous respiration has been re-established. Respiratory and cardiac stimulants are of little, if any, value until breathing has been established.

E. Immersion in fresh water for lengthy periods may result in massive hemolysis from the osmotic effect of fresh water. Transfusions of whole blood may be necessary.

13–3. **Heart-lung resuscitation by a single rescuer**

    A. Expired air respiration (Topic 17–1) 3 times (rate, 12 to 15 times per minute).

    B. Closed cardiac massage (Topic 17–2) 12 to 15 times (rate 40 to 50 times per minute).

    C. Alternate A and B, above, until assistance is available or until spontaneous and stable circulation and ventilation are present.

14. *SERUM SENSITIVITY AND DESENSITIZATION*

Although hypersensitivity of the skin to animal serum does not necessarily parallel systemic hypersensitivity, intradermal (intracutaneous) skin tests should always be done before tetanus antitoxin (TAT) injections, or injections of antisera of any type, are given. The injection must be made into, and not through, the skin and must not draw blood. A syringe containing 1 ml. of epinephrine (Adrenalin) hydrochloride should be available for immediate use; deaths have occurred from anaphylactic reactions (Topic 24–1) to the diluted antitoxin used for skin tests.

If an indurated wheal (with or without pseudopods) is present 20 minutes after intradermal (intracutaneous) injection of 0.1 ml. of 1:10 dilution, the test should be considered as positive and the need for the passive protection resulting from antitoxin should be re-evaluated. If indicated, the following desensitization procedure should be carried out as a considered risk:

Inject	0.01 ml. of antitoxin subcutaneously
20 minutes later	0.02 ml. of antitoxin subcutaneously
20 minutes later	0.04 ml. of antitoxin subcutaneously
20 minutes later	0.10 ml. of antitoxin subcutaneously
20 minutes later	0.25 ml. of antitoxin subcutaneously
20 minutes later	0.58 ml. of antitoxin subcutaneously
Total	1.00 ml.

Twenty minutes later 1 ml. of antitoxin may be injected subcutaneously or intramuscularly, accompanied by 0.5 to 1 ml. of a 1:1000 solution of epinephrine hydrochloride (Adrenalin) subcutaneously. This amount of tetanus antitoxin (3000 units of TAT given over about 2 hours) is generally considered to give adequate protection unless gross contamination is present.

Following this desensitization procedure, large amounts can be given with relative safety provided no local erythema, urticaria, asthmatic breathing, nausea, vomiting or chills have occurred. If such reactions develop at any time during the procedure outlined above, the last dose should be repeated after a 20-minute wait; two reactions make further attempts at administration of the particular antiserum (usually equine or bovine) inadvisable. Similar skin testing with available antisera derived from other animals (i.e., bovine instead of equine, etc.) may be practical, or the recently developed human TAT (human antitetanus serum) may be used. As an alternative, bicillin and tetracycline therapy, combined with a series of intracutaneous injections of small amounts of toxoid, have been reported as effective.

Ophthalmic tests for sensitivity to antisera should never be used in emergency situations—severe reactions may result in permanent eye damage. Scratch tests are of no value.

Oral administration of an antihistaminic (preferably in sustained action form) at the time the antitoxin is given and daily for 10 days thereafter may prevent, or decrease the severity of, serum sickness (Topic 59–66).

Provided it is not given in the same extremity as the antitoxin, active immunization by a series of toxoid injections [two subcutaneous injections of 0.5 ml. of precipitated toxoid or three of 0.5 ml. of plain (fluid) toxoid at 30-day intervals] may be begun concurrently with antitoxin therapy.

15. SHOCK

See also Topic 48–47 (*Shock in Children*).

15–1. **Definition**

Shock is a condition of collapse or prostration which is:

  A. Induced by any number of factors—blood loss, injury, fright, etc.

  B. Accompanied by signs and symptoms of peripheral circulatory impairment or failure—pallor, sweating, coldness, faint rapid pulse.

   C. *Characterized by* a progressive REDUCTION IN THE CIRCULATING BLOOD VOLUME indicated by vessel collapse, hypotension, etc.

15–2. **Types of shock**

15–3. **Primary ("neurogenic") shock.** In this condition there is a temporary depression of the sensorium resulting from sudden extreme emotion—fear, pain, tragic news—or the stunning effect of severe injury before blood volume loss has occurred.

15–4. **Secondary (surgical or traumatic) shock**

This is a severe disturbance of body function. The immediate cause is reduction in the volume of circulating blood which reduces venous pressure and diastolic filling of the heart. Cardiac output falls but immediate fall of blood pressure is prevented by reflex arteriolar constriction. As the blood flow progressively diminishes, maximal arteriolar constriction no longer suffices to maintain blood pressure. The resultant hypoxia is the most damaging feature of shock, as it increases the capillary permeability and impairs the function of the myocardium and brain. If these changes are severe or prolonged, irreversible and terminal tissue changes may develop.

15–5. **Factors in the production of shock**

   A. *Severe Trauma*
      1. MASSIVE HEMORRHAGE. Loss of 15 to 20% of total blood volume will result in mild shock; 40% or more will cause severe shock. The total blood volume of an average adult male is about 4900 ml.
      2. SEVERE CRUSHING INJURIES may cause extensive loss of blood and serous fluid with resultant hemoconcentration and renal failure.
      3. TRAUMATIC AMPUTATIONS.
      4. MAJOR FRACTURES, especially of the proximal half of the shaft of the femur.
      5. SEVERE MACERATING OR CRUSHING WOUNDS OF THE EXTREMITIES.
      6. CHEST WOUNDS which penetrate the pleura (Topic 31–10). These are often characterized by marked air hunger and cyanosis. Some develop acute pulmonary edema (Topic 52).
      7. ABDOMINAL WOUNDS. With peritonitis, hemoconcen-

tration may be present with resultant renal
failure from lower nephron nephrosis.

B. Loss of Plasma. Following severe burns (Topic 28) or
exposure to chemical or bacterial irritants, extreme
tissue anoxia may develop. Vasoconstriction may
cause the blood pressure in these patients to remain at a normal level.

C. Loss of Water and Electrolytes from loss of body fluids
or inadequate intake of water or salt (Topic 7).

D. Reflex Fall in Blood Pressure secondary to abdominal
manipulation, solar plexus blows, etc.

E. Collapse of Arterial Vasomotor Tone with resultant
syncope.

15–6. **Symptoms and signs of shock**

A. The patient is prostrated but usually conscious, with a
moist skin, circumoral pallor and sunken eyes.
Cyanosis may be marked.

B. The pulse is rapid, feeble and of small volume, and the
extremities are cold and clammy.

C. The patient is often depressed, restless and apprehensive, and complaining of severe thirst. The
urine is scanty or absent when measured with a
Foley catheter in place.

D. Progressive hypotension develops, with the systolic
pressure usually falling more rapidly than the
diastolic. Prolonged hypotension below adequate
perfusion levels may produce tissue damage of
varying degrees which may be permanent even if
the patient survives the initial period of shock.

E. Increasing acidosis due to progressive anoxia of the
tissues develops. This, in turn, results in decreased
cardiac muscle contractibility and more anoxia,
then increased acidosis, etc., etc.

15–7. **Treatment of shock**

The duration of the acute shock state is a reliable index to
prognosis. Therefore, TREATMENT OF SHOCK TAKES PRE-
CEDENCE OVER ALL OTHER EMERGENCY MEASURES EX-
CEPT CONTROL OF GROSS HEMORRHAGE AND INSUR-
ANCE OF ADEQUATE OXYGENATION. Any patient with a
systolic blood pressure of 80 or below should be considered to
be in shock and treatment instituted immediately. (Exception:

"pulseless disease" caused by blocking of the subclavian artery by atheromatous plaques—hence no peripheral pulses.)

A. General Measures
1. Position of comfort except in:
    a. Very severe shock, when the foot of the bed, stretcher or gurney should be elevated or the thighs flexed on the abdomen.
    b. Head injuries (Topic 43), respiratory distress or pulmonary edema (Topic 52), when the head may be raised slightly.
2. Conservation of body warmth WITHOUT OVER-HEATING.
3. Administration of oxygen under positive pressure by face mask and rebreathing bag.
4. Injection of caffeine sodiobenzoate, 0.5 gm., intramuscularly or intravenously.

B. Maintenance or Quick Restoration of Blood and Tissue Fluid Volume
1. BEFORE WHOLE BLOOD IS AVAILABLE
    a. Saline solution intravenously at once. If superficial veins are collapsed or unsatisfactory, it is simple and safe to use a femoral vein until a cutdown can be done.
    b. Plasma volume expanders (dextran, Plazmoid, etc.). These solutions can be given intravenously without blood typing. They are not intended to take the place of whole blood but they do act as satisfactory temporary substitutes. If a plasma volume expander is to be used, 10 ml. of whole blood should be collected in a test tube before the intravenous administration is started. This blood should be sent with the patient so that cross matching for later blood transfusions will be facilitated.
2. WHEN WHOLE BLOOD IS AVAILABLE
    Transfusion takes precedence over all other antishock measures. The blood volume of an average male is about 4900 ml.; as much as 1200 ml. can be lost without clinical signs of shock. Hematocrit determinations are of absolutely no value.

When blood bank blood (properly cross matched) is used, calcium gluconate should always be added to combat hypernatremia from the blood preservative. If Type O Rh negative blood is used, it must be continued.

a. In moderately severe shock the total blood transfusion volume should equal about ½ of the patient's estimated blood volume.

b. In severe shock 1½ to 2 times the estimated blood volume (up to 10,000 ml.) may be required over a 1½- to 2-hour period, using as many sites of transfusion as are necessary. Unless conditions such as central nervous system damage or severe heart disease are present, there is very little danger of overtransfusion.

c. Bleeding from major vessels must always be controlled as soon as possible (Topic 8).

C. Vasoconstriction. The vasoconstrictor drugs are invaluable adjuncts in treatment of shock, but because of their effect (they decrease visceral perfusion, particularly of the kidneys), their use should be deferred if possible until blood volume has been restored. As a rule, they should be given slowly in 500 to 1000 ml. of intravenous fluids. The most effective of the vasoconstrictors are:

1. Phenylephrine hydrochloride (Neo-Synephrine), 3 to 5 mg. added to 500 to 1000 ml. of solution.

2. Ephedrine sulfate, 10 to 25 mg. in 500 to 1000 ml. of solution.

3. Arterenol bitartrate (Levophed, norepinephrine), 4 mg., given slowly intravenously in 1000 ml. of 5% dextrose in water or saline and continued for as long as necessary. The speed of intravenous injection should be controlled by blood pressure readings every 2 minutes until a plateau with the systolic pressure slightly below normal has been reached. A plastic catheter inserted into a vein is preferable to a needle because extravasation of arterenol bitartrate into soft tissues will cause sloughing. If long-continued use is necessary and blanching along the course of the

vein develops, the site of injection should be changed at once. If extravasation into the soft tissues does occur, infiltration of the area through multiple punctures, using a fine (No. 26) needle, with 5 to 10 mg. of phentolamine methanesulfonate (Regitine) and 150 turbidity reducing units (TRU) of hyaluronidase dissolved in 15 ml. of normal salt solution may prevent extensive necrosis.

4. Metaraminol bitartrate (Aramine) subcutaneously, intramuscularly or intravenously.

Advantages

a. Ease of administration. Aramine can be injected subcutaneously or intramuscularly without danger; intravenously, a plastic catheter is not necessary since sloughing of the soft tissues does not follow extravenous infiltration.

b. Rapidity of action:

Subcutaneously—10 to 20 minutes (depending upon circulation)

Intramuscularly—7 to 10 minutes

Intravenously—1 to 2 minutes

Dose

a. Subcutaneously or intramuscularly—2 to 10 mg.

b. Intravenously:

Directly (in grave emergencies), 0.5 to 5.0 mg.

By infusion, 15 to 100 mg. in 500 ml. of 5% dextrose in saline. The rate of administration should be controlled by frequent blood pressure readings.

D. Corticosteroid Therapy. In cases of severe shock which do not respond satisfactorily to the measures outlined in C, above, corticosteroids may be tried. Hydrocortisone sodium succinate (Solu-Cortef), 100 mg. intravenously, repeated every 4 hours if necessary, may be lifesaving.

E. Control of Pain. Morphine sulfate intravenously may be used in small doses if the patient is in severe pain. For restrictions in the presence of head and chest injuries see Topic 43 and Topic 31.

15–8. **Pressure infusion of intravenous fluids** has no use under emergency conditions because of the danger from air embolism (Topic 60–8).

15–9. **Arterial administration of fluids** requires special training and equipment. The additional benefits in comparison with the intravenous method are not great enough to justify the additional risk.

15–10. **Conditions interfering with response to shock therapy**
Recognition and correction by treatment whenever possible of the following conditions is essential.

- A. Adrenal insufficiency, which usually causes an eosinophilia, requires hydrocortisone therapy.
- B. Aspiration of vomitus.
- C. Biochemical changes, especially acidosis.
- D. Coronary occlusion.
- E. Gram-negative sepsis.
- F. Head injuries.
- G. Hemopericardium.
- H. Hypernatremia.
- I. Massive hemorrhage from a major vessel or ruptured viscus.
- J. Mediastinal emphysema with resultant venous pressure.
- K. Previous corticosteroid intake.
- L. Tension pneumothorax.
- M. Urinary extravasation.

15–11. **Transportation** for hospitalization and definitive treatment should be arranged as soon as the patient is in condition to be moved. Speed of transportation is not important—care in transportation is. Intravenous fluids and oxygen therapy can be continued during transportation if necessary, preferably under the supervision of a physician or registered nurse.

15–12. **Responsibilities of the attending physician in cases of shock**

- A. To recognize the symptoms and signs promptly and to begin correct treatment at once.
- B. To guard against aggravation of the patient's condition by prevention of:
    1. Unnecessary moving for examination, x-rays or diagnostic procedures.
    2. Superimposing additional insult by wound repair, attempted reduction of fractures or dislocations and/or administration of prophylactic injections.
    3. Excitement caused by solicitous family or friends, or

by overenthusiastic law enforcement officers, newspaper reporters, cameramen, insurance representatives or other interested persons.

C. To record in detail all findings and treatment (and reasons therefor).

D. To make the decision regarding transfer for definitive care, and to make a permanent record of his reasons for such transfer.

E. To contact the hospital to which the patient is being sent so that proper equipment and personnel will be standing by and delay in definitive treatment minimized.

16. *SUICIDE*

All cases of attempted or successful suicide are reportable to the closest law enforcement agency. Any physician called upon to examine or treat this type of case should protect the hospital emergency department and himself by reporting any cases in which, in his opinion, self-destruction may have been attempted through asphyxiation, drowning, falls, poison, shooting, lacerations or other means. ANY PERSON KNOWN TO HAVE ATTEMPTED SUICIDE, OR SUSPECTED OF THE ATTEMPT, SHOULD BE KEPT UNDER CLOSE OBSERVATION, WITH A PHYSICALLY ABLE ATTENDANT IN THE ROOM AT ALL TIMES WHILE HE IS UNDER EMERGENCY MEDICAL CARE.

If toxic substances in any form are known or suspected as the means of attempted suicide, ALL BODY CAVITIES ACCESSIBLE TO THE PATIENT SHOULD BE EXAMINED AS SOON AS POSSIBLE AND EMPTIED IF INDICATED. A specimen of any suspect material obtained from each site (including the stomach and bladder) should be collected and placed in a labeled container for possible later toxicologic examination and identification.

17. SURGICAL AND EMERGENCY PROCEDURES AND TECHNIQUES

17–1. **Artificial respiration**
  A. *Mouth-to-Mouth* (preferred method) (See Fig. 3).
    1. Remove excessive mucus from mouth with fingers or handkerchief.
    2. Tilt the patient's head slightly backward.
    3. Support angles of jaw.
    4. Take a deep breath; then breathe directly between the patient's lips, compressing nostrils with cheek or with fingers of one hand. The lips must form an air-tight seal.
    5. Lift head; allow the patient to exhale.
    6. Repeat every 4 to 5 seconds in an adult, slightly faster in a child. Regular rhythm is not important.
    7. In a small child, cover the mouth and nose with lips—blow in very gently.
  B. *Mouth-to-Nose* (See Fig. 4). Same as A (above) except that the mouth is held closed with fingers of one hand.
  C. *Mouth-to-Airway* (See Fig. 5).
    1. Remove excess mucus from the patient's mouth and throat.
    2. Insert a proper size plastic airway ("Resusitube"). Avoid pushing the tongue backward during insertion.
    3. Pinch nose with thumbs while holding jaws up with fingers.
    4. Take a deep breath and blow into the airway mouthpiece—forcibly for an adult, gently for a child.
    5. Watch the chest. When it rises, allow the patient to exhale.
    6. Repeat every 4 to 5 seconds.
  D. *Mouth-to-Mask.* Success depends upon holding the mask firmly in place.

MOUTH-TO-MOUTH BREATHING
(Preferred Method)

REMOVE EXCESSIVE MUCUS.

TILT HEAD BACK

HOLD JAW UP

SEAL NOSTRILS BY DIGITAL
OR CHEEK PRESSURE.

BLOW FORCIBLY INTO MOUTH.

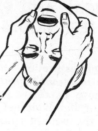

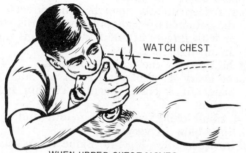

WATCH CHEST

WHEN UPPER CHEST MOVES
ALLOW THE PATIENT TO EXHALE.
REPEAT 10 TO 12 TIMES PER MINUTE.

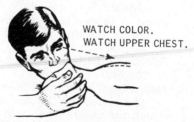

WATCH COLOR.
WATCH UPPER CHEST.

IN BABY BLOW GENTLY INTO MOUTH AND NOSE
- THE SMALLER THE CHILD THE FASTER THE RATE.

Figure 3. Modified from Safar, P., and McMahon, M. C.: *Resuscitation of the Unconscious Victim—A Manual for Rescue Breathing.* 2nd Ed. Charles C Thomas, 1961.

E. Manual Methods. All of the well-known manual methods are inefficient and unsatisfactory and should be used only if mouth-to-mouth or mouth-to-nose respiration is impractical (fastidiousness on the part of the rescuer; severe nasal or facial injuries) or mechanical equipment is not available. The only exception is in infants in whom the Rickard prone-tilting visceral shift ("teeter-board") method is of value.

TECHNIQUE

1. Place the child face down on the operator's supinated forearm flexed to 90 degrees at the elbow.
2. Insert the middle finger in the child's mouth to insure a clear airway by holding the tongue

MOUTH-TO-NOSE BREATHING

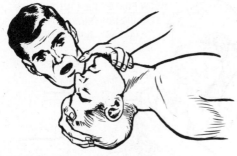

BE SURE NOSTRILS ARE PATENT.

TILT HEAD BACK.

HOLD CHIN UP - SEAL LIPS BY DIGITAL PRESSURE.

BLOW FORCIBLY INTO NOSTRILS (GENTLY IN CHILDREN).

WATCH UPPER CHEST.

ALLOW PATIENT TO EXHALE.

REPEAT 10 TO 12 TIMES PER MINUTE.

Figure 4. Modified from Safar, P., and McMahon, M. C.: *Resuscitation of the Unconscious Victim—A Manual for Rescue Breathing.* 2nd Ed. Charles C Thomas, 1961.

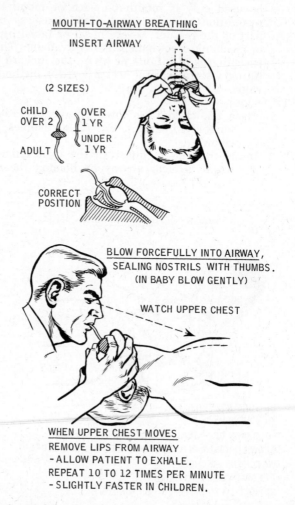

Figure 5. Modified from Safar, P., and McMahon, M. C.: *Resuscitation of the Unconscious Victim—A Manual for Rescue Breathing.* 2nd Ed. Charles C Thomas, 1961.

down and the jaw forward. The remaining
digits should be pressed against the child's
face for stability.
3. Hold the child on the forearm with the opposite
hand.
4. Alternately extend to 180 degrees and flex the arm
to 90 degrees at the elbow. The weight of the
child's abdominal organs will result in enough
tidal flow of air to insure adequate aeration of
the lungs and prevent irreversible central
nervous system changes from anoxia.

F. Mechanical Methods
1. Face mask and rebreathing bag (air).
2. Oxygen under intermittent positive pressure by face
mask or endotracheal catheter and rebreathing
bag (Fig. 6).
3. Intermittent pressure ventilatory apparatus (Bennett,
Bird, Pulmotor, "iron lung," etc.).

17–2. Cardiac massage
A. Closed Chest (External) Cardiac Massage
1. Start effective artificial respiration (17–1, above).
This is indicated by motion of the UPPER CHEST
and by improvement in color.
2. Place the patient on a firm surface. If the patient is
in bed, a bed board should be slid under him, if
possible, instead of pulling him to the floor.
3. Check the size of the pupils; even under heavy miotic
drugs such as morphine, the pupils dilate at the
terminal stage.
4. Check the pulse (palpation of the carotid or tem-
poral arteries is most convenient).
5. Start cardiac massage by placing the heel of one
palm over the distal (inferior) portion of the
sternum, covering it with the other hand and
making forcible downward pressure. Remove
hands; repeat compression of the chest at a rate
not to exceed 50 to 60 times per minute. Pressure
should be applied with a sudden thrust, followed
by quick release. In children, pressure should be
made with less force, with the hands near the
center of the sternum using the fingers only.
6. Check the pulse and pupillary size.

BAG-MASK-OXYGEN RESPIRATION

REMOVE EXCESSIVE MUCUS.

PLACE MASK SNUGLY OVER MOUTH AND NOSE.

SUPPORT ANGLES OF JAW - TILT HEAD BACK.

SQUEEZE BAG INTERMITTENTLY 10 TO 12 TIMES

PER MINUTE (FASTER IN CHILDREN).

LIFT MASK WHEN BAG IS TOO FULL.

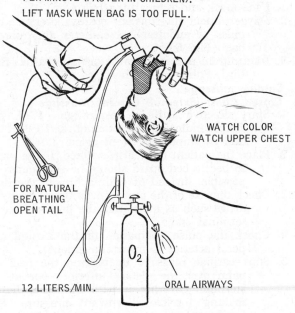

WATCH COLOR
WATCH UPPER CHEST

FOR NATURAL
BREATHING
OPEN TAIL

O_2

12 LITERS/MIN.   ORAL AIRWAYS

Figure 6.   Modified from Safar, P., and McMahon, M. C.: *Resuscitation of the Unconscious Victim—A Manual for Rescue Breathing.* 2nd Ed. Charles C Thomas, 1961.

7. Inject sodium bicarbonate solution (3.75 gm. in 50 ml. of saline) intravenously every 10 minutes to increase reactivity of heart muscle; use 50 ml. in adults, 25 ml. in children.

8. Dilute 1 ml. of 1:1000 epinephrine hydrochloride (Adrenalin) to 20 ml.; inject 2 ml. intravenously every 5 to 10 minutes. Do not use Adrenalin intracardially.

9. Recheck the pulse and pupils. Determine heart action clinically and confirm by ECG or cardiac monitor if available.

   a. If in standstill, continue measures outlined above.

   b. If fibrillating (or if fibrillation is suspected in the absence of monitoring equipment), proceed as follows:

   (1) Adjust the defibrillator controls for external defibrillation.

   (2) Apply electrolyte jelly (not K-Y jelly) to the electrodes and to the patient's chest. Press the electrodes firmly in place—one over the apex, the other over the base of the heart.

   (3) Stand clear of the patient.

   (4) Press switch for defibrillation charge; repeat two or three times if necessary. Check results by palpation of pulse or by monitor. For successful results at least 880 volts (A.C.) must be delivered. Poor electrode contact is the most common cause for failure.

   (5) Continue attempted defibrillation. A fibrillating heart is a strong heart, with a much better chance of recovery than an asystolic heart. WHEN IN DOUBT, DEFIBRILLATE!

10. When normal rhythm has been established, supportive massage and artificial respiration as needed should be continued for at least 5 minutes more. At the end of this period, the following measures to facilitate recovery can be begun:

    a. Determination and treatment of cause of cardiac arrest.

    b. Intravenous supportive or replacement therapy

(plasma, blood, plasma volume expanders, saline, etc.).

c. Vasopressor drugs.

d. Cardiac stimulants and pacemaker as needed.

B. Open Chest (Direct) Cardiac Massage (in the operating room with chest open)

1. RESPONSIBILITIES OF THE ANESTHESIOLOGIST

   a. To watch for, recognize, and notify the surgeon of, signs of incipient cardiac arrest.

   b. To apply a face mask and start administration of 100% oxygen under positive pressure by manual squeezing of the rebreathing bag, followed by insertion of an intratracheal catheter.

   c. To lower the head of table, and extend the patient's left arm if possible.

2. RESPONSIBILITIES OF THE SURGEON

   a. To attempt closed chest cardiac massage. If impractical or unsuccessful, to open the pericardium immediately through a longitudinal incision and squeeze the heart rhythmically with one or both hands, using enough pressure to force oxygenated blood throughout the circulatory system.

   b. To distinguish between cardiac standstill and ventricular fibrillation by observation and/or electrocardiogram.

3. TREATMENT TO RESTORE THE HEART BEAT. Direct manual massage may result in restoration of a normal heart beat without further measures. If it does not, insurance of oxygenation and blood circulation by adequate manual massage changes the problem from an acute emergency to a situation which will allow time for consultation and the assistance of special apparatus and instruments.

   a. IF THE HEART IS IN STANDSTILL

      (1) Continue manual massage. Dilute 1 ml. of 1:1000 epinephrine hydrochloride (Adrenalin) to 20 ml.; inject 2 ml. intravenously every 10 minutes. Larger doses may be given intravenously if necessary. Intracardiac injection is of questionable value.

       (2) Inject sodium bicarbonate (3.75 gm. in 50 ml. of saline) intravenously; repeat every 10 minutes if necessary.

       (3) Reinforce a feeble heart beat with synchronized manual compression every third or fourth beat as required.

  b. IF THE HEART IS FIBRILLATING

       (1) Continue manual massage until the defibrillator leads have been applied properly, using sterile saline in place of electrolyte jelly.

       (2) Check to be certain that the current specified by equipment's manufacturer is being used.

       (3) Apply the electrodes of the defibrillator and deliver a countershock. Repeat three or four times if necessary.

       (4) Resume manual massage.

       (5) Repeat the intravenous injection of sodium bicarbonate (3.75 gm. in 50 ml. of saline).

       (6) Repeat the defibrillating shocks and injections as often as necessary.

  c. When ventricular fibrillation has ceased proceed as given under standstill (17–2,B,3,a, above). WHEN IN DOUBT, DEFIBRILLATE!

 4. CLOSURE OF THE CHEST

  a. Postpone closure until the pulse and blood pressure have been stable for some time; then close the pericardium and anterior wall as rapidly as possible.

  b. Inject atropine sulfate, 0.6 mg., intravenously, followed by lantoside C (Cedilanid), 0.8 mg.

  c. Keep under constant close observation until there is no doubt of the stability of the heart beat. Personnel and equipment for external cardiac massage (17–2,A, above) should be available for immediate use. Open chest (direct) massage should not be repeated once the chest has been closed unless there are other indications.

 5. MEDICOLEGAL ASPECTS of closed and open cardiac massage. See Topic 29–2,E.

17–3. Catheterization

Insertion of any type of tube into the bladder invites serious infection; therefore, it should not be done to obtain specimens for routine examination. A "clean catch" or second glass specimen usually is satisfactory. If acute retention or need for determination of kidney function requires catheterization careful technique should be used.

A. Male

1. Cleanse the penis thoroughly with soap and water and place on a sterile towel.
2. Put on sterile gloves.
3. Insert a sterile catheter using gentle, steady pressure, holding the dorsum away from the body to straighten the urethral curve.
4. If any obstruction is encountered so that entry into the bladder cannot be made on two or three GENTLE attempts, or if there is bleeding, a sedative should be given and the patient referred at once for urologic care. As a rule, filiform or stylet-containing catheters should not be used except under the supervision of a urologist.

B. Female. In female patients, catheterization can be done very easily, preferably by a nurse, using sterile technique and a NONBREAKABLE catheter.

17–4. Gastric lavage

Since the object of lavage in acute poisoning is rapid removal of the contents of the stomach, as large a tube as possible should be used. Even small children will tolerate passage through the mouth of relatively large tubes. Attempted lavage through an intranasal tube is utterly unsatisfactory. A CHILD MUST BE "MUMMIFIED" BY BEING WRAPPED TIGHTLY IN A SHEET AND PLACED ON HIS BACK WITH THE HEAD TURNED TO ONE SIDE AND THE FEET SLIGHTLY ELEVATED. The lavage tube should be smooth and well lubricated with a water-soluble preparation. Either a large syringe or a large funnel or container raised above the patient's head, and equipped with a two-way stopcock for drainage, is satisfactory for introduction of the solution. Repeated washings with small amounts of solution should always be done until the return solution is clean. Overfilling of the stomach should be guarded against because of the danger of regurgitation and aspiration. The tube should be pinched off, or gentle suction retained during removal, to prevent aspiration.

In cases of suspected poisoning, a specimen of the stomach

washings should be collected, marked for identification, and saved for possible analysis.

Gavage-emesis methods are not suitable for emergency use.

17–5. Intraglossal injections

In unconscious patients whose veins are collapsed or impossible to locate without a cutdown, small amounts (up to 2 ml.) of medications are rapidly absorbed from the tongue without residual ill effects. If a vasopressor is used, enough effect can usually be obtained to allow location of a peripheral vein for insertion of a needle for conventional venous infusions.

Technique

1. Grasp the tongue by the tip and pull it upward toward the nose.
2. Using a short bevel, 20 or 22 gauge needle, inject the solution into the muscles on the underside of the tongue, avoiding the large veins on each side of the midline.
3. Only rapidly absorbable, nonirritating medications should be used except as a lifesaving measure.

17–6. Nasal packing

A. Anterior. Several methods are satisfactory.

1. Pack tightly with petrolatum gauze.
2. Pack firmly with a gauze strip moistened with 1:1000 epinephrine hydrochloride (Adrenalin).
3. Fill a rubber finger cot or glove finger loosely with gauze and insert into the nostril; then moisten the gauze. The resultant swelling of the gauze will cause uniform and even pressure.

   Topical anesthesia often is required. Medicated gauze (especially iodoform gauze) should not be used for nasal packing.

B. Posterior (Nasopharyngeal)

1. Give a preliminary injection of morphine sulfate or dihydromorphinone hydrochloride (Dilaudid) to older children and adults. To allay apprehension, a pentobarbital sodium (Nembutal) suppository should be substituted in children under 10 years of age. Topical anesthesia may be indicated in hypersensitive persons.
2. Pass a small, soft rubber catheter through the nostril and into the pharynx.

3. Grasp the slotted end of the catheter with forceps and bring it out through the mouth.

4. Attach to the slotted end of the catheter a 12-inch length of No. 30 or No. 40 cotton to which is fastened a piece of soft nonmedicated gauze, attached to another 12-inch length of cotton.

5. Pull the gauze gently but firmly into the posterior nares by withdrawing the catheter through the nose.

6. Unfasten the catheter and tie the cotton ligatures extruding from the nostril and mouth together loosely over a piece of gauze placed on the upper lip below the nostril, avoiding pressure on the columella.

7. Instruct the patient to report to a physician for recheck examination in 24 hours. He should NOT be told that the pack will be removed at that time.

17–7. Pericardial sac aspiration

The only equipment needed for this procedure, which may be lifesaving if cardiac tamponade (Topic 29–4) is present, is a large (18 or 20 gauge) hypodermic needle and a medium syringe.

A. Sites of Aspiration (in order of desirability)

1. Slightly to the left of the xiphoid process of the sternum with the needle directed superiorly.

2. Through the left fourth interspace ½ inch to the left of the sternocostal junction.

3. Through the posterior chest slightly to the right of the inferior angle of the left scapula. This method transverses the lung and should not be used if there is any possibility of pericardial sac empyema.

B. Technique

1. Cleanse the selected area thoroughly with soap and water and paint with merthiolate.

2. Insert a 2½ inch long 18 gauge needle with a short bevel attached to a 10 or 20 ml. syringe through the chest wall into the pericardial sac and aspirate gently. Either fresh or defibrinated blood may be obtained. Relief from tamponade may be obtained from removal of as little as 5 ml. The

procedure may be repeated as often as necessary for relief, but immediate thoractomy is indicated if:
  a. Aspiration gives no relief.
  b. If no blood is obtained.
  c. If signs and symptoms of tamponade recur in spite of repeated aspirations.

17–8.   Peritoneal aspiration

Using a small abdominal paracentesis trocar with obturator, or a large bore spinal puncture needle with stylet, abdominal aspiration can be performed safely and easily and is a valuable diagnostic procedure, especially in abdominal contusions (Topic 55–1). Fresh blood is an indication for immediate exploratory laparotomy. For details of insertion, see 17–9, below.

17–9.   Peritoneal dialysis

This very simple procedure is of great value in the treatment of severe poisoning and in certain systemic diseases such as hepatic coma (Topic 3–10).

Technique (See Fig. 7).

  1. Prepare a site in the abdomen by shaving and the usual presurgical skin preparation. The patient should be supine and, if necessary, in bed. The site of choice is in the midline 4 cm. below the umbilicus. Any scarred areas should be avoided because of the probability of adjacent intra-abdominal adhesions.
  2. After anesthetizing the area, insert a No. 22 paracentesis trocar through a stab wound. In the absence of ascites, 500 ml. of air should be pumped in preliminarily; if there is ascites, this is not necessary.
  3. Push the trocar with the obturator in place through the peritoneum; remove the obturator and substitute a previously prepared dialysis tube—a 12-inch section of plastic intravenous tubing with elliptical holes cut at frequent intervals in the distal 4 inches is satisfactory. Gently work the dialysis tube into the pelvis.
  4. Remove the trocar and suture the skin around the dialysis tube.
  5. Connect the dialysis tube to a piece of tubing at least 36 inches long. The tubing, in turn, should

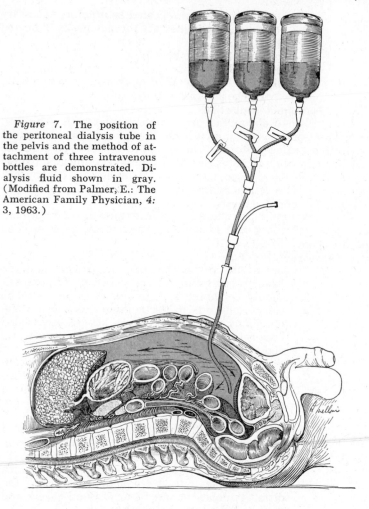

Figure 7. The position of the peritoneal dialysis tube in the pelvis and the method of attachment of three intravenous bottles are demonstrated. Dialysis fluid shown in gray. (Modified from Palmer, E.: The American Family Physician, 4: 3, 1963.)

be connected through a three-way stopcock or double Y connectors with flasks containing the following solutions:

   a. Normal saline, 1000 ml.
   b. Dextrose, 5% in water, 1000 ml.
   c. Sodium bicarbonate (100 ml. of 10% solution) in 5% dextrose in saline, 1000 ml.

6. With the solution bottles elevated on an intravenous stand, adjust flow from all 3 so that 1¼ to 1½ hours are required for all to empty into the abdomen.

7. When about 20 ml. remain in each bottle, remove them from the intravenous stand and place them on the floor and allow the fluid from the abdomen to run out by gravity.

8. Collect specimens of fluid for analysis as required.

9. Replace solution bottles and elevate to intravenous stand.

10. Repeat the procedure above as needed, governed by the patient's clinical condition and analysis of the returned dialysis fluid.

17–10. Reduction of dislocations

   A. Hip Dislocations require hospitalization for reduction under general anesthesia.

   B. Shoulder Dislocations

   1. ARM-WEIGHT TRACTION METHOD

      a. After preliminary administration of a narcotic, place the patient facedown on a narrow examination table with the arm on the injured side hanging down.

      b. Make firm but gentle traction on the wrist with gentle external rotation. If, after 15 to 20 minutes, reduction has not been accomplished, other methods should be tried, with hospitalization for reduction under general anesthesia if the heel-in-axilla and Kocher's methods are unsuccessful.

   2. HEEL-IN-AXILLA METHOD. With the emergency physician's heel in the axilla as a fulcrum, reduction can often be accomplished by traction and manipulation. If two attempts are unsuccessful, refer for hospitalization and general anesthesia.

3. KOCHER'S METHOD
    a. Traction on the elbow with lateral pressure on the humeral head.
    b. Adduction of the elbow with slow forcible external rotation of the forearm.
    c. Slow internal rotation of the forearm with the elbow held close to the body until the hand is on the opposite shoulder.
    d. Confirmation of reduction by x-rays or fluoroscopic examination (Topic 21).
    e. Application of a snug Velpeau bandage.

17–11. **Tracheotomy**
  A. Indications
    1. Angioedema (Topic 24–2 and Topic 48–4).
    2. Burns (usually of the flash type with flame inhalation (Topic 28–19,B).
    3. Cerebral vascular accidents with respiratory muscle involvement (Topic 60–2).
    4. Debilitated and severely ill persons with impaired respiratory function [Topic 3–6 (*Emphysema*)].
    5. Foreign bodies lodged above the second tracheal ring (Topic 38–4).
    6. Laryngeal paralysis, bilateral [Topic 32–4 (*Diphtheria*)].
    7. Poliomyelitis, bulbar type (Topic 32–21 and Topic 47–5).
    8. Poisoning resulting in coma (see under name of poison, Topic 49).
    9. Respiratory obstruction from any cause.
    10. Surgical procedures (jaw injuries, neck dissections, etc.), elective.
    11. Tetanus (Topic 32–31).
    12. Transverse myelitis, cervical, usually traumatic, high enough to affect respiratory muscles (Topic 47–5).
    13. TRAUMA
        a. Chest injuries (Topic 31–2,B).
        b. Facial injuries.
        c. Fractures and dislocations of the cervical spine.
        d. Head injuries (Topic 43 and Topic 48–28).
        e. Soft tissue injuries of the throat and neck with resultant edema (Topic 45–11).

f. Spinal cord injuries (cervical) (Topic 47–7).

B. Methods

1. CRICOTHYROID MEMBRANE PUNCTURE. This is a life-saving measure only and can be done with any sharp instrument, such as sharp-pointed scissors, knife blade, or nail file. It must be supplanted by a regular tracheotomy (17–11,B,2, below) within two days.

a. Locate the space between the two most prominent cartilages with the neck slightly hyper-extended.

b. Make a 1-inch long transverse incision in the soft space between the cartilages. This incision should go through the skin only (Fig. 8).

c. Stabilize the larynx between the left thumb and middle finger; press the index fingernail firmly into the exposed cricothyroid ligament.

d. Using the index fingernail as a guide and holding the instrument blade transversely, work the blade through the ligament and into the tra-

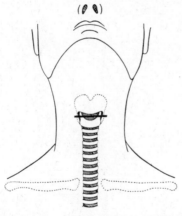

Figure 8. Drawing of cricothyroid membrane. Solid line shows incision. (Nicholas, T. H., and Rumer, G. F.: J.A.M.A., *179*:1933, 1960.)

chea (Fig. 9). Avoid excess pressure with damage to the posterior wall.

e. Spread by turning the blade through 90°.

f. If necessary, substitute a key or pen barrel for the blade. DO NOT USE SMALL OBJECTS WHICH MIGHT BE ASPIRATED.

2. LOW TRACHEOTOMY (method of choice except in extreme emergencies).

a. Place the patient on his back with his neck slightly hyperextended by a support under his shoulders.

b. Under local anesthesia, make a longitudinal incision through the skin and subcutaneous tissues from below the cricoid to just above the sternal notch.

c. Separate the muscles.

d. Locate the inferior border of cricoid with the

CRICOTHYROID MEMBRANE PUNCTURE

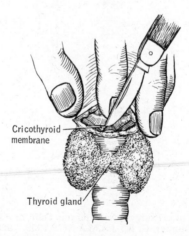

Cricothyroid membrane

Thyroid gland

Figure 9. To establish an emergency airway, a 1-inch transverse skin incision is made over the cricothyroid membrane. The larynx is stabilized between the thumb and middle finger of the left hand. A sharp instrument is then passed along the nail of the index finger, which is pressed firmly into the membrane. (Modified from Nicholas, T. H., and Rumer, G. F.: Modern Medicine, April 17, 1961.)

finger transversely. Avoid the inferior thyroid
veins. Clamp the thyroid isthmus and suture
after cutting between clamps.

e. Retract the isthmus stumps laterally and inject a
few drops of 10 per cent cocaine through
the tracheal wall.

f. Expose rings 1 to 5.

g. Incise the 3rd and 4th tracheal rings vertically
and pick up the edges with hooks.

h. Insert the cannula followed by the inner tube.
Complete hemostasis is important.

i. Suture the upper angles of the wound loosely to
allow escape of air.

j. Fasten the tapes snugly around the neck.

k. Arrange for frequent suction and aspiration
through the tube.

l. Check the position of the tracheotomy tube by
fluoroscopy or x-rays when the patient's condition will permit.

18. *TESTS APPLICABLE TO EMERGENCY CASES*

No attempt has been made in the following sections to list
or describe the numerous clinical and laboratory tests which
constitute an essential and invaluable part of the efficient
management of emergency cases. The six tests outlined below,
however, are peculiarly valuable in emergency situations, even
though their interpretations may be suggestive and not conclusive.

18–1. Alcohol intoxication tests

Measurements of the alcohol content of the breath and of the
blood can be made without difficulty and are of approximately
equal accuracy. The admissibility of blood alcohol tests as evidence is becoming more widespread year by year. The results
of breath analysis tests at the present time are not, as a general rule, accepted as legal evidence but may be of great value
to law enforcement officers.

A. Breath Analysis. The three types of equipment most frequently used are the Drunkometer (Harger), the Intoximeter (Forrester) and the Alcometer (Greenberg). All three depend upon the analysis of alveolar air collected in a small balloon. The expired breath forced into the balloon is generally considered to contain ⅝ alveolar air and ⅜ corridor air (from the nares, mouth and nasopharynx). Since the alveolar air–blood ratio for alcohol is known (about 1:2100) and the alveolar air contains about 5.5% carbon dioxide, by weighing the amount of carbon dioxide and determining the amount of alcohol in a given specimen, the blood alcohol concentration can be determined very accurately.

B. Blood Analysis. All tests for alcohol in the blood depend upon a complex chemical analysis of blood obtained from a vein by a technique which avoids possible contamination with alcohol from outside sources.

METHOD OF OBTAINING BLOOD SPECIMEN

1. On request of a patient, his legal guardian or a law enforcement officer, blood may be drawn by a physician for blood alcohol determination, provided the permission of the patient or his legal guardian is obtained in writing without misrepresentation or coercion. For a satisfactory permit form, see Topic 70–4. Before the permission is signed the patient or his guardian should be informed in simple nontechnical language of the purpose of the test. It is the physician's responsibility to determine that the patient is sufficiently in possession of his faculties at the time of signature to understand the reason for, purpose of, and possible consequences of, the test. Tacit permission for withdrawal of blood for the test is assumed if the patient, after having been given the information above, makes no active attempt to prevent completion of the procedure.

2. No alcohol, or substance containing alcohol, can be used in cleansing the skin.

3. Syringes, needles and vials used in collecting the blood specimen must have been sterilized by a non-alcohol technique.

4. Special containers, marked for identification, must be used. These should be labeled carefully for identification and initialed by at least two witnesses before being sent to the laboratory for analysis.

5. The exact time that the specimen is taken should be indicated on the container.

C. Clinical Examination for Alcoholic Intoxication

1. HISTORY AND HABITS

a. Occupation (deep-sea or sport diver, caisson worker, exposure to narcotic or inebriating gases at work, etc.).

b. Injuries or diseases which might modify interpretation of results of tests.

c. Medications, especially narcotics, hypnotics, sedatives, "mood modifiers," muscle relaxants and antihistaminics.

d. Consumption of alcoholic beverages:

(1) Daily or periodic drinker.

(2) Average daily amount.

(3) Time, kind and amount of last drink.

(4) Companions or witnesses—name of bar, etc.

e. Treatment in past for acute or chronic alcoholism, delirium tremens, addiction to any substances, or neuropsychiatric complaints.

2. PHYSICAL EXAMINATION. A fair and accurate conclusion regarding alcohol intoxication requires comparison of the original examination findings with the results of previous examination or of re-examination several hours later, preferably by the same physician.

The following points should be covered:

a. Odor of alcoholic beverages on the breath. In spite of the claims of the manufacturers of various proprietary compounds, this odor cannot be masked or dissipated by any known method.

b. Red ("bloodshot") or watery eyes.

c. Impairment of speech (indistinctness, slurring).

d. Unbuttoned or disarrayed clothing.

e. Evidence of vomiting, bowel or bladder incontinence, or seminal emission.

      f. Mental alertness and attitude (euphoria, sullenness, belligerence, depression, etc.).

      g. Evidence of recent trauma—especially head injuries (Topic 43).

      h. Muscular coordination:

          (1) Gait—broad base, straddling, unsteady.

          (2) Balance—ability to walk a straight line and to execute rapid turns.

          (3) Joint sense—finger to nose or ear, foot to opposite knee, etc.

          (4) Specialized motions—picking up pins or coins, comparison of handwriting with previous or subsequent samples.

      i. Evidence of unrelated injuries or of local or systemic conditions which could be mistaken for alcoholic intoxication.

D. Interpretation of Results of Blood Alcohol Tests

Per Cent Alcohol in Blood (by Weight)	Milligrams of Alcohol per Milliliter of Blood	Clinical Effect (Average)	Slowing of Reaction Time (Average)	Legal Interpretation: Under Influence of Alcohol?
0.01 to 0.05	10 mg./100 ml. 50 mg./100 ml.	None	Possibly slight	No
0.06 to 0.10	60 mg./100 ml. 100 mg./100 ml.	Decreased coordination and visual fields, blurring of vision, impaired control and restraint, euphoria, slurring of speech, impairment of special senses	2 ×	Possibly
0.11 to 0.30	110 mg./100 ml. 300 mg./100 ml.	Staggering, mental confusion, stupor	4 ×	Definitely
0.31 to 0.45	310 mg./100 ml. 450 mg./100 ml.	Respiratory and circulatory impairment, subnormal temperature, coma, sometimes death	Total loss	Completely
0.46 up	460 mg./100 ml.	Complete respiratory and circulatory paralysis, death	Total loss	Irreversibly, often terminally

E. Modifying Factors. The amount of alcohol necessary
to produce the different stages of alcoholism outlined in D (above) may be modified by:

1. Individual sensitivity (constitutional tolerance, age,
   sex).
2. Acquired tolerance (habituation).
3. Mental condition.
4. Environment and circumstances (climate, temperature, exercise, type of work).
5. Diet—recent intake of food.
6. Medications.
7. Unrelated organic pathology. Among these diseases
   and pathologic conditions are:
   a. Metabolic disturbances such as diabetic hypogly-
      cemia, acidosis, uremia, effects of increased
      barometric pressure, etc.
   b. Pulmonary diseases, such as emphysema with car-
      bon dioxide retention.
   c. Myocardial infarction; angina pectoris.
   d. Hypertension.
   e. Senility.
   f. Postsurgical and postanesthetic reactions.
   g. Intracranial pathology.

18–2. Cervical spine injury test

Determination of the possibility of cervical spine injury in the
presence of other injuries which may mask discomfort in the
neck is often very important since presence of cervical injuries
makes modifications in handling and transportation essential.
The patient must be conscious for this test to be of value.

A. Gently move the head so that the neck is comparatively
straight (NOT in the presence of obvious deformity
or malalignment or of evidence of cord injury).

B. Place one hand on the top of the head and tap it
lightly with the other, with the force in the long
axis of the spine.

If cervical pathology is present, the patient will show subjective signs of discomfort by protest, objection or facial
grimace.

18–3. Narcotic addiction test

A. For Clinical Signs of Addiction, see Topic 2–4.

B. For Signs and Symptoms of Acute Intoxication from Overdosage, see Topic 49–370 (*Morphine*).

C. Nalorphine Hydrochloride (Nalline) Test

1. Have the patient (or his legal guardian if a minor or mentally incompetent) give written permission for the test in the presence of two witnesses. The permission form must include a statement that the purpose of the test has been explained to, and is understood by, the signer and that no coercion has been used in obtaining the signed permission.

2. Measure the size of the patient's pupils, using a piece of cardboard pierced or marked in 0.5 mm. gradations from 0.5 mm. to 3 mm.

3. Inject 3 mg. of nalorphine hydrochloride (Nalline) subcutaneously, with means at hand for combatting sudden severe withdrawal symptoms (6, below).

4. Wait 30 minutes.

5. Re-measure the size of the pupils with exactly the same amount of light present as in 2, above.

6. Treat withdrawal symptoms if necessary by subcutaneous or intravenous injection of an effective amount of morphine sulfate or dihydromorphinone hydrochloride (Dilaudid).

7. Interpret the results of the test as follows:

Pupillary Size	Using Addictive Narcotics?
Decreased	No
No change	Occasionally (or normally has small pupils)
Increased	Yes (addict)

The injections suggested in steps (3) and (6) must be performed by a licensed physician.

18–4. Pelvic-femoral integrity test

Determination of the possibility of bony injury to the femur and pelvis is of extreme importance, especially in elderly or debilitated persons with impaired stability.

A. With the patient supine press a stethoscope firmly against the exact center of the symphysis pubis.

B. With the legs straight and the quadriceps completely relaxed, tap firmly against the anterior surface of each patella and listen for a difference in sound intensity between the injured and uninjured side. Suggestive findings are as follows (NOT conclusive):

   1. Same intensity, both sides—no bony injury.

   2. No transmittal on one side—fracture, probably displaced, of femur or pubic rami.

   3. Decreased intensity, one side—suggestive of fracture with impaction, such as of the femoral neck.

Emergency handling can be tentatively based on the results above, with diagnostic x-rays as soon as possible.

18–5. Salicylate ingestion test

Because of the delay in the development of symptoms and signs such as hyperpnea after ingestion of salicylates, and because of the too frequent uncertainty on the parts of parents as to what their child may have swallowed, the following simple, rapid test is of value for emergency use.

A. Heat a specimen of urine gently to rule out presence of acetone bodies.

B. To 5 ml. of urine, add 1 ml. of 10% ferric chloride solution.

C. Shake gently and observe color. Development of a purple color indicates presence of one of the following:

   1. Acetylsalicylic acid (aspirin).

   2. Methyl, phenyl or sodium salicylate.

   3. Phenol derivatives.

Presence of a purple color indicates the ingestion of as little as one 0.3 gm. aspirin tablet between 30 minutes and 12 hours before examination. The test is not quantitative.

18–6. Ventilation test (Snider)

As a rough index of expiratory volume and flow rate, the following match test is of value in estimating changes in respiratory physiology in potentially progressive conditions.

A. Have the patient remove dentures if present.

B. Hold a lighted, ½ burned, book-type match 6 inches from his mouth.

C. Instruct the patient to blow out the match. (Several positions should be used to compensate for facial weakness, etc.).
D. Inability to blow out the flame indicates (roughly):
   1. Forced expiratory volume—less than 1000 ml.
   2. Flow rate—less than 120 liters per minute.

19. TETANUS IMMUNIZATION

See also Topic 14 (*Serum Sensitivity and Desensitization*); Topic 32–31 (*Tetanus*); and Topic 48–55 (*Tetanus in Children*).

Because the mortality from established tetanus (Topic 32–31) is extremely high, protective injections should be given without hesitation after as efficient a wound toilet as possible (Topic 55–20). Failure to recognize the need for active or passive immunization against tetanus and to institute the proper protective measures could be (and should be) actionable (Topic 69–1 and 3).

19–1. **Conditions requiring protection against tetanus**
   A. All puncture wounds, even if minute (Topic 55–27).
   B. All animal, bat, human, snake, or spider bites (Topic 27).
   C. All open (compound) fractures (Topic 45–8).
   D. All wounds grossly contaminated with dirt, dust, soil or animal excreta.
   E. All friction and pavement burns (Topic 28–21).
   F. All gunshot wounds (Topic 55–26).
   G. All wounds (including minute abrasions and superficial lacerations) in which firearms or explosives of any kind (dynamite, firecrackers, fireworks, gunpowder, cap pistol ammunition) may have been factors.
   H. All wounds in which adequate debridement has not been possible because it would involve sacrifice of essential structures (nerves, major blood vessels, tendons, joint cartilages, etc.), or in which complete obliteration of all dead spaces has not been accomplished.

I. All wounds for which treatment has been delayed beyond the safe time limit (Topic 55–20,B).

19–2. **Indication for use of tetanus antitoxin** (Passive Protection)

Tetanus antitoxin in doses of 3000 to 30,000 units, depending upon the extent and character of the wound (19–1, above),
should be given intramuscularly [after a skin test and desensitization if necessary (Topic 14)] in the following circumstances:

A. If there is no history of previous active immunization
(series of toxoid injections).
B. If active immunization by a series of two or three
toxoid injections at 4- to 6-week intervals is incomplete, has been completed within 6 months, or
was completed more than 10 years previously with
no interval boosters.
C. If IMMEDIATE protection is required. Since passive
protection from antitoxin lasts for a limited period
only (not over 10 days), further injections of antitoxin may be necessary if gross infection is present.

19–3. **Indications for use of tetanus toxoid** (Active Protection)

A booster injection of 0.5 ml. of tetanus toxoid will result in
an increase of antibody titer to a protective level in 14 to 21
days. It should be given if:

A. Active immunization by injections of toxoid has been
completed not less than 6 months or more than
10 years previously.
B. The original active immunization has been followed
every 5 years by boosters of 0.5 ml. of toxoid.
C. The patient has never been actively immunized and is
acutely sensitive to available animal serum antitoxins and no human antitetanus serum is available.

19–4. **Indications for tetanus antitoxin and toxoid concurrently**

A. Immediate protection is required (19–2,C, above).
B. Strong indications for protection (19–1, above) are
present but active immunization has been completed more than 10 years previously with no interval booster.
C. No previous active immunization at any time. The first
of the series of two or three toxoid injections should

be given on the first visit and the patient given specific instructions regarding completion of the series and subsequent interval boosters.

D. Tetanus antitoxin and toxoid injections should never be given at the same time in the same extremity.

20. URGENCY EVALUATION

Classification of emergency cases by the urgency with which treatment is required is one of the most important functions and responsibilities of a physician called upon to treat such cases (Topic 1–2 and Topic 72). Rapid and accurate urgency evaluation, often complicated by the presence of multiple serious conditions in the same individual and almost always in an unstable, excited environment, not only calls for thorough knowledge of surgery, medicine, toxicology, psychology (especially crowd psychology) and psychiatry, but also for the ability to translate this knowledge into immediate effective action under stressful circumstances.

In contrast to many of the conditions encountered on a busy emergency service, IMMEDIATE recognition and prompt, effective and correct management of the conditions listed below may be lifesaving.

A. Massive hemorrhage from major vessels (Topic 8–1 and Topic 60–1).

B. Cardiac arrest (Topic 29–2).

C. Cessation or acute embarrassment of respiration (Topic 13).

D. Profound shock from any cause (Topic 15).

E. Rapidly acting poisons (Topic 49).

F. Anaphylactic reactions (Topic 24).

G. Acute epidural hemorrhage (Topic 43–20 and Topic 48–22).

H. Acute overwhelming bacteremia and toxemia (Topic 32–16 and Topic 48–38 and 59).

I. Severe head injuries with rapidly degenerating vital signs (Topic 43–2).

J. Penetrating wounds of the pleura or pericardium (Topic 31–9).

    K. Rupture of an abdominal viscus (Topic 8–3,I, and Topic 55–1).

    L. Acute maniacal states (Topic 51).

Only through experience and complete confidence in his own knowledge and judgment will the emergency physician develop the ability to distinguish between an individual dying from an uncontrollable irreparable condition and a less spectacularly injured or sick person for whom his knowledge and skill may be life or function saving.

21. X-RAYS

21–1. Indications

A surprisingly large percentage of injury cases requiring emergency care are potentially medicolegal problems, especially if industrial coverage (Topic 76) or liability or subrogation factors (Topic 68) are involved. Malpractice actions (Topic 69) are all too frequently based on the first treatment received by the patient. Therefore, to protect the patient, the hospital and the attending physician, x-rays should be taken whenever bony injuries, or any conditions demonstrable roentgenologically, are suspected, provided moving and positioning the patient will not be harmful. Normal ("negative") x-rays may have as much medicolegal value as those showing traumatic or other pathology. The attending physician's interpretation of the recently developed films can often be used as a basis for emergency therapy. In many instances, the presence or absence of pathology can be determined from wet films with a reasonable degree of accuracy and a working diagnosis established. This original interpretation of the x-rays should be confirmed by a qualified roentgenologist as soon as possible and a report incorporated in the patient's record.

21–2. Transferral of x-rays

X-rays essential to definitive care should be sent with the patient whenever transfer to any hospital is arranged. If referral to another physician's office is made, the films should be held awaiting his request except in those instances when adequate treatment requires their immediate presence (fractures, dislocations, head injuries, etc.). If x-ray films leave the direct control of the physician by whom they are ordered for any reason, a receipt should be signed by the person to whom they are consigned for transportation, and return of the x-rays as soon as possible should be requested, with careful follow-up in a reasonable time.

21–3. **Ownership of x-rays**

No matter who pays for them, x-rays are the property of the physician who orders them and not of the patient, the hospital or laboratory where they are taken, other medical attendants, attorneys, insurance companies or other interested persons. Since the films (NOT the reports based on them) must be produced when designated by due process of law [Topic 74 (*Subpoenas*)] they must be safeguarded in the same manner as the clinical record.

21–4. **Fluoroscopic examination**

If fluoroscopic equipment is available it will be found to be of assistance in some instances in the reduction of fractures and dislocations. An x-ray technician should be present if possible whenever the fluoroscope is used but, TO PROTECT HIMSELF AND THE PATIENT, any physician using the equipment should personally, carefully and invariably observe the following safety factors:

A. Always wear a protective apron and, if possible and practical, lead-impregnated gloves.

B. Never use more than 5 milliamperes (5 ma).

C. Never use more than 80 kilovolts (80 kv).

D. Always limit each exposure time to not more than 3 seconds.

E. Never use more than 10 exposures.

21–5. **Protection of gonads**

Although the danger from gonadal radiation has been greatly overemphasized in the lay press, shielding of the lower abdomen and external genitalia is a simple procedure and should be done whenever practical, especially in children, males in the reproductive age, and women during the first trimester of pregnancy.

21–6. **X-ray burns.** See Topic 28–31.

EMERGENCY TREATMENT
OF SPECIFIC CONDITIONS

22. ABDOMINAL PAIN

See also Topic 55–1 (*Abdominal Injuries*) and Topic 55 under specific abdominal viscera.

Distinguishing between an acute surgical abdomen and other less serious or less fulminating conditions may require blood counts and other laboratory procedures not available in an emergency situation. However, in a high percentage of cases a tentative diagnosis can be made from the history and physical examination; certainly, from the history and clinical picture, the attending physician should be able to determine whether or not immediate hospitalization is indicated. UNLESS A DEFINITE DIAGNOSIS OF A NONDANGEROUS CONDITION HAS BEEN ESTABLISHED, any person with persistent or recurrent severe pain should be hospitalized as soon as possible for thorough examination, diagnosis and treatment.

Some of the numerous conditions which may cause acute abdominal pain are included in the following list:

Aneurysm, dissecting (Topic 60–2,D).
Angina, intestinal—caused by mesenteric vascular insufficiency (Topic 39–2,B).
Appendicitis, acute (Topic 39–7).
Black widow spider bites (Topic 27–5).
Bowel obstruction, acute (Topic 39–2).
Caisson disease (Topic 26–3).
Cholecystitis, acute (Topic 39–8).
Coronary disease (Topic 29–5).
Cystitis, acute (Topic 40–12).
Decompression sickness (Topic 26–3).
Diabetes (hyperglycemia) (Topic 3–3).
Diaphragmatic rupture (Topic 31–6).
Diverticulitis (Topic 39–10).
Ectopic pregnancy, ruptured (Topic 50–3).
Enteritis, acute bacterial or regional (Topic 39–2,B).
Epilepsy, abdominal (Topic 33 and Topic 51–9).
Gallbladder disease (Topic 39–8) or trauma (Topic 55–17).
Hepatitis, acute (Topic 63–8,A) or traumatic (Topic 55–21).
Herpes zoster (Topic 47–4,E).
Kidney stones (Topic 40–22).
Lead colic [Topic 49–313 (*Lead Salts*)].
Liver disease (Topic 3–10) and trauma (Topic 55–21).

Mesenteric lymphadenitis (in children), thrombosis and embolism (Topic 39–24,B).
Migraine (Topic 30–21 and Topic 48–39).
Mittelschmerz (Topic 41–8).
Myocardial infarction (Topic 29–5).
Ovarian cyst with torsion of the pedicle (Topic 41–13).
Pancreatitis, acute (Topic 39–19) or traumatic (Topic 55–24).
Parathyroid crises (Topic 35–3,B).
Peptic ulcer with or without perforation (Topic 39–3,B).
Peritonitis, acute (Topic 55–27,B,7).
Pleurodynia (Topic 63–16).
Pneumonia [Topic 53–14 and Topic 48–41 (*Pneumonia in Children*)].
Poisoning, acute (Topic 49 under entries listed below unless otherwise noted) from:

Antimony (49–57)	Lead [under *Lead Salts* (49–313)]
Arsenic trioxide (49–63)	Methyl alcohol (49–358)
Aspidium (49–68)	Morphine (49–370)
Barium (49–77)	Mushrooms (49–373)
Bichloride of mercury (49–87)	Parathion [under *Organic Phosphates* (49–421)]
Cadmium (49–106)	Phenolphthalein (49–451)
Carbon tetrachloride (49–120)	Physostigmine (49–463)
Chromates (49–145)	Solanine (49–553)
Colchicine (49–154)	Spider venom (Topic 62)
Copper salts (49–157)	Squill (49–557)
Croton oil (49–166)	Sulfapyridine [under *Sulfonamides* (49–569)]
Cyanides (49–170)	Tetraethyl pyrophosphate (TEPP) [under *Organic Phosphates* (49–421)]
Diethylstilbestrol (49–190)	
Ergot (49–218)	Thallium (49–597)
Fluorides (49–242)	Tung nuts (49–632)
Formaldehyde (49–246)	Turpentine (49–633)
Gasoline (49–254)	Veratrum viride (49–640)
Kerosene (49–303)	Viosterol (49–644)

Porphyria (Topic 44–20).
Rupture of a viscus (Topic 55–1,A and B).
Salpingitis (Topic 41–9).
Tabes dorsalis (Topic 61–9 and 10).
Trauma, direct—especially to the liver (Topic 55–21) and spleen (Topic 55–30).
Tubo-ovarian abscess (Topic 41–9).
Uremia (Topic 3–15).
Ureteral stones (Topic 40–22).

If by a careful history and physical examination and utilization of available laboratory tests the emergency physician is unable to determine the cause of persistent or recurrent abdominal distress, the patient should be hospitalized at once. Because of the possibility of masking signs and symptoms, no opiates or synthetic narcotics of any kind should be given for control of pain or relief of apprehension until a definite diagnosis has been established; even then, barbiturates or phenothiazines in small doses are preferable.

A detailed summary of all findings, ESPECIALLY CHANGES IN CONDITION, and of all treatment, should be sent with any patient with abdominal pain who is referred for diagnosis and treatment to a hospital or private physician's office.

23. ABSCESSES

GENERAL CONSIDERATIONS
23–1. **Early abscesses** without localization or fluctuation should be treated expectantly by local application of heat. Many will be absorbed under this regimen; others will localize in a short time.

23–2. **Small superficial abscesses** may be incised and drained under ethyl chloride spray or procaine or lidocaine (Xylocaine) block anesthesia.

23–3. **Large deep abscesses** should be treated conservatively by application of heat until localization occurs, then referred for hospitalization and wide drainage, usually under a general anesthetic.

ABSCESSES REQUIRING SPECIAL CARE
23–4. **Alveolar abscesses** arise from infection at a tooth root and are often exquisitely painful [Topic 58 (*Toothache*)].

   Treatment
   A. Early Cases
   1. Codeine sulfate and acetylsalicyclic acid (aspirin) for pain.
   2. Penicillin intramuscularly and/or tetracyclines by mouth.
   3. Reference to a dentist for drilling (not extraction).
   B. Late Cases with fluctuation at the gingival margin ("gum boils").
   1. Drainage through a small incision parallel to the border of the gum. No anesthetic is required and relief is immediate.
   2. Reference for dental care.

23–5. **Anorectal abscesses** may be superficial or deep but all require incision and drainage under general or low spinal anesthesia.

Control of pain while hospitalization is being arranged is the only emergency treatment required.

23–6. **Apical abscesses.** See 23–4, above (*Alveolar Abscesses*).

23–7. **Bartholin abscesses.** See Topic 41–3.

23–8. **Boils**

Treatment

1. Application of local heat until localization and fluctuation develop or spontaneous resolution takes place.
2. Incision and drainage under ethyl chloride spray anesthesia, with insertion of a rubber dam drain and application of an absorbent dressing after obtaining material for cultures.
3. Ringing of the draining sinus with petrolatum gauze to minimize mechanical spreading.
4. Reference for further medical care.

23–9. **Brain abscesses** may follow head injuries (especially fractures), otitis media and mastoiditis. Suspicion of the presence of a brain abscess is an indication for immediate hospitalization.

23–10. **Breast abscesses** may give severe pain, with general malaise and elevated temperature.

Treatment

1. Start local heat at once.
2. Have the patient wear an oversize brassiere for support.
3. Refer for surgical drainage and cultures, with antibiotic therapy if indicated.

23–11. **Carbuncles** are multilocular abscesses with multiple individual compartments.

Treatment

1. Avoidance of incision and drainage if possible by:
   a. Control of pain by acetylsalicylic acid (aspirin), and/or small doses of narcotics.
   b. Application of local heat.
   c. Limitation of activity.
   d. Search for, and treatment of, underlying metabolic abnormalities such as diabetes mellitus and Cushing's syndrome.

    2. Reference for hospitalization if surgical drainage becomes necessary.

23–12. **Cold abscesses** are usually due to attenuated organisms following antibiotic therapy or to tuberculosis and are rarely encountered as an emergency unless sudden spontaneous drainage occurs. Fluctuation may be present, but the usual signs of inflammation (redness, local heat, tenderness) are absent.

No emergency treatment is needed, but the importance of adequate medical care should be stressed to the patient.

23–13. **Collar-button abscesses** are infections in the webs between the fingers which cause acute palmar tenderness and swelling but which point on the dorsal surface.

Treatment

A. Early
1. Immobilization with a splint and sling.
2. Frequent hot soaks.
3. Control of pain by elevation, anodynes and, if necessary, small doses of narcotics.

B. Advanced
1. Incision and drainage through two incisions, a curved incision along the edge of the volar swelling and a small incision over the dorsal web. This procedure should be done under nerve block or general anesthetic, preferably in a hospital. Culture should be obtained.
2. Insertion of a rubber dam drain.
3. Application of a hand splint and sling.
4. Administration of antibiotics if indicated.
5. Careful and frequent follow-up care.

23–14. **Dental abscesses.** See 23–4, above (*Alveolar Abscesses*), and Topic 58 (*Toothache*).

23–15 **Epidural abscesses** are characterized by low back pain, progressive flaccid weakness of the legs and urinary retention, and represent an acute emergency. IMMEDIATE hospitalization for drainage is mandatory.

23–16. **Felons (whitlows)** require immediate drainage through an extensive fish-mouth or through-and-through incision of the fingertip. Care must be taken to open every infected compartment. Digital nerve block at some distance above the infected area is usually adequate, but in some cases a general anesthetic may be necessary.

23–17. **Gas abscesses.** Development of crepitus, foul odor and tenderness with severe systemic signs and symptoms in a previously comfortable wound 2 to 4 days after injury requires immediate hospitalization for exploration and removal of necrotic tissue.

Penicillin in massive doses (up to 12 million or more units a day) is indicated, with large doses of tetracyclines. Treatment with gas gangrene antitoxin is of no value.

23–18. **Ischioanal abscesses** develop suddenly with extreme pain, fever and chills, a feeling of fullness in the rectum, and urinary retention.

    Treatment

       1. Superficial ischioanal abscesses:

         a. Preliminary sedation with sodium phenobarbital (Luminal) or a small dose of morphine sulfate.

         b. Intracutaneous infiltration of a local anesthetic over the point of localization between the anus and the ischial tuberosity.

         c. Incision and drainage with insertion of a drain.

         d. Reference for follow-up care. Late fistulectomy is often necessary.

       2. Deep or extensive abscesses with severe toxic symptoms and signs:

         a. Control of pain by morphine sulfate or dihydromorphinone hydrochloride (Dilaudid).

         b. Hospitalization for drainage under general anesthesia. Cultures should be obtained and antibiotics given if indicated.

23–19. **Middle ear abscesses.** See Topic 34–12,B.

23–20. **Nasal septum abscesses** may follow trauma or operative procedures.

    Treatment

       1. Start antibiotic therapy at once.

       2. Refer to an otolaryngologist for incision and drainage.

23–21. **Palmar space abscesses.** See Topic 42–2 and 23–13, above (*Collar-button Abscesses*).

23–22. **Paronychia.** Throbbing pain accompanied by redness and swelling adjacent to the border of a finger- or toenail can be relieved only by incision and drainage.

23–23. **Perianal abscesses.** See 23–18, above (*Ischioanal Abscesses*).

23–24. **Perineal abscesses** require emergency care only if pressure causes partial or complete urinary retention. All cases should be referred to a urologist for care.

23–25. **Peritonsillar abscesses (quinsy)**

A. Signs and Symptoms

1. Severe agonizing pain on one side of throat, with acute dysphagia.
2. High temperature.
3. Extreme general malaise.
4. Bulging in the supratonsillar fossa.

B. Treatment

1. If the abscess is fluctuant and can be accurately localized:
   a. Infiltration of the mucous membrane only with 1% procaine or lidocaine (Xylocaine).
   b. Incision with a sharp knife with adhesive tape wrapped around the blade ⅜ inch from the point as a guard against too deep penetration.
   c. Irrigation with warm saline.
   d. Administration of antibiotics if indicated by cultures.
   e. Reference to an otolaryngologist for follow-up care.
2. If the abscess is deep and no area of fluctuation can be determined:
   a. Control of pain by adequate doses of morphine sulate or dihydromorphinone hydrochloride (Dilaudid).
   b. Reference to an otolaryngologist for further care.

C. Do Not Attempt to "Explore" the Throat. Deaths have occurred from uncontrollable hemorrhage from the ascending pharyngeal, external carotid and internal carotid arteries and from the internal jugular vein.

23–26. **Periurethral abscesses** arise from acute urethritis or from infection of the glands in the area and usually point near the base of the shaft of the penis.

Treatment

1. Incision and drainage under local anesthesia.
2. Antibiotic therapy based on sensitivity tests.
3. Reference to a urologist for further care.

23–27. **Pilonidal abscesses**
   Treatment
      1. Control of pain by anodynes or narcotics as required.
      2. Hospitalization for incision and drainage under spinal or general anesthesia.

23–28. **Psoas abscess.** See 23–12, above (*Cold Abscesses*).

23–29. **Retroperitoneal** [anterior, posterior (perinephric) and retrofascial] abscesses require immediate hospitalization for surgical drainage.

23–30. **Stitch abscesses** may be superficial or deep and can be drained easily by removal of the offending stitch (cutting it close to the uninfected side). Spreading of the incision may be necessary.

23–31. **Suburethral abscesses.** These abscesses should not be opened externally if this can be avoided. Reference to a urologist is indicated as soon as the diagnosis has been made.

23–32. **Tendon sheath abscesses (tenosynovitis).** See Topic 42–2 (*Cellulitis of the Hand*).

23–33. **Tubo-ovarian abscess.** See Topic 41–9 (*Pelvic Inflammatory Disease*)

23–34. **Whitlows.** See 23–16, above (*Felons*).

24. ALLERGIC REACTIONS

See also Topic 59–66 (*Serum Reactions*).

Three types of acute allergic reactions require immediate, sometimes lifesaving, emergency measures.

24–1. **Anaphylactic shock** usually develops within a few seconds or minutes of exposure to the allergen but may be delayed for a few hours. Its onset may be overwhelming, and death may occur from rapid respiratory and circulatory collapse before any treatment can be given.

   Treatment
      1. Immediate injection of epinephrine hydrochloride (Adrenalin), 0.5 to 1.0 ml. of 1:1000 solution intravenously, repeated in 20 minutes if necessary. Infiltration of the site of entrance of the allergen with 0.3 ml. of 1:1000 epinephrine

hydrochloride (Adrenalin) should be done as soon as possible.

2. Insurance of a clear airway by suction, positioning and support of the angles of the jaw.

3. Administration of oxygen under positive pressure by face mask or endotracheal catheter and rebreathing bag.

4. Removal or neutralization of allergen if known or suspected.

5. Intramuscular or intravenous injection of ephedrine sulfate, 0.25 to 0.5 ml., or caffeine sodiobenzoate, 0.5 gm., followed by arterenol bitartrate (Levophed) or metaraminol bitartrate (Aramine) intravenously (Topic 15–7).

6. Intravenous injection of 100 mg. of hydrocortisone sodium succinate (Solu-Cortef) or of 50 mg. of prednisolone sodium hemisuccinate (Meticortelone). Repeat if necessary in 4 hours.

7. Intramuscular or intravenous injection of antihistaminic drugs.

8. Hospitalization after the above measures.

24–2. Angioedema. In addition to the measures outlined under *Anaphylactic Shock* (24–1, above), *tracheotomy* (Topic 17–11) may be necessary as a lifesaving measure.

24–3. Asthma with acute bronchospasm. See Topic 53–1,A.

24–4. Less serious allergic reactions are common and may cause varying degrees of edema, urticaria and pruritus.

Treatment

1. Remove from contact with, or stop intake of, the offending agent if known or suspected.

2. Inject epinephrine hydrochloride (Adrenalin), 0.5 to 1 ml. of 1:1000 solution, intramuscularly. For home use, a 1:100 solution used with a nebulizer may be prescribed.

3. Prescribe tripelennamine hydrochloride (Pyribenzamine), 50 mg., by mouth three times a day for swelling and wheals and trimeprazine tartrate (Temaril), 2.5 mg., four times a day for severe itching [unless the offending drug is an antihistaminic (Topic 59–14)].

4. Apply calamine lotion to the itching areas.

5. Refer severe or stubborn cases to an internist or
   allergist for follow-up care.
24–5. **Serum sickness.** See Topic 59–66.

25. *ASPHYXIATION*

See also Topic 3 (*Coma*) and Topic 13 (*Resuscitation*).
Asphyxia, or suffocation, is caused by lack of oxygen and
accumulation of carbon dioxide in the blood and is characterized by signs and symptoms of air hunger (acute anxiety,
increasing lividity and cyanosis), coma and death.

25–1. **Causes**
   A. Mechanical obstruction of the respiratory passages by
      edema (Topic 24–2) and foreign bodies (Topic
      38–4 and Topic 48–25 and 40).
   B. Paralysis of the respiratory center by drugs such as
      morphine (Topic 49–370).
   C. Filling of the alveolar air space with fluid [Topic 52
      (*Pulmonary Edema*)], products of infection [Topic
      53–14 (*Pneumonia*)] or blood [Topic 31 (*Chest
      Injuries*)].
   D. Disturbances in the oxygen carrying ability of the red
      blood cells—for example, carbon monoxide poison-
      ing (Topic 49–119).
   E. Paralysis of the muscles concerned with respiration by
      disease [Topic 32–21 (*Poliomyelitis*)], by drugs
      which act on the motor end-plates [Topic 49–168
      (*Curare*)], or by cervical trauma (Topic 47–5,B).

25–2. **Treatment**
   A. Removal from exposure.
   B. Provision of an adequate airway by postural drainage,
      suction and support of the angles of the jaw.
   C. Removal of foreign bodies blocking the airway (Topic
      38–4).
   D. Formation, if necessary, of an emergency airway by a
      tracheotomy (Topic 17–11).
   E. External cardiac massage (Topic 17–2) if indicated.
   F. *Immediate Expired-Air Respiration* (Topic 17–1). Other

methods of nonmechanical artificial respiration are less efficient but should be made use of if for any reason mouth-to-mouth, mouth-to-nose or mouth-to-adjunct techniques (Topic 17–1) cannot be used. Of these, the Holger Nielsen chest-pressure arm-lift method is the most effective for adults; the Rickard prone-tilting visceral shift (Topic 17–1,E), for infants and small children.

G. Mechanical Artificial Respiration as soon as equipment is available. Air or oxygen under intermittent positive pressure should be administered by one of the following methods:

1. Face mask and rebreathing bag.
2. Endotracheal catheter and rebreathing bag.
3. Mechanical respirators of various types.

H. Avoidance of Dependence on Analeptics. Drugs such as alphalobeline, caffeine sodiobenzoate and pentylenetetrazol (Metrazol) are of no value until respiration has been re-established.

26. BAROTRAUMA

Changes in atmospheric pressure—both decreases and increases—can cause numerous conditions which may require emergency care.

26–1. Altitude sickness [to be distinguished from *Air Sickness* (Topic 44–4)].

A. Signs and Symptoms

1. Anoxia of varying degrees ranging from increase in pulse and respiration rate and euphoria to gradually decreasing mental and physical efficiency with eventual loss of consciousness.
2. Postanoxial symptoms such as persistent headache, nausea and vomiting, tinnitus and deafness.

B. Treatment

1. Return to an accustomed atmospheric pressure.
2. Oxygen inhalations under positive pressure by face mask and rebreathing bag.

3. Dimenhydrinate (Dramamine), 50 to 100 mg. by mouth.

4. Circulatory stimulation by caffeine sodiobenzoate, 0.5 gm., intramuscularly.

5. Reference for care by an otolaryngologist if ear symptoms persist.

26-2. **Bends.** See 26-3, below.

26-3. **Caisson disease** ("bends," Compressed Air Sickness, Decompression Sickness)

A. Causes. This condition may occur in divers who breathe air or oxygen through any type of mechanical equipment (26-5, below) and in persons who work in air locks under increased atmospheric pressure. If decompression is not gradual, bubbles of nitrogen are released into the blood and produce a variety of signs and symptoms. The most common of these are:

1. SEVERE PAIN, usually of a throbbing type which shifts its location frequently. Muscles, joints and bones may be the sites of the pain; abdominal pain may be acute enough to be confused with an acute surgical abdomen.

2. VERTIGO (Topic 47), often severe enough to cause staggering. If the patient has alcohol on his breath his condition may be mistaken for drunkenness (Topic 2-1 and Topic 18-1,C).

3. CUTANEOUS MANIFESTATIONS—pruritus, mottling and erythema.

4. NERVOUS SYSTEM SYMPTOMS
   a. Numbness and tingling of the extremities; bizarre paresthesias.
   b. Bladder and bowel incontinence.
   c. Hemiplegia, paraplegia, quadriplegia, strabismus, nystagmus, diplopia and paresis.

5. ACUTE DYSPNEA. This may occur several hours after apparently successful recompression and decompression.

6. COLLAPSE AND UNCONSCIOUSNESS.

B. Treatment. Recompression and gradual decompression is the only treatment of any value. While this is being arranged the following supportive measures may be necessary:

1. Continuous artificial respiration by any feasible method—mouth-to-mouth or mechanical are the most satisfactory.
2. Inhalation of pure oxygen or oxygen-helium mixtures.
3. Injection of caffeine sodiobenzoate, 0.5 gm., intramuscularly.

26–4. **Compressed air sickness.** See 26–3, above.

26–5. **Diving hazards**

The problems, limitations and hazards of deep-water diving with airhose, suit and metal helmet have long been recognized. Commercial divers are required to be in excellent physical condition and are trained and instructed in accordance with government and other regulations designed for their safety. In contrast, the recent development, commercial exploitation and wide use of various types of self-contained underwater breathing apparatus (commonly abbreviated to SCUBA) by inexperienced, untrained, unsupervised and unlicensed persons diving for sport has resulted in the need for recognition and treatment of various physical, metabolic and mental disturbances resulting from exposure to an unfamiliar and potentially dangerous environment.

"Skin divers" (who can remain under water only as long as they can hold their breath) are subject only to the usual well-known hazards of diving and swimming. "Snorkel" divers are exposed to these hazards plus the additional danger of thoracic squeeze if an overly long (more than 18 inch) breathing tube is used.

A. General Principles of Management and Care

1. Knowledge of the location of, and shortest route to, and indications for the use of the closest pressure chamber equipped for recompression and gradual decompression.
2. Recompression and slow, supervised decompression of any seriously ill, stuporous or comatose diver who has been 30 feet or more under water using any type of air- or gas-filled diving apparatus no matter how long an interval has elapsed since the dive. Recompression and gradual controlled decompression in a pressure chamber is harmless not only to the diver, but also to an attendant, and under certain circumstances may prevent serious, permanent—even terminal—

aftereffects. WHEN IN DOUBT, RECOMPRESS!
3. ARTIFICIAL RESPIRATION [Topic 13 (*Resuscitation*)
   and Topic 17–1]. Mouth-to-mouth respiratory assistance to dyspneic, cyanotic, unconscious or
   "drowned" divers at the earliest possible moment,
   continued without interruption not only during
   rescue and en route to the pressure chamber but
   also in the chamber during recompression may
   be lifesaving.
4. The conditions listed in the table are related directly
   or indirectly to underwater pressure or subsur-
   face environment and may require emergency
   management.

Condition	Skin Divers (Breath-holding)	Snorkel Divers (Tube-to-Surface)	SCUBA Divers	Helmet-Suit-Air Hose Divers	Cause	Signs and Symptoms	Recompression in Pressure Chamber?	Artificial Respiration	Other Treatment and Comments
Air embolism	No	No	Yes	Yes	Holding breath during ascent	Any picture—indistinguishable from decompression sickness	Yes	Yes	Sedatives and anodynes for pain. Permanent sequelae may require symptomatic therapy
Anoxia	No	No	Closed circuit only	Air supply cut off	Failure of breathing apparatus	Unconsciousness without warning	Yes	Yes	Failure of oxygen supply is often associated with air embolism and/or decompression sickness caused by too rapid rescue
"Bends"	No	No	Yes	Yes	Decompression sickness	Pain in legs and/or abdomen	Yes	No	Sedatives and narcotics for pain. See 26–3, above (Caisson Disease)
Carbon dioxide poisoning	No	No	Yes, closed circuit	No	CO_2 absorbent inadequate	Rapid breathing, unconsciousness	Yes	Yes	Prevention—avoidance of deep breathing exercises before starting dive

Condition	Skin Divers (Breath-holding)	Snorkel Divers (Tube-to-Surface)	SCUBA Divers	Helmet–Suit–Air Hose Divers	Cause	Signs and Symptoms	Recompression in Pressure Chamber?	Artificial Respiration	Other Treatment and Comments
Carbon monoxide poisoning	No	No	Yes, open circuit	No	Impure air in cylinder	Sudden loss of consciousness	Yes	Yes	See Topic 49–119
"Chokes"	No	No	Yes	Yes	Decompression sickness	Dyspnea, cough, chest pain	Yes	Yes	Must be adequately recompressed immediately. (See 26–3, above (*Caisson Disease*)
Cold	Yes	Yes	Yes	Yes	Low water temperature	Slowing of functions, shivering	Often	Often	Shivering makes holding mouthpiece impossible, or slowed mental and physical responses may lead to other complications
Conjunctival hemorrhage	No	No	Yes	No	Tight goggles—excessive depth	Bleeding may be retrobulbar	No	No	Symptomatic treatment only. Recovery complete

Decompression sickness	No	No	Yes	Yes	Rapid ascent from deep dives	May give any picture. Onset may be delayed for many hours	Yes	Often	Sedatives and anodynes for pain. See 26-3, above (*Caisson Disease*)
Drowning	Yes	Yes	Yes	Yes	Water in lungs	Unconsciousness, absent vital signs (see Topic 4)	Often	Yes	Any "drowned" diver using any type of gas-containing breathing apparatus requires recompression at once
Ear drum rupture	Yes	No	Yes	Yes	Barotrauma, previous disease	Pain	No	No	Shrinking of eustachian tubes. Nothing into ear. Antibiotics may be necessary
Emphysema (subcutaneous, mediastinal)	No	No	Yes	Yes	Air embolism	Crepitus of soft tissues, dyspnea	Yes	Often	Subcutaneous emphysema usually clears; mediastinal often recurs after decompression
Epistaxis	Yes	Yes	Yes	Yes	Barotrauma, previous disease	May vary from slight oozing to severe hemorrhage	No	No	Symptomatic treatment only

Condition	Skin Divers (Breath-holding)	Snorkel Divers (Tube-to-Surface)	SCUBA Divers	Helmet-Suit-Air Hose Divers	Cause	Signs and Symptoms	Recompression in Pressure Chamber?	Artificial Respiration	Other Treatment and Comments
External ear squeeze	No	No	Yes	Yes	Nonequalizing air-containing apparatus	Redness, bleb formation, bleeding	No	No	Symptomatic only—recovery complete in short time
Hemoptysis	Yes	Yes, if tube too long	Yes	Yes	Usually air embolism; occasionally too long snorkel or barotrauma	Bloody froth indicative of lung sinus, or middle ear damage from attempts to equalize pressure on descent	Yes	Often	In snorkel or skin divers, supportive therapy only; in SCUBA or helmet-suit-air hose divers immediate recompression and slow decompression may be lifesaving

Neurologic disturbances	No	No	Yes	Yes	Air embolism or decompression sickness	Yes	All types. Onset may be deferred many hours or occur after apparent recovery from other conditions	May be necessary	Neurologic abnormalities in a diver who has descended more than 30 feet using any type of breathing apparatus requires recompression and slow decompression at once
Otitis externa	Yes	Yes	Yes	Yes	Water in external canal	No	See *External ear squeeze* (above)	No	If irritation or maceration of canal is present, drying after each dive is indicated. Also see Topic 34–12,A
Otitis media	Yes	Yes	Yes	Yes	Frequent wetting, chilling	No	Pain, tinnitus	No	See Topic 34–12,B
Oxygen poisoning	No	No	Yes	Yes	Excessive depth, inadequate lung ventilation	Yes, usually	Vertigo, nausea, muscle twitching, followed by convulsions	Yes, usually	Usually complete recovery if rescued before drowning, air embolism, or decompression sickness occurs

Condition	Skin Divers (Breath-holding)	Snorkel Divers (Tube-to-Surface)	SCUBA Divers	Helmet-Suit-Air Hose Divers	Cause	Signs and Symptoms	Recompression in Pressure Chamber?	Artificial Respiration	Other Treatment and Comments
Paralysis	No	No	Yes	Yes	Air embolism	Any part of body may be involved. Onset may be deferred many hours	Yes	May be necessary	Permanent paralysis may remain in spite of recompression and controlled decompression
Pneumothorax	No	No	Yes	Yes	Usually air embolism and/or decompression sickness, but may occur independently	Dyspnea, cyanosis, and/or chest pain	Usually	Occasionally	After re-expansion in pressure chamber symptoms may recur when pressure is lowered
Respiratory arrest	Yes	Yes	Yes	Yes	Air embolism, decompression sickness, CO or CO_2 intoxication	Not breathing	Often	Yes	Immediate oxygenation by mouth-to-mouth, or mechanical artificial respiration continued during transportation to, or institution of, other therapy

Thoracic squeeze	Yes	Yes	Yes	Yes	Holding breath on descent, or too long snorkel tube	Bloody froth from pulmonary congestion and edema	Often	Often	Breath-holding or snorkel divers require only supportive treatment, SCUBA and helmet-suit–air hose divers require pressure chamber therapy because condition may be due to air embolism or decompression sickness
Unconsciousness	Yes	Yes	Yes	Yes	Air embolism, decompression sickness, O, CO or CO_2 excess trauma	Depending on cause	Often	Yes	Loss of consciousness during or after a dive in any diver using any type of gas-filled apparatus requires pressure chamber treatment as soon as possible with artificial respiration (Topic 13) and shock treatment (Topic 15–7) en route to chamber

26–6. Mountain sickness

Acute mountain sickness, characterized by sleeplessness, lethargy, poor appetite, nausea and vomiting is common among mountain climbers above 17,000 feet altitude. The condition is self-limiting and clears slowly under symptomatic treatment or on descent to a lower altitude. Frequent complications are pulmonary edema (Topic 52) and thrombophlebitis (Topic 60–10).

26–7. Restrictions on air travel

Although modern commercial airlines are equipped with pressurized cabins which limit the effects of barotrauma to those caused by ascent to, and descent from, a maximum of 8000 feet, persons with certain physical limitations should not travel by air. Among these limitations are:

A. Conditions such as valvular heart disease, extreme hypertension, angina pectoris and coronary disease which could be seriously aggravated by air sickness (Topic 44–4) or altitude sickness (26–1, above).

B. Conditions in which the normal expansion of body gases (1.75 at 8000 feet as compared to 1.0 at sea level) might be detrimental. Among these are acute or chronic sinusitis, nasopharyngitis, and otitis; large unsupported hernias, acute appendicitis and peptic ulcers or other conditions in which increased gas volume might cause perforation.

C. Fractured jaw patients. Unless some method of quick release in case of vomiting has been substituted for the usual wiring, persons with broken jaws should not travel by air.

D. Conditions in which slight hypoxia (90% arterial oxygen saturation at 8000 feet as compared to 96% at sea level) might be detrimental; among these are status asthmaticus and pulmonary emphysema with very small respiratory reserve.

E. Conditions associated with profound anemia. This includes Negroes with S and C hemoglobins; sickling and hemolysis may occur.

27. BITES

Also see Topic 56 (*Stings*) and Topic 62 (*Venoms*).

27–1. **Animal bites** are notorious for causing severe infections and require energetic treatment. Bites on the face are especially dangerous. Lacerations and deep puncture wounds may require debridement, irrigation and primary closure. All cases should be given tetanus antitoxin or toxoid (Topic 19) and antibiotics, and follow-up care in 24 hours should be arranged. CAUTERIZATION WITH FUMING NITRIC ACID—as suggested in some first-aid texts—SHOULD NEVER BE DONE. For details of prophylactic treatment following bites of non-rabid and rabid animals see Topic 63–19.

27–2. **Ant bites** (see also 27–10, below, and Topic 56–2).

Although the bites of many common varieties of ants can cause transient discomfort and occasional allergic reactions, the venom of the fire ant is injected not by its jaws but by an abdominal stinger, causing severe localized reactions and systemic effects which may be dangerous (Topic 56–2).

27–3. **Barracuda bites**

These voracious fish have tremendously long jaws armed with large, serrated, sharp teeth which can inflict serious lacerations requiring extensive debridement and repair. Pound for pound, they are much more dangerous than any variety of shark.

27–4. **Bat bites**

Certain varieties of carnivorous and insectivorous bats may be rabid. In addition, they may carry other infectious viruses in their salivary glands. Orchitis, oophoritis and aseptic meningitis have been reported following bat bites.

27–5. **Black widow spider bites**

The female of this species (*Latrodectus mactans*)—easily identifiable by a bright orange, hour-glass-shaped coloration of the abdomen—is responsible for many of the severe toxic effects following spider bites. The bite of the very drab male is harmless.

In spite of wide publicity to the contrary, black widow spider bites are rarely fatal in adults unless an exceptionally vascular part of the body is bitten. However, in infants the mortality rate is very high; it decreases progressively with age.

  A. Toxic Picture (developing from 1 to 2 hours after the bite)

    1. Severe headache.

    2. Nausea and vomiting, associated with intense local and abdominal pain which is severe enough to be mistaken for an acute surgical abdomen.

    3. Very severe cramping of the extremities.

    4. Shock (Topic 15)

  B. Treatment

    1. Treat shock at once (Topic 15–7).

    2. Relieve apprehension and pain with rapid-acting barbiturates or opiates. Sodium pentobarbital, 0.2 to 0.3 gm., intramuscularly, should be given first; if no relief, morphine sulfate, 10 to 15 mg., should be given very slowly intravenously.

    3. Give 500 to 1000 ml. of 5% dextrose in saline intravenously. Force fluids by mouth.

    4. Control the characteristic acute myalgia by intravenous injection of 10 ml. of 10% calcium gluconate solution. Ten ml. of a 25% solution of magnesium sulfate given slowly intravenously is also of value for this purpose.

    5. Transfer to a hospital as soon as the shock and acute pain have been controlled.

    6. Antiserum may be necessary in severe cases but should not be given as a part of emergency therapy unless a long delay before hospitalization is anticipated. If antiserum is to be given, inject 0.02 ml. intracutaneously to test for sensitivity. If no wheal or indurated area is present after 20 minutes, give 2.5 ml. intramuscularly. If the intradermal test is positive, administration should be postponed until the patient has been hospitalized.

27–6.   Brown spider bites

Volume for volume the venom of *Loxosceles reclusa* (brown spider, false hackled band spinner) is much stronger than that of a rattlesnake, and of about the same potency as the female black widow spider (27–5, above). The venom contains levarterenol and a powerful hemolysin.

    A. *Mild Reactions* to brown spider bites are characterized by:

      1. Slight discomfort (less than a bee sting) at the time of the bite, gradually increasing over a period of 8 hours to agonizing pain.

      2. Bleb formation surrounded by an area of intense ischemia.

      3. Development in 24 to 48 hours of a tough black eschar surrounded by purplish induration which on removal bares a deep irregular, necrotic-based ulcer which heals very slowly with extreme scarring and (usually) surrounding pigmentation.

B. *Severe Reactions*

    1. Generalized morbilliform eruption.

    2. Severe shock.

    3. Fever up to 40° C. (104° F).

    4. Recurrent fainting spells.

    5. Severe arthralgia.

    6. Hemoglobinuria.

C. *Treatment*

    1. MILD CASES

      a. Antihistaminics.

      b. Anodynes for severe pain. Narcotics may be necessary.

      c. Calcium gluconate, 10 ml. of a 10% solution, intravenously for arthralgia.

      d. Local infiltration of phentolamine (Regitine) to limit necrosis.

    2. SEVERE CASES

      a. Treatment of shock (Topic 15–7).

      b. Administration of antivenin, used with excellent results against *L. rufescens* and *L. rufipes* in South America (no antivenin for the North American variety, *L. reclusa*, is as yet available).

D. *Prognosis.* Good for recovery unless a massive dose of venom has been received. Repeated bites apparently cause immunity. Disfiguring scarring and pigmentation are common.

27–7. Camel bites

Because of the tremendous leverage resulting from the unusual shape of the jaws and the peculiar dentition (long incisors in the upper jaw which imbricate with the canines) of these vicious animals, camel bites usually result in fractures and dislocations in addition to extensive crushing, tearing and avulsion of soft tissues. Extensive reconstruction surgery is often required.

27–8. Cat bites

In addition to the care outlined under *Animal Bites* (27–1, above), cat bites and scratches unless thoroughly cleansed and treated at once may cause a relatively benign low-grade infection, cat scratch fever.

27–9. Chigger bites

The small larvae of trombiculid mites ("chiggers")—often parasitic to birds and reptiles—may cause uncomfortable but rarely serious local irritation, especially in children. Infestation usually occurs from playing in damp swampy areas of scrub vegetation.

A. Signs and Symptoms

1. Papules and vesicles at the site of the bite, especially around the genitalia, sometimes causing difficulty in voiding.
2. Itching, redness and swelling lasting 3 to 5 days.
3. Secondary infection with cellulitis and lymphadenitis (occasionally bacteremia) from scratching.

B. Treatment

1. Scrubbing with soap and water.
2. Trimming fingernails.
3. Application of a lotion containing 1% gamma benzene hexachloride.
4. Antipruritic ointments and lotions.
5. Antibiotics for secondary infection.

27–10. Fire ant bites

Over 20,000,000 acres of land in the southern part of the United States are useless because of infestation with these ants which first appeared, apparently from South America, in 1918 and which kill small animals and fowl. For human toxicity see 27–2, above; and Topic 56–2.

27–11. Flea bites may cause a severe local reaction with surrounding edema, wheals, cellulitis and intense itching.

Treatment

1. Cold compresses.
2. Application of sodium bicarbonate paste or calamine lotion.

     3. Tripelennamine hydrochloride (Pyribenzamine), 30 to 50 mg., by mouth.

     4. Referral to a dermatologist for possible desensitization in extreme cases.

27–12. **Gila monster bites** cause severe local reactions but are rarely dangerous except in infants and small children.

    Treatment

     1. Immediate use of ice packs.

     2. Application of a tourniquet proximal to the bite if on an extremity, with slow release over a period of one hour.

     3. Thorough cleansing, with debridement and primary closure under local anesthetic if necessary.

     4. Protection against tetanus (Topic 19).

     5. Administration of prophylactic antibiotics.

27–13. **Human bites** often result in severe infections. Treatment as outlined under *Animal Bites* (27–1, above) is in order except that prophylaxis against rabies is not necessary.

27–14. **Llama bites** have the same peculiarities and characteristics as *Camel Bites* (27–7, above).

27–15. **Mosquito bites.** The treatment is the same as that given for *Flea Bites* (27–11, above). See also Topic 63–24 (*Yellow Fever*).

27–16. **Sandfly bites.** (See also Topic 63–20.)

Sandfly fever is caused by a virus transmitted to humans by sandfly bites. Its course is brief and never fatal.

27–17. **Snake bites**

"Bites" of poisonous snakes are not caused by closing of the jaws, but by strikes or thrusts with the mouth open, with introduction of the venom through needle-like hollow fangs.

Of the four species of poisonous snakes inhabiting North America (rattlesnake, copperhead or highland moccasin, water moccasin or cottonmouth, and coral or harlequin snake), by far the most common is the rattlesnake (*Crotalus*), which may vary in length from 6 inches to over 7 feet, and in color and markings with its environment. The fer-de-lance group (*Bothrops*), the tropical rattler (*Crotalus terrificus*), the cantril, and the bushmaster are common in tropical Central and South America. Many varieties of poisonous snakes have thick bodies and blunt tails but this is not an invariable rule. Snake venoms contain hemotoxic and neurotoxic substances in varying proportions and amounts, depending on the species (Topic 62).

A. Symptoms and Signs

1. Typical fang marks—two distinct punctures. A row of small superficial wounds from the lower teeth may be present.
2. Local pain may be absent, mild or very severe.
3. Ecchymosis, edema and local hemorrhage may be present with some varieties, absent with others.
4. Progressive respiratory and circulatory depression and neurologic signs and symptoms, depending upon the toxic properties of the venom (Topic 62).

B. Treatment

1. Apply a tourniquet about 2 inches proximal to the bite or swelling (if on an extremity), tight enough to partially occlude the lymphatics and venous return but not tight enough to shut off the arterial blood supply. Packing an extremity in ice may be of value.
2. Keep the patient as quiet as possible. Excessive activity may result in more rapid spread of the venom.
3. Give morphine sulfate or dihydromorphinone hydrochloride (Dilaudid) subcutaneously, intramuscularly or intravenously *cautiously* for severe pain and apprehension. The smallest possible effective doses should be used because of the danger of increasing respiratory depression.
4. Excise the bite (including the fang marks) under 1 or 2% procaine or lidocaine (Xylocaine) injected around, not into, the site of the bite. This central area should be surrounded by multiple cruciate, superficial incisions, repeated as necessary around the advancing edge of the swelling to allow removal of lymph by suction, preferably by means of a breast pump, cupping glass or empty antivenin syringe, although mouth suction may be used without danger—the venom is harmless if swallowed.
5. Support the circulation. Large amounts of black coffee by mouth, or caffeine sodiobenzoate, 0.5 gm., intramuscularly or intravenously, usually are effective. If circulatory depression is acute,

support by administration of vasoconstrictor drugs may be necessary (Topic 15–7).

6. Inject antisnakebite serum, if available, in adequate amounts as soon as possible—even if the victim is moribund. The usual North and South American antiserum (antivenin) is polyvalent for every variety of rattlesnake, copperhead, moccasin, fer-de-lance group, cantril and bushmaster. It is not effective against the coral snake. In other parts of the world special types of antisera effective against indigenous poisonous snakes are prepared and available, usually through local public health authorities. After testing for sensitivity to horse serum (Topic 14), 5 ml. of antivenin (or appropriate antiserum) should be injected subcutaneously and intramuscularly around the bite to prevent sloughing and necrosis. The remainder of the ampule should then be injected intramuscularly at some distance from the bite. This initial injection of antiserum represents only a small fraction of the total amount required for adequate treatment. Four or 5 ampules may be required to adequately neutralize the venom of large or tropical species. Children require two to three times the adult dose. If coma or paralysis is present, intravenous injections of antivenin may be necessary.

7. Inject tetanus antitoxin, 3000 or more units, after testing for sensitivity and desensitization if necessary (Topic 14). Tetanus toxoid should be substituted if the patient has ever been actively immunized.

8. Transfer all patients to a hospital as soon as possible for further antivenin, necessary supportive therapy, and close observation for at least 4 days. Dangerous relapses may occur after apparent marked improvement as long as 3 days after the bite, and less serious complications may require medical care for 2 weeks or more.

9. DO NOT cauterize the punctured area with acids, potassium permanganate crystals, iodine or hot metallic objects. Whiskey, locally or internally,

is of no therapeutic value although it may result in a beneficial temporary decrease in anxiety and activity.

27–18. Spider bites

Except for the 3 varieties listed below, spider bites result in mild local reactions only and require no specific therapy.

> **A. Black Widow Spider.** Characterized by an hour-glass shaped, bright orange marking on the belly (27–5, above).
>
> **B. Brown Spider.** Characterized by a violin-case shaped darker brown colorature on the back (27–6, above).
>
> **C. Tarantulas.** Characterized by large size and hairiness of legs and body (27–19, below).

27–19. Tarantula bites cause no systemic reactions, but locally the reaction may be very severe especially in children. Thorough cleansing followed by debridement of the wound under procaine or lidocaine (Xylocaine) infiltration anesthesia often is necessary. Tetanus antitoxin or toxoid (Topic 19) should be given routinely.

27–20. Tick bites are characterized by burying of the head of the tick.

> **A. General Principles of Treatment**
>
> > The following procedures may be necessary to release the head from the tissues:
> >
> > 1. Gentle rotation of the body.
> > 2. Application of kerosene, turpentine or gasoline.
> > 3. Careful approximation of the glowing end of a cigarette close to the body of the tick.
> > 4. Excision of the buried head under local anesthesia (see 27–20,C, below).
>
> **B. Rocky Mountain Spotted Fever**
>
> > This rickettsial disease, transmitted by both the wood tick and the dog tick, is endemic in the United States and represents an often overlooked cause of severe cutaneous and general symptoms.
>
> **Treatment**
>
> > 1. Frequent inspection for, and removal of, ticks, especially from the scalp.
> > 2. Hospitalization for agglutination tests and definitive therapy if the clinical picture is suggestive of Rocky Mountain spotted fever. If a delay in

hospitalization is anticipated, large doses of broad spectrum antibiotics are indicated.

C. Tick Paralysis

Bites of certain varieties of wood ticks (*Dermacentor andersoni*) and dog ticks (*Dermacentor variabilis*) may cause severe, even fatal, paralysis. Some type of powerful neurotoxin absorbed from the head of the gravid female tick is apparently the toxic agent. The paralysis is often ascending and progressive and can be distinguished from that of anterior poliomyelitis and Guillain-Barré syndrome only by the absence of fever and spinal fluid changes.

Treatment

1. Surgical removal of the buried head. Except in moribund patients, this will result in progressive improvement starting 2 to 3 days after excision, with ultimate complete recovery.
2. Energetic supportive therapy until improvement begins.

27–21. **Bites of unidentified etiology** suspected of being dangerously toxic should be treated as follows:

1. Application of a tourniquet if on an extremity.
2. Chilling of the site of the bite by ice packs.
3. Control of severe pain by appropriate anodynes.
4. Intravenous injection of 10 ml. of 10% calcium gluconate for acute myalgia. If relief is obtained, this injection can be repeated as needed; if not, the tourniquet and ice packs with symptomatic measures should be continued until the patient can be hospitalized for observation.

28. BURNS

See also Topic 48–10 (*Burns in Children*).

28–1. **Principles of evaluation**

Emergency therapy, disposition and prognosis in all types of burns are based on five basic factors which must be considered at the first evaluation of the patient.

A. Per Cent of Body Surface Affected

The body surface of an average-sized (70 kg. or 154 lb.) adult is about 1.72 square meters or 18½ square feet. Disposition, treatment and prognosis depend upon estimation of the amount of body surface involved.

The "Rule of Nines" is sufficiently accurate for emergency use. (For variations in infancy and childhood, see Topic 48–10,A.)

PART OF BODY	% OF BODY SURFACE
Head, face and neck	9
Right arm, forearm and hand	9
Left arm, forearm and hand	9
Thorax—front	9
Thorax—back	9
Abdomen—lower ribs to inguinal creases	9
Back—lower ribs to subgluteal creases	9
Right thigh, leg and foot—front	9
Right thigh, leg and foot—back	9
Left thigh, leg and foot—front	9
Left thigh, leg and foot—back	9
Genitalia	1
	100%

B. Depth

1. SUPERFICIAL (FIRST DEGREE). Erythema only.
2. PARTIAL SKIN THICKNESS (SECOND DEGREE). Bleb formation.
3. DEEP (THIRD DEGREE). Involvement of the full thickness of the skin and the subcutaneous and deeper tissues with discoloration, charring and loss of substance.

C. Location

1. Shock is much more common if the head, face, hands, genitalia and feet are damaged.
2. Severe pain may be present if highly specialized areas such as the face or hands, or freely movable areas such as flexion creases or joints, are involved.

D. Time Elapsed Since the Burn.
The danger of shock and infection varies directly with the interval between injury and treatment.

E. Age and General Physical Condition.
Children under 5, elderly persons, and all individuals whose re-

sistance is below normal for any reason are especially susceptible to the systemic effects of burns.

28–2. **Principles of treatment**

   A. Superficial (First Degree)

1. LOCALIZED, involving less than 35% of body surface in adults. (For children, see Topic 48–10.)

   Treatment

   a. Wash thoroughly with nonmedicated white soap and water.

   b. Apply a petrolatum gauze dressing; or, in very mild cases, a soothing lotion.

   c. Prescribe sedatives for restlessness and/or acetylsalicylic acid (aspirin) for pain.

   d. Arrange for follow-up care.

2. EXTENSIVE, involving more than 35% of body surface in adults, less in children (Topic 48–10).

   Treatment

   a. Wash thoroughly with a mild detergent followed by soap and water.

   b. Apply petrolatum gauze dressings or wrap in sterile towels or sheets.

   c. Control apprehension, restlessness and pain, using narcotics if necessary. In infants and children under 4 a pentobarbital sodium (Nembutal) suppository should be substituted for narcotics.

   d. Hospitalize if the location of the burn makes ambulatory or home care impractical.

   B. Partial Skin Thickness (Second Degree) or Deep (Third Degree) Burns

   Treatment

1. Control apprehension, restlessness and pain by subcutaneous, intramuscular or intravenous barbiturates and/or narcotics as indicated.

2. Combat shock (Topic 15–7).

3. Gently remove all clothing from the involved areas.

4. Using aseptic technique cleanse the burned areas thoroughly with a mild detergent followed by soap and water and irrigation with sterile saline solution. Gross contamination and loose devitalized tissue should be removed but no attempt at thorough debridement should be made. Blebs should NOT be opened or drained.

5. Apply a sterile dressing of one of the following types:
   a. Petrolatum gauze held in place by bias-cut stock-inette or loosely wrapped elastic bandage.
   b. A cellulose pad faced with fine mesh gauze held in place by bandage or adhesive.
   c. Pads of gauze, sterile towels or sheets saturated with sterile saline if immediate hospitalization has been arranged.
6. Apply splints if necessary to prevent motion of the burned areas.
7. Administer tetanus antitoxin or toxoid (Topic 19).
8. Hospitalize as soon as possible if:
   a. More than 35% of body surface is involved. (For children, see Topic 48–10.)
   b. The patient has been, or remains, in severe shock (Topic 15).
   c. The head, eyes, face, respiratory tract, hands, feet or genitalia are extensively involved.
   d. The areas involved, or other factors, preclude ambulatory or home care.

28–3. **Burns requiring special management**
28–4. **Acid burns**
   Treatment
   1. Wash thoroughly in running water for a lengthy period as soon as possible after contact with acid.
   2. Control restlessness and pain by administration of barbiturates and narcotics as needed. Combat shock if present (Topic 15–7).
   3. Manage as indicated under *Principles of Treatment* (28–2, above). See also *Eye Burns* (28–14, below); Topic 37–31,C, and 32,C; and Topic 49–19 (*Acids*).

28–5. **Alkali burns**
   Treatment
   1. Wash thoroughly and for a lengthy period with running water.
   2. Control restlessness and pain by administration of barbiturates and narcotics as needed. Treat shock if necessary (Topic 15–7).
   3. Manage as outlined under *Principles of Treatment* (28–2, above). See also 28–14, below (*Eye*

Burns); Topic 37–31,C; Topic 49–28 (*Alkalies*); and Topic 49–323 (*Lye*).

28–6. **Asphalt or tar burns**
Treatment

1. Control apprehension and pain by barbiturates and narcotics as indicated. Combat shock if necessary (Topic 15–7).
2. Wash thoroughly with soap and warm water.
3. Remove adherent congealed asphalt or tar if the area involved is relatively small, and the site permits, by:
   a. Soaking with solvents such as skin cleanser, ether, mineral oil or Scriptoil. Certain substances can be removed most easily by freezing with ice or an ethyl chloride spray.
   b. Peeling off with forceps.
4. Wash thoroughly with soap and warm water, followed by irrigation with sterile saline.
5. Apply a petrolatum gauze dressing and hold in place by bias-cut stockinette or a loosely applied elastic bandage.
6. Splint if necessary.
7. Give tetanus antitoxin or toxoid if indicated (Topic 19).
8. Hospitalize if the congealed asphalt or tar covers a large portion of the body, or involves an area which will not permit removal without anesthetic. Hot asphalt and tar burns are usually much deeper than first examination would seem to indicate.

28–7. **Atomic energy burns.** See Topic 64–4,B.

28–8. **Caustic burns.** See *Alkali Burns* (28–5, above).

28–9. **Cement or concrete burns.** See *Alkali Burns* (28–5, above).

28–10. **Chemical burns.** See 28–4, above (*Acid Burns*); 28–5, above (*Alkali Burns*); and under the chemical involved under this topic and Topic 49.

28–11. **Ear burns**

A. **Of the Soft Tissues.** Treat as outlined under *Principles of Treatment* (28–2, above) except that open treatment without bandaging is often practical.

B. **Of the Canals,** usually from hot slag or metal. No treat-

ment is required except removal of the foreign body
(Topic 38–1). The patient should be warned
against putting medications or plugs of any type
into the ear canal.

C. *Of the Ear Drums.* If slight, removal of the foreign body
(Topic 38–1) is all that is required. If the foreign
body is buried in, or has perforated through the
drum:

1. Control pain.
2. Apply a pad over the ear.
3. Refer at once for specialist care.

28–12.   Electrical burns

Passage of an electrical current through living tissues often
does far more damage than is apparent on superficial examination. Immediate death from ventricular fibrillation may occur
(Topic 3–5). Respiratory failure requiring artificial respiration
(Topic 17–1) is common. Low voltage currents are more dangerous than high tension and alternating currents more lethal
than direct.

Treatment

1. If the patient is in coma or in circulatory or respiratory collapse defer all local treatment until the
measures outlined in Topic 3–5 have been carried
out and the patient's condition has stabilized.

2. Identify the points of entrance and exit of the current (the latter is often overlooked). By estimating the path of the current some idea of the
organs which may have been damaged can be
obtained.

3. Debride both the entrance and exit wounds thoroughly under local anesthesia, removing all
charred or devitalized structures. Close with
loose, interrupted, nonabsorbable sutures and apply sterile dressings. Relaxing incisions and skin
grafting may be necessary.

4. Hospitalize for observation for at least 48 hours if the
patient has been unconscious, if cardiac irregularities have been noted, or if the burned areas
are deep or extensive or involve important structures.

28–13.   Esophageal burns. See 28–19 (*Mucous Membrane*

Burns) and Topic 49–323 (*Lye*). Strictures requiring dilatation may occur.

28–14. **Eye burns.** (Also see Topic 37–31,C.)

A. If caused by acids, alkalies, caustics or other irritant chemicals:

1. Irrigate for at least 15 minutes with tap water, sterile water or normal salt solution. Never attempt to use neutralizing solutions in the eyes.
2. Instill 2 drops of 0.5% tetracaine (Pontocaine) solution to control pain, and apply an eye patch.
3. Refer at once to an ophthalmologist.

B. If caused by hot asphalt, tar, slag or metal:

1. Instill 2 drops of 0.5% tetracaine (Pontocaine) solution.
2. Remove any loose or superficially embedded foreign bodies (Topic 37–31,C, and 32,C). If deep or firmly adherent do not attempt removal. DO NOT attempt to use the solvents for asphalt and tar previously recommended (28–6, above).
3. Apply an eye patch.
4. Refer at once to an ophthalmologist.

28–15. **Flash burns**

A. *Atomic (Hydrogen) Bomb Flash Burns* are characterized by involvement of the side of the body toward the point of explosion and by bizarre patterns of several depths resulting from the varying absorbability of different clothing fabrics. The treatment is the same as outlined under *Principles of Treatment* (28–2, above) and under Topic 64–4 (*Wartime Emergencies*).

B. *Welder's Flash Burns (Photophthalmia).* See Topic 37–31,D.

28–16. **Friction burns** usually involve the palmar surface of the hands ("rope burns") or those portions of the body not protected by heavy clothing [*Pavement Burns* (28–21, below)]. Friction burns may range in severity from slight superficial abrasions to shredding and avulsion of charred and blackened tissues. For treatment see 28–2, above; Topic 55–2 (*Abrasions*); and Topic 42 (*Hand Injuries*).

28–17. **Gasoline (distillate, fuel oil, kerosene) burns**
      Treatment

1. Remove all contaminated clothing at once.

2. Wash the affected areas thoroughly with mild soap and water.

3. Apply a bland ointment to areas of erythema. Second degree burns are not common but if present should be dressed with petrolatum gauze.

4. Watch carefully for evidence of upper respiratory tract irritation caused by aspiration or inhalation of fumes or flames; if present, antibiotics followed by hospitalization are indicated.

28–18. **Magnesium burns.** (Also see Topic 49–325.)

Treatment

1. Paint the burned area with copper sulfate solution.

2. Irrigate with large amounts of saline solution.

3. Remove superficially embedded particles of metal by sharp dissection, using local anesthesia or regional nerve blocks if necessary.

4. Apply a petrolatum gauze dressing.

5. Give broad spectrum antibiotics.

6. Watch carefully for development of crepitation, ulceration or sloughing.

28–19. **Mucous membrane burns** are usually mild but in some instances may result in extreme edema and severe pain. Three sites are common:

A. The Mouth and Throat. Except for *Acid Burns* (28–4, above) and *Alkali Burns* (28–5, above), these burns are usually caused by swallowing too hot foods or drinks and, as a rule, are more uncomfortable than serious. Symptomatic treatment only is required.

B. The Upper Respiratory Tract, caused by the inhalation of flame or hot gases.

Treatment

1. Administration of sedatives. In severe cases, narcotics for control of reflex spasm may be necessary.

2. Prescription of a soothing cough mixture.

3. Insurance of an adequate airway by removal of secretion by postural drainage and suction. If marked edema, dyspnea and/or cyanosis is present, emergency tracheotomy (Topic 17–11) may be necessary.

4. Immediate hospitalization if evidence of lung damage

is present. Terminal pulmonary edema (Topic 52) may occur, usually as a delayed development.

C. The Vagina. Use of strong caustic medications as douches or in attempts to induce abortions [see Topic 49–476 (*Potassium Permanganate*)] may cause mucous membrane injury ranging from slight edema to necrosis and perforation.

Treatment
  1. Mild cases require only sedation and copious, frequent, nonirritating douches.
  2. Moderate cases require adequate frequent cleansing to prevent secondary infection.
  3. Severe cases with extreme edema, ulceration and, sometimes, perforation must be hospitalized at once. Surgical debridement and repair under general anesthetic may be necessary.

28–20. **Mustard gas burns.** See Topic 49–648 and Topic 64–11 (*Poison Gases*).

28–21. **Pavement burns**

Persons thrown from moving vehicles often slide along abrasive surfaces with considerable momentum. Friction and abrasion, with grinding into the skin, subcutaneous tissues and underlying structures of multiple small foreign bodies, can result in injuries peculiarly susceptible to infection, tattooing and permanent scarring.

Treatment. See 28–16, above (*Friction Burns*) and Topic 55–2 (*Abrasions*).

28–22. **Phosphorus burns.** (See also Topic 49–462.)
  Treatment
  1. Flood with large quantities of water—keep wet until the burned areas can be bathed with 2% sodium bicarbonate solution.
  2. Coat with 1% copper sulfate solution.
  3. Remove all particles of phosphorus with forceps.
  4. Debride all necrotic or loose tissue, under local or regional block anesthesia if necessary.
  5. Apply a petrolatum gauze dressing with slight pressure.
  6. Arrange for adequate follow-up medical care.

28–23. **Radiation burns.** See 28–31, below (*X-ray Burns*) and Topic 64–4,B.

28–24. Respiratory tract burns. See 28–19, above (*Mucous Membrane Burns*).

28–25. Scalp burns

Mild cases require only application of a soothing lotion. In severe cases, after clipping the hair and shaving the area around the burn, treat as outlined under *Principles of Treatment* (28–2, above).

28–26. Slag burns

    A. In the Ear. See 28–11, above.

    B. In the Eye. See 28–14, above; Topic 37–31,C, and 32,C.

28–27. Sunburn

    A. Mild cases require only sedatives and anodynes, with local application of a soothing lotion.

    B. Severe cases with bleb formation should be treated as outlined under 28–2, above (*Principles of Treatment*). Hospitalization may be required if over 40% of the skin surface (less in children—see Topic 48–10,A) is affected. Death can occur from extensive severe sunburn with involvement of a large percentage of the body surface.

28–28. Titanium tetrachloride burns. DO NOT USE WATER for original treatment. (See Topic 49–608.)

28–29. Vaginal burns. See 28–19,C, above and Topic 49–476 (*Potassium Permanganate*).

28–30. War gas burns. See Topic 49–648. Tear gas burns respond well to early use of topical steroids, especially ACTH.

28–31. X-ray burns. Roentgen therapy in large doses may result in an uncomfortable erythema.

    Treatment

      1. Sedation by barbiturates, preferably by mouth.

      2. Control of pain by acetylsalicylic acid (aspirin), 0.6 gm., with codeine sulfate, 0.03 gm., by mouth every 4 hours.

      3. Limitation of painful motion by splinting.

      4. Application of petrolatum gauze dressings.

29. CARDIAC EMERGENCIES

See also Topic 48–11 (*Cardiac Emergencies in Children*).

The definitive treatment of acute cardiovascular pathology varies, of course, with the etiologic background of the illness or injury and usually requires more than brief treatment under emergency conditions. There is, however, a distinct group of acute cardiac emergencies in which PROMPT AND RATIONAL ACTION ON THE PART OF THE ATTENDING PHYSICIAN MAY BE THE DECIDING FACTOR IN THE PATIENT'S CHANCE FOR SURVIVAL.

29–1. Auricular fibrillation, rapid, with failure

The treatment for this emergency cardiac condition is the same as that outlined for acute pulmonary edema from ventricular failure (29–6, below) except that rapid intravenous digitalization with ouabain (G-strophanthin), 0.6 to 1.0 mg., may be the prime therapeutic agent.

29–2. Cardiac arrest

Characterized by loss of arterial pulse, pulse pressure and respiration, arrest may be due to cardiac standstill or to ventricular fibrillation (asystole cordis, convulsion of the heart). It represents one of the most urgent conditions which may be encountered in the practice of medicine (Topic 20). Rapid recognition of the condition and prompt re-establishment of adequate oxygenation and circulation represent the only possible chance of saving the patient's life. Because anoxia for more than 5 minutes will result in irreparable damage to the higher centers of the brain, success depends upon carrying out AN ALREADY PLANNED COURSE OF ACTION WITHOUT DELAY.

A. Causes of Cardiac Arrest

1. TOO RAPID OR CARELESS ADMINISTRATION OF, or overdosage of, any anesthetic (inhalation, intravenous, spinal or local), with lack of close observation for, and recognition of, changes in condition.

2. OBSTRUCTION OF THE RESPIRATORY TRACT (mucus, vomitus, foreign bodies, trauma, angioedema, bronchospasm).

3. PRE-EXISTENT CONDITIONS (acute anxiety states, anemia, cardiac disease, dehydration, hyperpyrexia, pulmonary edema, shock).
4. "SHOTGUN" PREOPERATIVE MEDICATIONS.
5. INSUFFICIENT PREOPERATIVE ADMINISTRATION of atropine sulfate.
6. MECHANICAL ERRORS (faulty gauges, mislabeled tanks, poor valves, etc.).
7. POSITION OF THE PATIENT. The sitting position (sometimes used for throat operations) and the deep Trendelenburg are the most dangerous. Rapid shifting on the operating table may precipitate cardiac arrest.
8. AIR EMBOLI—rare (Topic 60–3,B,4).

B. Preliminary Warning Signs of Incipient Cardiac Arrest
1. Signs of respiratory obstruction (cyanosis, gasping respiration, tracheal tug, increased rate and shallowness of respiration).
2. Pulse irregularities and rate changes with a fall in pulse pressure. A pulse rate above 120 suggests shock; below 50, decreased cardiac output.
3. Early cardiac decompensation—auricular fibrillation.
4. Dilation of the pupils; coldness and clamminess of the skin.
5. Muscular twitching.

C. Treatment of the Acute Emergency Occurring in the Operating Room
1. RESPONSIBILITIES OF THE ANESTHESIOLOGIST. If cardiac arrest develops in the operating room, see Topic 17–2,B.
2. RESPONSIBILITIES OF THE SURGEON IF THE CHEST IS ALREADY OPEN. To proceed with direct cardiac massage as outlined under Topic 17–2,B.
3. RESPONSIBILITIES OF THE SURGEON IF THE CHEST IS NOT OPEN.
   a. To take any steps necessary to prevent irreparable damage to the patient during closed chest cardiac massage (application of pressure, insertion of packs, control of bleeding, temporary occlusive dressings, etc.).
   b. To apply, or assist in applying, closed chest cardiac massage as outlined under Topic 17–2,A.

    c. *After satisfactory circulation and respiration have been re-established*: To complete the operative procedure if necessary for survival of the patient—otherwise to close as soon as possible.

    d. To be immediately available during the patient's recovery period.

D. Treatment of the Acute Emergency Outside of the Operating Room

1. See Topic 17–2,A, for technique of closed chest cardiac massage.
2. Treatment should, whenever possible, be directed and supervised by a qualified anesthesiologist.

E. Medicolegal Aspects of Cardiac Arrest

1. Failure to recognize the preliminary warning signs of incipient cardiac arrest (29–2,B, above) and to institute prompt and proper treatment (Topic 17–2) has been held to constitute negligence (Topic 69–1).
2. Closed chest cardiac massage is now accepted as the proper resuscitative measure unless the chest is already open and the heart readily accessible for direct open chest manual massage.
3. Delay in recognition and treatment, with resultant permanent nervous system damage on recovery, has been held to constitute negligence (Topic 69–1).
4. Lack of constant attendance during the recovery period from cardiac arrest has been construed as indicating negligence on the part of the attending physician.

29–3. **Heart block (complete) with Stokes-Adams syncope**

Stokes-Adams syncopal attacks can be caused by ventricular standstill or by ventricular tachycardia.

A. With Ventricular Standstill

Treatment

1. Elevate the foot of the bed.
2. Inject epinephrine hydrochloride (Adrenalin) (1 : 1000 solution), 0.5 ml., intramuscularly. Intracardiac injection of the same dose can be tried but is rarely successful.
3. Give oxygen by face mask and rebreathing bag, using positive pressure.

4. Inject atropine sulfate, 0.4 to 0.6 mg., subcutaneously or intravenously.

B. With Ventricular Tachycardia. Abolition of ventricular tachycardia as soon as possible is imperative to prevent the occurrence of ventricular fibrillation.

Treatment
1. Enforce absolute rest.
2. Inject morphine sulfate, 10 to 15 mg., subcutaneously or intravenously.
3. Administer procainamide (Pronestyl) intravenously. The maximum dose is 1 gm. given slowly at a rate of not more than 200 mg. per minute. The oral preparation may be substituted: 1 gm. at once, followed by 0.5 to 1.0 gm. every 2 to 4 hours. If no procainamide (Pronestyl) is available, quinidine sulfate, 0.6 gm. every 2 hours by mouth, can be substituted.
4. DO NOT administer epinephrine hydrochloride (Adrenalin) if ventricular tachycardia is present.

29–4. Hemopericardium (traumatic) with cardiac tamponade
This condition may be encountered following penetrating wounds of the chest (gunshots, stab wounds). It is characterized by venous back pressure with distention of the neck veins, dusky cyanosis and progressive decrease of pulse pressure, even before the systolic pressure falls to shock level. The heart sounds are generally distant or not audible. The most reliable sign is the absence of pulsation of the cardiac silhouette on fluoroscopic examination.

Treatment
A. Immediate pericardial sac aspiration with a 2½ inch, 16 or 18 gauge, short-bevel needle. Removal of relatively small amounts of blood may be lifesaving. Because of the potential danger of cardiac arrest (29–2, above), this procedure should, if possible, be done in a fully equipped operating room with an anesthesiologist in attendance. However, if the patient is in extremis, or rapidly becoming worse, the attending physician has a definite positive obligation to aspirate the pericardial space, even in an emergency setting, as soon as he recognizes the condition. For technique of pericardial sac aspiration see Topic 17–7.

B. Supportive Measures

1. TREATMENT OF SHOCK (Topic 15–7). Plasma volume expanders and 5% dextrose in saline intravenously will usually support the circulation adequately, although addition of metaraminol bitartrate (Aramine), 100 mg., or arterenol bitartrate (Levophed), 4 ml. of 0.2% solution to 1000 ml. of 5% dextrose in saline, may be necessary.

2. INJECTION OF MORPHINE SULFATE, 10 to 15 mg., combined with atropine sulfate, 0.4 to 0.6 mg., intravenously.

3. ADMINISTRATION OF OXYGEN under positive pressure by face mask and rebreathing bag.

4. TRANSPORTATION to the closest surgical facilities equipped for thoracic surgery at the earliest possible time but not before aspiration has been done. The hospital should be notified in advance so that a thoracotomy can be done without delay.

29–5. Myocardial infarction, acute

Persons with suspected or proved myocardial infarction should receive the following emergency therapy while awaiting hospitalization:

Treatment

1. Absolute rest in a position of comfort.

2. Morphine sulfate, 10 to 15 mg., subcutaneously or intravenously for relief of pain and apprehension.

3. Atropine sulfate, 0.4 to 0.6 mg., subcutaneously to prevent reflex vagal vasoconstriction of the coronary arteries.

4. Oxygen under positive pressure by face mask and rebreathing bag if cyanosis is present.

5. Small (250 ml.) transfusions of plasma volume expanders if the patient is in shock. Early signs of pulmonary edema (Topic 52) should be watched for very carefully and appropriate treatment given. To combat shock associated with myocardial infarction with low venous pressure, small doses (0.2 to 0.3 ml.) of 1:1000 solution of epinephrine hydrochloride (Adrenalin) can be given subcutaneously. Phenylephrine hydrochloride (Neo-Synephrine), 1 to 3 mg., intravenously is even more effective.

6. With high venous pressure, plasma volume expanders, epinephrine hydrochloride (Adrenalin), and phenylephrine hydrochloride (Neo-Synephrine) are definitely contraindicated. Instead, rapid digitalization should be accomplished by intravenous injection of 0.8 mg. of lanatoside C (Cedilanid), repeated in 1 hour.

7. Treatment of shock (Topic 15–7) should be instituted before moving the patient for any reason.

8. Transportation of proved or suspected cases to hospital facilities BY AMBULANCE—never by private automobile. If cyanosis or evidence of shock is present, oxygen therapy by face mask and intravenous support should be continued in the ambulance.

29–6. Pulmonary edema (acute) from sudden ventricular failure. [See also Topic 52 (*Pulmonary Edema*).]

Treatment

1. Morphine sulfate, 10 to 20 mg., subcutaneously or intravenously, according to the urgency of the situation.

2. Atropine sulfate, 0.4 to 0.6 mg., subcutaneously or slowly intravenously if tachycardia is not a prominent feature.

3. Oxygen inhalations under positive pressure, preferably by face mask and rebreathing bag.

4. Allowance of a position of comfort. The patient may be placed in semi-Fowler position or permitted to sit on the edge of the bed (provided an attendant is present at all times).

5. Application of tourniquets serially to all four extremities with alternate regular periods of release.

6. Phlebotomy with removal of 250 to 500 ml. of blood [except in pulmonary edema associated with acute myocardial infarction (29–5, above)].

7. Rapid digitalization by intravenous injection of an initial dose of 0.8 mg. of lanatoside C (Cedilanid), repeated in 1 hour.

30. CEPHALGIA

Many types of headache may be severe enough to cause the sufferer to seek emergency medical care. Although the etiology in many instances is obscure and requires more thorough study for determination than is practical in an emergency setting, there are certain types which can be recognized and given at least temporary relief on an emergency basis.

30-1. **Alcoholic excess ("hangover") headaches.** [Also see Topic 2-1 and Topic 49-227 (*Ethyl Alcohol*).] Inhalations of oxygen and administration of fluids may help as may acetylsalicylic acid (aspirin). Barbiturates and all types of opiates and synthetic narcotics should be avoided.

30-2. **Altitude sickness** (Mountain Sickness). See Topic 26-1 and 6.

30-3. **Arthritis of the cervical spine** (with or without aggravation by trauma) may cause severe headaches, usually localized to the distribution of the greater or lesser occipital or the posterior auricular nerves on one or both sides. Occasionally the pain may be frontal or postorbital.

> *Treatment* consists of salicylates, muscle relaxants and sedation. Application of a Thomas collar or cervical traction may be necessary. (See also Topic 45-1.)

30-4. **Asthenia due to Addison's disease.** See Topic 35-1.

30-5. **Brain tumors** may cause frontal or generalized headaches, aggravated by changes in position.

> *Treatment.* Acetylsalicylic acid (aspirin), with or without codeine sulfate, may give temporary relief. If a brain tumor is suspected, referral to a neurologist for thorough investigation and definitive treatment is mandatory.

30-6. **Caffeine-withdrawal headaches.** In habitual coffee drinkers, abstinence may cause severe, often completely disabling, headaches.

> *Treatment.* Coffee by mouth, caffeine sodiobenzoate, 0.5 gm., intramuscularly, amphetamine sulfate, 5 mg., orally, or oxygen inhalations will give immediate relief.

30–7. Concussion headaches follow direct trauma to the head, but the severity of the headache has little, if any, relationship to the intensity of the trauma. In mild cases rest, reassurance and acetylsalicylic acid (aspirin) are all that is necessary. Severe cases require treatment as outlined under *Head Injuries* (Topic 43–1).

30–8. Constipation. The remedy is obvious.

30–9. Eclampsia. See Topic 50–9.

30–10. Epilepsy. See Topic 3–7 and Topic 33 (*Convulsive Seizures*).

30–11. Eye strain

> *Treatment* consists basically of avoiding excessive use of the eyes, especially at close or fine work. Dark glasses may be of assistance if photophobia is present. Acetylsalicylic acid (aspirin) will often give temporary relief. The patient should be instructed to see an ophthalmologist as soon as possible.

30–12. Febrile headaches may be caused by any condition which results in a high fever. Administration of acetylsalicylic acid (aspirin), antibiotics, cold packs or other measures to bring the fever down should be postponed until serious conditions such as meningitis (Topic 32–16), poliomyelitis (Topic 32–21) and pneumonia (Topic 53–14) have been ruled out by careful examination.

30–13. Food allergy headaches may occur following the ingestion of almost any kind of food by susceptible individuals. The most common offenders, especially in children, seem to be cabbage, chocolate, garlic, green peppers and peanuts. Antihistaminics give rapid relief.

30–14. Hemorrhage from a peptic ulcer may be accompanied by a very severe headache which disappears with supportive therapy or cessation of bleeding.

30–15. Herpes of the posterior auricular or greater or lesser occipital nerves may cause severe localized headache with or without severe burning. The diagnosis can usually be made from the distribution of the lesions and by the type of pain.

> *Treatment*
>
> 1. Protection of the herpetic lesions from infection by petrolatum gauze or butacaine (Butyn) and nitromersol (Metaphen) ointment dressings. If the lesions are on the scalp above the hair line,

chlortetracycline (Aureomycin) ointment, rubbed
in gently, is effective.
2. Control of pain:
   a. If moderate, by acetylsalicylic acid (aspirin) and
      barbiturates.
   b. If severe, by:
      (1) Codeine sulfate, 0.03 to 0.06 gm., orally or
          intramuscularly.
      (2) Meperidine hydrochloride (Demerol), 50 to
          100 mg., intramuscularly.
   c. If exquisite, by
      (1) Morphine sulfate, 10 to 15 mg., intramuscu-
          larly or, in extreme cases, intravenously.
      (2) Methadone (Amidon, Dolophine), 10 mg.,
          orally. The analgesic effect of this drug
          given by mouth lasts from 8 to 12 hours.
      (3) Hospitalization in severe or stubborn cases, or
          if the eyes are involved (Topic 37–14).

30–16. **Histamine headaches** (Cluster Headache, Horton's
Cephalgia) are severe, throbbing, and often associated with
unilateral redness and lacrimation of the eye. They may be
precipitated or aggravated by alcohol ingestion. Measures, such
as jugular pressure, which raise the spinal fluid pressure and
decrease the blood supply will temporarily relieve the cephalgia.
Severe cases require hospitalization.

30–17. **Hunger headaches** are usually hypoglycemic and are
relieved by food, especially proteins. There may be enough time
lag to require acetylsalicylic acid (aspirin).

30–18. **Hypertensive headaches** are usually present in the
morning and "wear off" by noon. Acetylsalicylic acid (aspirin)
will give temporary relief. Sleeping with the head elevated may
prevent attacks.

30–19. **Hypotensive headaches** are caused by any of the many
conditions which produce a drop in blood pressure and often
are accompanied by vasodepressor syncope (Topic 60–4).

30–20. **Meningeal irritation**

Severe and persistent headaches associated with fever and a
stiff neck require an immediate spinal puncture to determine
the etiology (Topic 32–16; Topic 48–38; and Topic 63–1).

30–21. **Migraine**

   A. In Adults. Relief from the acute discomfort of migraine

type head pain in adults can sometimes be obtained through a combination of the following measures:
1. Absolute rest in a darkened room.
2. Oxygen inhalations.
3. Ergotamine tartrate (Gynergen), 3 to 6 mg., by mouth, or 0.5 mg., subcutaneously. In addition, 2 mg. may be given every 2 hours by mouth. The sublingual method also can be used with an initial dose of 3 to 4 mg. dissolved under the tongue, followed by 1 to 2 mg. every hour. By either method, THE TOTAL DOSE SHOULD NEVER EXCEED 10 MG. A slower effect can be obtained by 2 tables of Cafergot (Ergotamine tartrate, 1 mg., with caffeine sodiobenzoate, 100 mg.) orally, repeated in 2 hours (once only).

   Ergot in therapeutic doses has many undesirable side effects (Topic 49–218), including myalgia, fatigue, nausea, vomiting, and tingling and numbness of the hands and feet, or even myocardial infarction. Atropine sulfate, 0.4 mg., subcutaneously, will neutralize some of these side effects; calcium gluconate, 10 ml. of a 10% solution intravenously, will decrease muscle pain. Numbness or tingling of the extremities calls for immediate discontinuance of ergot in any form; so does a cold feeling or cyanosis.
4. Nicotinic acid, 50 to 75 mg., orally.
5. Amphetamine (Benzedrine) sulfate, 10 to 15 mg., orally.
6. Dimenhydrinate (Dramamine), 50 to 100 mg., intramuscularly. The same dose by slow intravenous injection will give almost immediate relief. For intravenous use, each ml. (50 mg.) of dimenhydrinate must be diluted with 10 ml. of normal salt solution.
7. Methyliso-octenylamine (Octin) 50 mg., subcutaneously. If a rise in blood pressure occurs, Octin therapy must be stopped at once; if there is no rise in ½ hour, 250 mg. by mouth, repeated once, may be given.
8. Hospitalization in severe or intractable cases.

B. In Children. See Topic 48–39.

C. Prophylaxis. Although it is of no value in treatment, methysergide maleate (Sansert), 2 mg., three times a day by mouth may prevent the development of migraine.

30–22. **Myofibrositis** of the upper portion of the neck from trauma (30–3, above) postural strain ("television headache") or infection (especially viral) may cause severe unilateral or bilateral headache, usually occipital but sometimes localized to the distribution of the posterior auricular or greater or lesser occipital nerves on one or both sides. Treatment of the underlying cause is necessary for permanent relief. Symptomatic relief can be given by the measures outlined for *Whiplash Injuries* (Topic 45–11,B).

30–23. **Orthostatic headaches.** See *Hypotensive Headaches* (30–19, above).

30–24. **Poliomyelitic headaches.** See *Meningeal Irritation Headaches* (30–20, above).

30–25. **Psychoneurotic headaches** are characterized by complaints of a tight band around the head or a pulling sensation over the vertex. Also see *Tension Headaches* (30–33, below).

30–26. **Relaxation** *("Sunday morning")* **headaches** are probably due to peripheral vasodilation. They can usually be relieved by small doses of acetylsalicylic acid (aspirin) or by activity, mental or physical.

30–27. **Sinus headaches** often can be relieved temporarily by shrinking the nasal mucous membranes and postural drainage. The patient should be referred to an otolaryngologist for definitive care.

30–28. **Spinal puncture headaches** occur in 10 to 20% of cases whether or not local anesthetics or the preventive measures outlined below are used.

A. Cycle of Development
1. The cerebrospinal fluid pressure is decreased by puncture.
2. The difference between the spinal fluid pressure and intracranial venous pressure is increased.
3. Dilation of the intracranial venous structures results in increased volume of the brain with resultant stimulation of the intracranial pain centers.

B. Preventive Measures
1. Use of a small needle with the bevel parallel to the long axis of the body to minimize dural tears.

  2. Avoidance of any motion of the spine while the needle is in place.
  3. Limitation of amount of fluid removed to not more than 6 ml.
  4. Intravenous administration of 5% dextrose in water (unless contraindicated by some systemic condition). Caffeine sodiobenzoate, Pituitrin, ergotamine and nicotinic acid have been used empirically but probably are of no value. Contrary to general belief, keeping the patient flat after the procedure does not decrease the incidence of postpuncture headaches. It does, however, decrease the intensity after cephalgia has developed.

C. Symptomatic Treatment
  1. Acetylsalicylic acid (aspirin) in mild cases; codeine sulfate in small doses if the discomfort is acute. The drugs listed under *Tension Headaches* (30–33, below) may be of benefit.
  2. Application of a tight abdominal binder, especially following puncture for obstetric spinal anesthesia.
  3. Hospitalization if the headache persists or is unaffected by postural changes.

D. Prognosis.
Complete recovery is the rule although in some cases 7 to 10 days may be required for complete relief of symptoms. The patient may or may not develop symptoms if spinal puncture is repeated at a later date.

30–29. Spontaneous rupture of an intracranial artery (Topic 60–2,C) is characterized by sudden onset of very severe occipital pain following extensive subarachnoid hemorrhage. Progressive involvement of the vital centers, which may be fatal, often occurs.

30–30. Starch or sugar headaches
Ingestion of excessive amounts of sweet or starchy foods may cause severe headaches which persist until the dietary imbalance is corrected. No emergency treatment except advice is necessary.

30–31. Sunlight headaches are caused by peripheral vasodilation from unaccustomed exposure to bright sunlight and often precede heat cramps (Topic 57–2), heat stroke (Topic 57–4) and sunstroke (Topic 57–8).

30–32. **Syphilis** (cerebral). See Topic 61–9, 10 and 11.

30–33. **"Tension headaches"** is an overworked catch-all for many cases of mixed etiology. Although extreme mental stress and strain may cause severe headaches in certain individuals, a thorough history and examination will usually disclose a specific causative factor. Administration of some of the following drugs may give relief:

1. Acetylsalicylic acid (aspirin), 0.6 gm., by mouth every 4 hours.
2. Meprobamate (Miltown, Equanil), 400 mg., orally three times a day.
3. Valoctin [a combination of methyliso-octenylamine (Octin), 0.06 gm., and monobromisovalerylurea (Bromural), 250 mg.] 1 tablet by mouth, repeated in 4 hours.
4. Reserpine, 0.25 to 0.8 mg., orally.
5. Chlorpromazine hydrochloride (Thorazine), 10 to 25 mg., orally three times a day. See also 30–21, above (*Migraine*) and Topic 48–39 (*Migraine in Children*).

30–34. **Toothaches** (Topic 58) or **earaches** secondary to middle ear infection (Topic 34–12,B) may cause severe generalized headaches.

30–35. **Toxic headaches**

Ingestion, inhalation or absorption through the mucous membranes or the intact skin of many substances may cause severe headaches, usually frontal in location, but sometimes orbital, occipital or diffuse. Among the more common toxic substances are:

Alcohol—amyl (Topic 49–48); ethyl (Topic 49–227); and isopropyl (Topic 49–300).

Ammonia fumes (Topic 49–42).

Benzene—inhalation or ingestion (Topic 49–80).

Chlorine (Topic 49–133).

Epinephrine hydrochloride (Adrenalin)—from overzealous use of a nebulizer or from hypodermic administration. See Topic 49–214 and Topic 59–26.

Hydrochloric acid vapors. See *Acids* (Topic 49–19).

Iodine—inhalation of the fumes (Topic 49–292).

Kerosene fumes (Topic 49–303).

Lead and its salts—inhalation of the fumes or dust, or ingestion, may be the mode of entry. Chronic lead poisoning (plumbism) is often characterized by severe headaches (Topic 49–313).

Metal fumes (Topic 49–348).

Methyl acetate fumes (Topic 49–357).

Naphthalene fumes (Topic 49–381).

Nicotine (Topic 49–389).

Nitrites (Topic 49–393).

Ozone—in certain hypersensitive persons inhalation of even minute concentrations of this gas will cause very severe frontal headache (Topic 49–429).

Phosphorus pentachloride fumes (Topic 49–462).

Pyrethrum dust or powder (Topic 49–483).

Tobacco—inhalation of dust or ingestion. See *Nicotine* (Topic 49–389).

Zinc oxide—inhalation of dust. See *Metal Fumes* (Topic 49–348).

30–36. Traumatic headaches. See *Concussion Headaches* (30–7, above).

30–37. Trigeminal neuralgia ('tic douloureux"). See Topic 47–4,J.

30–38. Uremia (Topic 3–15) may be accompanied by a very distressing type of headache which will persist until the causative condition is remedied. Sedatives and anodynes are of very little value in treatment.

30–39. Vasopressor headaches may be caused by administration of phenylephrine hydrochloride (Neo-Synephrine) or epinephrine hydrochloride (Adrenalin) (Topic 49–214). Unless excessively large doses have been given or individual hypersensitivity is present, the effect is transient only and requires no emergency treatment.

31. CHEST INJURIES

31–1. Nonperforating injuries to the chest

Acute restlessness and apprehension in a patient who gives a history of severe rib cage compression are often the only indications of intra-alveolar or mediastinal bleeding. Even in the absence of external evidence of trauma, supportive therapy should be begun at once.

Respiratory depressants, especially opiates and synthetic narcotics, should never be administered to a patient with any type of chest injury until the nature and extent of the injury have been definitely determined.

31–2. **Fractures**

   A. *Simple Fractures of Ribs or Sternum* usually require no treatment except limitation of activity and control of pain. Local application of cold will often decrease immediate discomfort; after 24 hours heat may give relief. Blocking of the intercostal nerves proximal to the fractures with a local anesthetic may be necessary for relief if overriding, depression or displacement is present. Binding or strapping the chest may be dangerous because it limits to some extent the aeration of the lungs and increases the possibility of the development of a traumatic pneumonitis. This is especially true in elderly persons. Marked sternal depression requires immediate hospitalization.

   B. *Multiple Rib Fractures* with loss of ability of the thorax to expand on inspiration may result in "paradoxical respiration," often associated with severe shock. Insertion of towel clips into the rib fragments, with overhead suspended weights attached to the clips for countertraction, may be lifesaving. Immediate hospitalization is always required if paradoxical respiration is present.

31–3. **Contusions—crushing and compression injuries.**

Especially in children, sudden forcible compression of the chest may cause serious intrathoracic damage without external evidence of injury. Slowly progressive bleeding due to alveolar rupture may result from the "accordion action" of the resilient rib cage. Plasma volume expanders intravenously should be started if a young patient with a history of possible thoracic compression is acutely and persistently apprehensive and restless, even if signs and symptoms of hemorrhagic shock (Topic 15–6) are absent and there are no other indications of intrathoracic injury. Hospitalization for careful and frequent observation for changes in vital signs and hematocrit levels is indicated for at least 24 hours after injury.

31–4. **Traumatic pneumothorax** should be ruled out by careful clinical and x-ray examination. Its presence requires hospitalization after careful observation for, and treatment of, latent or delayed shock (Topic 15).

31–5.   Tension pneumothorax, caused by leakage of air from the lung into the pleural cavity with an intact chest wall, is a very serious condition which requires hospitalization as soon as possible for water-seal drainage. Before transportation of the patient, a large bore (No. 16 or 18) hypodermic needle with a rubber glove finger or finger cot with a small hole in the tip fastened to the needle base should be inserted into the pleural cavity between the second and third ribs in the midclavicular line to act as a flutter valve.

31–6.   Rupture of the diaphragm may be caused by direct non-penetrating trauma over the lower ribs on either side or, less commonly, by penetrating wounds. Dyspnea and cyanosis may be acute. Shock, usually the result of mediastinal shift, may require treatment (Topic 15–7) before and during transportation to a hospital equipped for open chest surgery. Small defects in the diaphragm are very difficult to detect and are potentially more dangerous than large rents because of the increased chances of obstruction and strangulation.

31–7.   Thoracic squeeze occurs in underwater swimmers using a snorkel tube. See Topic 26–5,A,4.

31–8.   Costochrondal separation

The treatment is the same as outlined for *Fractures* (31–2, above).

31–9.   Penetrating injuries of the chest

31–10.   Lacerations through the pleura (stab and knife wounds, etc.)

  Treatment

1. Cover the surface laceration with petrolatum gauze and a pressure bandage.
2. Treat shock (Topic 15–7).
3. If dyspnea or cyanosis is marked, give air or oxygen under positive pressure by face mask or intra-nasal catheter and rebreathing bag after cleansing the airway by suction.
4. Use gentle restraint as needed. Opiates or synthetic narcotics are contraindicated.
5. As soon as possible transfer by ambulance for hospitalization, continuing respiratory assistance and restraint in the ambulance if necessary.

31–11.   Open (compound) fractures of ribs

Treatment is the same as outlined for penetrating injuries

(31–9, above); use towel-clip countertraction if paradoxical respiration (31–2, above) is present.

31–12. Bullet wounds

Treatment

1. Cover the wound of entry (and of exit if present) with sterile petrolatum gauze; apply a firm pressure bandage.
2. Give oxygen inhalations after determining that the airway is clear.
3. Institute shock therapy (Topic 15–7).
4. Apply gentle manual restraint as needed.
5. When the patient's condition has stabilized, transfer by ambulance—continuing oxygen and intravenous therapy if needed—to a hospital equipped for major chest surgery.
6. DO NOT
    a. Probe for a foreign body (bullet, shot, etc.).
    b. Give excessive amounts of intravenous fluids—pulmonary edema may result (Topic 52).
    c. Administer morphine sulfate, synthetic narcotics or other respiratory depressants.

31–13. Traumatic hemopericardium. See Topic 29–4. For technique of pericardial sac aspiration, see Topic 17–7.

32. CONTAGIOUS AND COMMUNICABLE DISEASES

32–1. Anthrax (Malignant Pustule, Wool Sorters' Disease)

Usually occurs in industry [Topic 76 (*Industrial Cases*)] in persons who handle, cure or process animal hides. The incubation period is 1 to 7 days. No quarantine is required, but the patient should be isolated until any drainage from superficial lesions clears.

Treatment. Symptomatic only.

32–2. Chancroid. See Topic 61–2.

32–3. Chickenpox (Varicella)

Usually occurs in fall or winter in children over 6 months

old. Incubation period—12 to 21 days; usually 14 to 16. Very contagious; spread by direct and indirect contact.

Treatment

1. Isolation for 10 days.
2. Bed rest and sedatives, with close observation regarding development of interstitial pneumonia (Topic 48–41).
3. Dressings to prevent scratching.
4. Trimeprazine tartrate (Temaril), 2.5 mg., by mouth every 4 to 6 hours for relief of itching.

32–4. **Diphtheria**

Affects chiefly children between 1 to 10 years, mostly 2 to 5 years. Incubation period—2 to 5 days. Average mortality, 5%. Spread by direct and indirect contact; carriers common.

Treatment

1. Immediate administration of adequate doses of diphtheria antitoxin is imperative if the clinical findings are suggestive of diphtheria. This applies even if smears are negative or inconclusive. Infants should be given 5000 units of diphtheria antitoxin; older children, 8000 to 20,000 units. Before administration 0.1 ml. of undiluted serum should be injected intramuscularly. If no wheal appears in 20 minutes, the whole dose can be given. If a wheal does develop, 0.05 ml. of a 1:100 solution should be injected intradermally, followed by desensitization if necessary (Topic 14).
2. Serious cases require hospitalization. Mild cases may be treated at home, with quarantine until two consecutive nose and throat cultures taken at 24-hour intervals show no diphtheria bacilli.
3. Emergency intubation or tracheotomy (Topic 17–11) may be indicated. Marked respiratory difficulty from edema must be relieved BEFORE TRANSFER OF THE PATIENT. Although in extreme emergencies a tracheotomy may be performed by simply passing a knife-blade in the middle between the cricoid and thyroid cartilages (Topic 17–11,B,1), this method may cause severe laryngeal damage. A more satisfactory method, which is easy to perform, avoids important structures

and allows introduction of the tube under visual control, is at the level of the third, fourth and fifth tracheal rings. For technique see Topic 17–11,B,2.

32–5. **Dysentery (bacillary)**

This disease which affects persons in all age groups is spread by indirect contact. Incubation period—1 to 9 days (usually less than 4). Isolation is indicated until stool cultures no longer show the bacilli responsible.

32–6. **German measles.** See *Rubella* (32–24, below).

32–7. **Gonococcus infections.** See Topic 61–3.

32–8. **Granuloma inguinale.** See Topic 61–4 (*Lymphopathia Venereum*).

32–9. **Hemolytic streptococcal infections**

These organisms may cause septic sore throat, scarlet fever (32–27, below) and various other serious conditions. Incubation period—1 to 5 days; spread by both direct and indirect contact. Since communicability lasts from first symptoms until complete recovery, patients should be isolated until afebrile and all discharges have cleared—usually about 14 days in uncomplicated cases. (Recovery from a condition caused by one type of hemolytic streptococcus does not result in immunity to other types.)

> *Treatment*
> 1. Bed rest under isolation precautions and symptomatic care.
> 2. Penicillin and sulfonamides in large doses, continued for at least a week after the acute picture has cleared.

32–10. **Hepatitis.** See Topic 63–8.

32–11. **Influenza.** (See also Topic 63–10.)

A viral disease which is usually characterized by high fever, coryza, myalgia and tonsillitis, but delirium, convulsions and coma may simulate meningitis, especially in children (Topic 48–37). The incubation period is 1 to 5 days.

> *Treatment.* Symptomatic treatment only is indicated. Extremely severe cases should be hospitalized to prevent complications, but the usual case does very well on home care. No quarantine is required.

32–12. **Leprosy**

Incubation period—very long; method of transmittal not

fully known. Quarantine in specially designed hospitals required.

32–13. Lymphopathia venereum. See Topic 61–4.

32–14. Malaria

No quarantine or isolation required. Incubation period 14 days.

> *Treatment.* Quinine, atabrine and other antimalarial drugs.

32–15. Measles (Rubeola)

Most common between the ages of 3 and 5 years. Children under 5 months are generally immune. The incubation period is 7 to 15 days (usually about 10). The eruption appears on the third to fifth day and lasts about 6 days. Koplik's spots, which appear on the third or fourth day, are pathognomonic. Very contagious by both direct and indirect contact from about 4 days before appearance of the rash to 5 days afterward. Isolation required during this period.

> *Treatment*
> 1. Complete isolation for 2 weeks.
> 2. Rest in a darkened room or protection of the eyes by dark glasses.
> 3. Steam inhalations; ear drops.
> 4. Early recognition and treatment of complications such as otitis media, bronchopneumonia and encephalitis.
> 5. Prophylactic injection of gamma globulin for contacts under 2, pregnant women and elderly or debilitated persons.

32–16. Meningitis. [See also Topic 48–38 (*Meningococcemia in Children*); Topic 48–59 (*Waterhouse-Friderichsen Syndrome in Children*); and Topic 63–1 (*Arbovirus Infections*).]

The incubation period of epidemic (meningococcal) meningitis is 2 to 10 days; quarantine period, 21 days or longer.

Evidence indicative of meningococcal septicemia requires immediate administration of large doses of penicillin and readily absorbable sulfonamides, preferably intravenously.

32–17. Mumps

The incubation period is 12 to 26 days, usually 16 to 18.

> *Treatment*
> 1. Bed rest in isolation until the fever and glandular swelling subside.
> 2. Hot compresses to swollen areas.
> 3. Careful mouth hygiene.

    4. Early recognition and treatment of complications
       (orchitis, pancreatitis, meningoencephalitis).
       Early administration of corticosteroids (Pred-
       nisone) orally, 60 mg. at once; then 20 mg.
       three times a day may prevent sterility from
       pressure necrosis of the testicles. Gradual taper-
       ing off of the steroid should accompany decrease
       of edema.

32–18. **Paratyphoid fever.** See *Typhoid Fever* (32–32, below).

32–19. **Pertussis.** See *Whooping Cough* (32–37, below).

32–20. **Plague**

The incubation period for both the bubonic and pneumonic
forms is 3 to 7 days. Quarantine until complete recovery is
mandatory.

32–21. **Poliomyelitis** (*Infantile Paralysis*). [See also Topic
47–5 and Topic 48–45 (*Respiratory Paralysis in Children*).]

Three causative viral strains have been identified. Spread is
by both direct and indirect contact. Incubation period—from
3 to 35 days (usually 7 to 14 days).

   Treatment
    1. Immediate hospitalization for spinal puncture to es-
       tablish the diagnosis if the history and clinical
       examination suggest the possibility of poliomye-
       litis [also see Topic 27–20,C (*Tick Paralysis*)].
       The puncture may be done by the attending
       physician if equipment and laboratory facilities
       are available.
    2. Isolation for one week from onset of first symptoms
       or while febrile.
    3. Control of pain by sedatives and anodynes. Narcotics
       are contraindicated if there is any respiratory
       weakness.
    4. Artificial respiration by mechanical or other methods
       if respiratory difficulty is present. Emergency
       tracheotomy (Topic 17–11) may be necessary
       before or after transfer for hospitalization.
    5. Orthopedic support of paralyzed parts to prevent con-
       tractures and other deformities.

32–22. **Psittacosis.** (Ornithosis, Parrot Fever). See Topic
63–18.

32–23. **Rabies.** See Topic 63–19.

32–24. **Rubella** (German Measles)

Incubation period—10 to 21 days. Very contagious; spreads by direct and indirect contact.

Treatment
1. Bed rest until acute symptoms subside.
2. Symptomatic care. Complications are rare, although an uncomfortable polyarthritis with fibrositis, paresthesias, myalgia and muscle weakness lasting as long as 2 weeks may occur.

32–25. **Rubeola.** See *Measles* (32–15, above).

32–26. **Salmonella infections.** See *Typhoid Fever* (32–32, below); and Topic 49–245 (*Food Poisoning*).

32–27. **Scarlet fever**

Incubation period—2 to 7 days. Quarantine for 21 days or longer is required.

Treatment
1. Simple cases may be cared for at home.
2. Toxic or septic cases require immediate hospitalization. Delirium and convulsions are the only complications which may require emergency treatment before transfer.

32–28. **Septic sore throat.** [See also *Hemolytic Streptococcal Infections* (32–9, above).]

Incubation period—1 to 5 days, usually 2 to 3 days. No quarantine is necessary.

32–29. **Shigella infections.** See *Dysentery* (*Bacillary*) (32–5, above).

32–30. **Smallpox**

Incubation period—7 to 16 days; commonly, 12; rarely, 21. Very contagious, especially in early stages. Spread by direct and indirect contact.

Treatment
1. Immediate hospitalization for isolation, with sterilization of the examination room and its contents after the patient has been transferred.
2. Immediate vaccination of all persons who have come in contact with the case.

32–31. **Tetanus** (Lockjaw)

(See Topic 14 for tests for sensitivity to antitoxin and Topic 19 for immunization.) The incubation period is from a few hours in infants to 3 weeks in older children and adults.

Treatment
1. Protection from external stimuli in a darkened room.

    2. Minimal handling.

    3. Sedatives to diminish spasm; large doses are generally necessary. Opiates and synthetic narcotics should not be used.

    4. Artificial respiration if necessary (Topic 17–1).

    5. Immediate transfer to a hospital equipped for care of acute contagious disease.

    Prognosis. Very poor if the disease has become established.

32–32. Typhoid fever

Incubation period—10 to 15 days.

    Treatment. As soon as the diagnosis is established or suspected, the patient should be hospitalized for confirmatory diagnosis and treatment. Severe epistaxis may require packing before transfer. Quarantine is required until two consecutive negative stool cultures have been obtained.

32–33. Typhus fever

Incubation period—12 days. Contacts must be quarantined for 14 days.

32–34. Undulant fever

Incubation period—5 to 21 days, occasionally longer. Quarantine is not required.

32–35. Varicella. See *Chickenpox* (32–3, above).

32–36. Variola. See *Smallpox* (32–30, above).

32–37. Whooping cough (Pertussis)

Incubation period—usually 7 to 10 days, but sometimes up to 21 days. Spread by direct and indirect contact. Communicable from about 7 days after exposure (when symptoms appear to be those of a common cold) until 3 weeks after onset of typical spasmodic cough. Exclusion from schools, theaters and other public places required, but usually no strict quarantine.

    Treatment

    1. Control of paroxysmal cough by:

        a. Codeine sulfate by mouth or subcutaneously.

        b. Chloral hydrate by mouth or retention enema.

        c. Ether, 25 per cent in 30 ml. of oil, as a retention enema.

        d. Paraldehyde orally or intramuscularly.

        e. Pentobarbital sodium (Nembutal) by rectal suppository.

    2. Early recognition and treatment of complications.

The following complications may require hospitalization:
a. Bronchopneumonia (Topic 63–11).
b. Gastric tetany, rectal prolapse, etc., following paroxysms of coughing or vomiting.
c. Meningitis or encephalitis (Topic 48–20 and 37).

32–38. Yellow fever
(See also Topic 63–24.) Incubation period—3 to 5 days.
   Quarantine
   1. Patient—3 to 5 days after development of acute symptoms.
   2. All contacts—6 days.

33. CONVULSIVE SEIZURES

See also Topic 48–14 (*Convulsions in Children*).

Persons of any age may develop convulsive seizures either for the first time or on a recurrent basis. Subsequent episodes are frequently though not invariably related to prior causes.

33–1. Incidence by age
The most common underlying factors responsible for convulsions vary with age.

A. Neonatal and Infant Age Group
   1. Birth injury.
   2. Developmental abnormalities.
   3. Bacterial and viral central nervous system infections.

B. Children and Adolescents. Same as 33–1,A, above, with addition of
   1. Trauma.
   2. Idiopathic causes.

C. Adults
   1. Trauma.
   2. Idiopathic causes.
   3. Metabolic abnormalities (Topic 44).
   4. Effects of drugs (Topic 49), including addiction (Topic 2).
   5. Toxemias of pregnancy (Topic 50–6).
   6. Vascular conditions (Topic 60).
   7. Neoplasms.

33–2. **Treatment**

The vigor with which emergency treatment is applied will depend largely on the state of the patient at the time the physician arrives, since frequently the acute episode will have subsided.

A. Protection from injury by:
1. Gentle restraint.
2. Maintenance in a lying position at a safe level.
3. Insertion of a rolled handkerchief, washcloth or padded mouth gag to prevent tongue biting and tooth damage.

B. Maintenance of an unobstructed airway during the postictal state. The patient should be placed in a prone or semiprone position with the head turned to one side.

C. Institution of cooling measures by sponging, tepid tub baths and cool water enemas.

D. Administration of:
1. Salicylates when the convulsive seizures are associated with hyperpyrexia.
2. Sodium amobarbital (Amytal), 200 to 500 mg., given intravenously at a rate not to exceed 30 mg. per minute until some decrease in intensity of the convulsive seizure occurs. Sodium phenobarbital, 200 to 300 mg., intramuscularly will usually prevent recurrence after the seizure has stopped.
3. Inhalation anesthesia in very severe cases. This must always be followed by hospitalization.
4. Paraldehyde, 1.0 to 3.0 gm., intramuscularly or orally, or chloral hydrate, 0.5 to 1.0 gms., orally or by retention enema. These drugs are particularly valuable if respiratory depression must be avoided.
5. Diphenylhydantoin sodium (Dilantin), 200 mg., intramuscularly. This is given for prophylaxis against further episodes and should be followed by oral use. Dilantin has no effect on the immediate seizure.

E. Treatment of causative condition. Some of the most common causes encountered are:
1. Acute infections [Meningoencephalitis (Topic 32–16; Topic 48–38 and 59; and Topic 63–1)].

2. Delirium tremens (Topic 36–3).
3. Eclampsia (Topic 50–9).
4. Epilepsy (Topic 3–7).
5. Heat stroke (Topic 57–4).
6. Hyperventilation (Topic 36–6).
7. Hypoglycemia (Topic 35–2, C and D, and Topic 44–16).
8. Poisoning, acute (Topic 49). For treatment see under the specific cause.
   F. Ultimate Management. Any person with convulsions of undetermined origin should have a thorough investigation including:
   1. History of medications and alcoholic intake.
   2. Family history of convulsions.
   3. Complete neurologic examination.
   4. Lumbar puncture (unless contraindications exist).
   5. Electroencephalograms.
   6. Blood should be drawn AT TIME OF THE CONVULSION for blood glucose and calcium determinations.
   7. Definitive care. This will depend upon type and cause of the convulsion and may require trial of several regimens for control.

34. EAR CONDITIONS

34–1. **Abscesses of middle ear.** See 34–12,B, below (*Otitis Media*).

34–2. **Burns.** See Topic 28–11.

34–3. **Cold injuries.** See Topic 57–1.

34–4. **Contusions**

The marked cosmetic blemishes caused by auricular contusions ("cauliflower ears") can often be prevented by immediate aspiration or surgical drainage of the hematoma, followed by application of pressure.

34–5. **Deafness**

   A. If caused by an upper respiratory infection with eustachian salpingitis, the underlying condition should be treated. Shrinking of the nasal mucous membrane by 0.25 per cent phenylephrine hydrochloride

(Neo-Synephrine) drops or spray may give marked relief. COCAINE SOLUTIONS AND NAPHAZO-LINE HYDROCHLORIDE (PRIVINE) SHOULD NOT BE USED OR PRESCRIBED, because of the relatively high incidence of untoward effects. [See Topic 49–477 (*Privine*) and Topic 59–10 (*Anesthetics, Local*).]

B. If due to impacted cerumen, the ear may be syringed, provided the condition of the drum is known. Any evidence of perforation is an absolute contraindication to irrigation or instillation of any substance into the canal. If removal of the wax is incomplete or unsuccessful, the patient should be given oily base ear drops to use at home and referred to an otolaryngologist.

C. If caused or aggravated by concussion (explosions, etc.) or by sudden or prolonged exposure to intense noise (jackhammers, riveting, etc.), symptomatic treatment only is indicated. The patient should be referred to an otolaryngologist for examination and care.

34–6. Earache

Acute earache requires care by an otolaryngologist after the acute symptoms have been relieved by:

1. Anodynes.
2. Antipyrine ear drops.
   Also see 34–12, below.

34–7. Eustachian salpingitis. See 34–12, below.

34–8. Foreign bodies. See Topic 38–1.

34–9. Lacerations. See Topic 55–20.

34–10. Mastoiditis

This complication of otitis media became rather rare for several years following the advent of the sulfonamides and antibiotics. Recently, however, an increase in cases has become apparent, probably as a result of inadequate treatment of otitis media with antibiotics. If mastoiditis is proved or suspected, immediate hospitalization is indicated.

34–11. Meniere's disease. See Topic 47–4,F.

34–12. Otitis. [Also see Topic 26–5 (*Diving Hazards*).]

A. Otitis Externa. Inflammation of the external auditory canal requires no emergency treatment and should be distinguished from middle ear involvement. The patient should be advised to consult an otolaryngologist if the irritation of the canal persists.

B. Otitis Media. Formerly uncommon in adults, acute inflammation of the middle ear is now a fairly common occurrence in sport divers. It is often encountered as an emergency in children.

Treatment

1. Penicillin in large doses intramuscularly or orally according to age (Topic 5). Tetracyclines by mouth may be given in addition.

2. Hot compresses. NO MEDICATION SHOULD BE GIVEN INTO THE CANAL unless there has been rupture of the drum with drainage of frank pus; in this case hydrogen peroxide ear drops may be of benefit.

3. Acetylsalicylic acid (aspirin), 0.06 to 0.3 gm., depending on age (Topic 5), every 4 hours. Codeine sulfate orally or subcutaneously may be necessary for control of severe pain.

4. Paracentesis of the drum under emergency conditions is rarely necessary. Whenever possible, the patient should be hospitalized if the bulging of the drum is acute and indicates the possibility of the need for this procedure. If paracentesis is done, the incision should be limited to the postero-inferior segment of the drum and cultures and sensitivity tests obtained from the drainage.

5. COMPLETE control of the infection is essential in all cases of otitis media. Inadequate therapy—especially with antibiotics—may result in apparent alleviation of acute symptoms but later development of a suppurative mastoiditis.

34–13. Otorrhea

Drainage of cerebrospinal fluid from the ears is prima facie evidence of basal skull fracture (Topic 43–16).

34–14. Tinnitus may be severe enough to require the emergency administration of anodynes. All cases of severe or persistent tinnitus require thorough examination and care by an otolaryngologist.

35. ENDOCRINE EMERGENCIES

35–1. **Adrenal**
  A. Acute Adrenal Cortical Insufficiency. This severe life-threatening situation manifested by shock, stupor, nausea, vomiting and, frequently, high fever occurs in persons with chronic adrenal insufficiency who omit their maintenance dose or whose requirements increase because of stress of some type. Primary acute cases may be associated with rampant infections and adrenal hemorrhage.

Treatment
  1. Inject 50 to 100 mg. of hydrocortisone hemisuccinate directly intravenously in severe cases.
  2. Give 100 to 300 mg. of hydrocortisone in 1000 ml. of 5% dextrose in normal saline at a rate of 250 to 500 ml. per hour.
  3. Treat shock with pressor amines (Topic 15–7).
  4. Prescribe cortisone or hydrocortisone, 50 mg., orally every 6 hours.
  5. Treat contributing causes.

  B. Pheochromocytoma. The urgent hypertensive complications that occur with this tumor are usually related to investigation of, or surgical procedures for, the tumor.
  1. A histamine test may elicit a profound hypertensive episode and may be treated by 5 mg. of phentolamine (Regitine) intravenously, repeated in equal or smaller doses at 10 to 20 minute intervals as needed.
  2. During surgical excision of the tumor, epinephrine or norepinephrine may be released. The resultant hypertension is treated expectantly with intravenous phentolamine (Regitine).
  3. Following surgical removal of the tumor, severe hypotension may develop.

TREATMENT

    a. Levarterenol bitartrate (Levophed), 4 mg. of 2% solution in 1000 ml. of 5% dextrose in water, intravenously.

    b. Whole blood transfusions.

    c. Phenylephrine hydrochloride (Neo-Synephrine) or mephentermine (Wyamine)* subcutaneously in milder cases.

35–2. Pancreas

  A. Diabetic Coma. See Topic 3–3, A, B and C.

  B. Insulin Shock. See Topic 3–3, A, B and D.

  C. Hypoglycemia Secondary to Islet Cell Tumor manifested by coma with or without convulsions, prior increase in appetite, and increase in body weight.

    1. Acute treatment—see insulin shock (Topic 3–3,D).

    2. High protein, low carbohydrate diet in frequent feedings.

    3. Referral for definitive work-up and treatment.

  D. Hypoglycemia Secondary to Insulin Rebound in post-gastrectomy patients.

35–3. Parathyroid

  A. Hypoparathyroidism. The neuromuscular excitability shown by carpopedal spasm, facial muscle twitching following tapping, convulsions and laryngeal stridor are due to low serum calcium concentrations. The occurrence of this condition is usually a complication of thyroidectomy. Signs and symptoms may become evident hours or months after the surgery.

  Treatment

    1. Collection of a blood specimen for serum calcium prior to administration of 1.0 gm. of calcium gluconate intravenously (give cautiously if the patient is digitalized).

    2. Sedation with barbiturates.

    3. Referral to a hospital for stabilization and institution of a long-range program (dihydrotachysterol, calciferol and low phosphorus, high calcium diet).

  B. Acute Parathyroid Intoxication. This uncommon emergency in hyperparathyroid patients is characterized by marked hypercalcemia, profound weakness, severe nausea and vomiting, and lethargy progressing to coma.

1. DEFINITIVE TREATMENT. Emergency exploration for removal of the parathyroid tumor.
2. INTERIM MEASURES are:
    a. Hydrocortisone, 100 mg., intravenously.
    b. 1000 ml. normal saline intravenously.
    c. Potassium salts intravenously to neutralize the effects of hypercalcemia on the heart.
    d. Low calcium-phosphorus intake.
    e. Acidification of urine with measures to insure a large output.
    f. Use of chelating agents may be considered.

35–4. Pituitary

Emergencies related to the pituitary gland are usually related to:

A. Hypofunction of the various target organs (particularly the adrenal and thyroid) following surgical or radiation ablation of the pituitary.

B. Destruction or damage of the posterior pituitary with resultant diabetes insipidus characterized by high urine volume of low specific gravity, polydypsia and dehydration.

Treatment

1. Aqueous Pitressin, 0.5 ml. (10 I.U.), subcutaneously or 0.4 ml. of Pitressin tannate in oil intramuscularly.
2. Correction of dehydration (Topic 7).
3. In new cases, hospitalization for evaluation and determination of Pitressin requirements.

35–5. Thyroid

A. Hypothyroid Emergencies

1. MYXEDEMA COMA. These patients have the classical picture of myxedema plus hypothermia and stupor or unconsciousness.

    TREATMENT
    a. Artificial ventilation as needed for respiratory depression.
    b. Triiodothyronine, 25 mcg., every 6 hours parenterally.
    c. Hydrocortisone, 50 mg., intramuscularly every 6 hours.

    d. Hypothermia is partially protective to tissues; elevation to normal body temperature must be accomplished slowly and with caution.

  2. MYXEDEMA COMPOUNDED BY NARCOTICS. Patients with myxedema are extremely sensitive to narcotics; ordinary doses may cause coma and shock.

  TREATMENT

    a. Treat as outlined under 35–5,A, above, plus
    b. Nalorphine hydrochloride (Nalline), 5 to 10 mg., intravenously, repeated as necessary.

B. Hyperthyroid Emergencies (Thyroid Storm). Hyperpyrexia, coma and marked tachycardia characterize this very serious condition, usually precipitated by stress or by overzealous palpation and manipulation of the gland of a hyperthyroid patient. Thorough preoperative preparation of hyperthyroid patients with antithyroid medications will usually prevent occurrence of thyroid storm.

Treatment

1. Propylthiouracil, 250 mg., orally every 6 hours.
2. Sodium iodide, 1.0 gm., intravenously.
3. Thiamine, 30 to 50 mg. in 1000 ml. of 10% dextrose in normal saline, intravenously.
4. Hydrocortisone, 100 mg., intravenously.
5. Reserpine, 2.0 mg., intramuscularly.
6. Reduction of hyperpyrexia.
7. Placement in an oxygen tent.
8. Minimal handling.
9. Hospitalization for close observation and definitive therapy.

36. EXCITEMENT STATES

Also see Topic 48–21 (*Excitement States in Children*); and Topic 51 (*Psychiatric Emergencies*).

The most common causes for acute excitement states in adults are:

36–1. **Alcoholism**

An acute excitement state may precede the onset of coma (Topic 3); therefore, care should be used in administering sedation for control. Chlorpromazine hydrochloride (Thorazine), 100 mg., intramuscularly, or 100 to 150 mg. by mouth, is rapid, effective and safe, provided barbiturates or opiates have not been given previously. Paraldehyde intramuscularly is also of value. Physical restraint should be used only while sedation is taking effect. Syrup of ipecac, 8 to 12 ml., by mouth if the patient will swallow, or apomorphine hydrochloride, 5 mg., subcutaneously if he will not, will usually induce vomiting and, in addition, have a delayed sedative effect. Gastric lavage should not be attempted unless the cooperation of the patient can be obtained except when emetics do not result in satisfactory emptying of the stomach. Other causes for acute excitement must be ruled out in all cases of alcoholism.

36–2. **Chest injuries**

Air hunger following penetrating chest wounds (Topic 31–9 to 12) and severe crushing injuries of the thorax (Topic 31–1 and 3) may cause acute excitement states. Unless cardiac tamponade (Topic 29–4) is present, gentle manual restraint, with cleansing of the airway, administration of oxygen by face mask and rebreathing bag, and treatment of shock (Topic 15–7) are generally adequate until transfer for hospitalization can be arranged.

36–3. **Delirium tremens**

This acute type of insanity may be precipitated in heavy drinkers by:

1. A prolonged alcoholic spree.
2. An acute infectious disease.
3. Trauma, especially fractures and severe crushing injuries.
4. Sudden withdrawal of alcoholic drinks.

There is usually a prodromal period of 1 to 2 days characterized by depression, uneasiness and insomnia and followed by development of a coarse tremor and hallucinations, usually of sight.

Treatment

1. Paraldehyde, 10 to 15 ml. by mouth, or 5 to 10 ml. intramuscularly, is the drug of choice for sedation. It may be given with safety 3 or 4 times

a day. Chloral hydrate by mouth or as a retention enema may be necessary.

2. Chlorpromazine hydrochloride (Thorazine), 50 to 100 mg., or prochlorperazine (Compazine), 10 to 15 mg., intramuscularly, is safe and very effective.
3. Hydration with normal salt solution.
4. Restraint may be necessary but should be avoided if possible.
5. Opiates, synthetic narcotics and alcohol should never be used.
6. Hospitalization in an institution equipped for the care of such cases is often necessary.

36–4. Head injuries. (Also see Topic 43–11 and Topic 48–8 and 28.)

Injury to the head can cause symptoms ranging from slight restlessness to homicidal mania. Physical restraint should be kept to a minimum, but to prevent further injury to the patient, or injuries to attendants, it may be necessary until adequate sedation has been accomplished. Rapid-acting barbiturates, chloral hydrate, chlorpromazine hydrochloride (Thorazine), paraldehyde or prochlorperazine (Compazine) may be given with caution to quiet the patient, but OPIATES OR SYNTHETIC NARCOTICS SHOULD NEVER BE USED unless other severe injuries make their use imperative.

36–5. Heart failure. See Topic 29 (*Cardiac Emergencies*).

36–6. Hyperventilation

Rebreathing into a paper bag held over the face, or inhalations of Carbogen by face mask and rebreathing bag, usually will result in complete recovery in a short time. In severe cases with profound alkalosis (Topic 44–5), the following measures should be kept in mind:

1. Copious fluids by mouth if patient will cooperate; if not, normal salt solution intravenously.
2. Ammonium chloride, 1 gm., orally.
3. Weak hydrochloric acid, 0.6 ml. in a glass of water, by mouth.
4. Calcium gluconate, 10 ml. of 10 per cent solution, intravenously.

In most cases the signs and symptoms subside rapidly and the patient can be given a sedative and sent home with a member of the family. If the history suggests mental stress as a causative factor, psychiatric evaluation should be recommended.

36–7. Infections

Sedatives should be given before any attempt is made to treat the underlying acute condition. Pentobarbital sodium (Nembutal) suppositories, 0.03 to 0.06 gm., are very effective in infants and children under 4 years of age. Older children tolerate other sedatives very well, provided the dosage is adjusted to age (Topic 5).

36–8. Manic-depressive psychosis. [Also see Topic 51–1,B,1 (*Psychiatric Emergencies*).]

During the excitement stage, physical restraint until control by adequate doses of rapid-acting barbiturates, chloral hydrate, chlorpromazine hydrochloride (Thorazine), paraldehyde or prochlorperazine (Compazine) may be required. An attendant must be with the patient AT ALL TIMES until transfer for psychiatric evaluation and care has been completed. No patient who shows evidence of an actual (or impending) excitement state should ever be left alone.

36–9. Phenothiazine extrapyramidal reactions. (Also see Topic 59–53.)

Idiosyncrasy to these drugs is relatively common, especially in children and elderly persons. Rapid subsiding of the acute excitement state occurs as soon as the offending medication is discontinued.

36–10. Thyrotoxicosis ("Thyroid Storm"). See Topic 35–5,B (*Hyperthyroid Emergencies*).

37. EYE CONDITIONS

An estimate of the vision of each eye should be recorded in the patient's record before examination is performed for any eye condition.

Vision should be tested, if possible, by the Snellen or Jaeger test charts; if these charts are not available, finger perception or reading tests are satisfactory.

NONTRAUMATIC CONDITIONS

37–1.   Angioedema. [See also Topic 24 (*Allergic Reactions*).]
Treatment
  1. Apply cold or heat, whichever is more comfortable for the patient.
  2. Inject epinephrine hydrochloride (Adrenalin) (1:-1000 solution), 0.5 to 1 ml., subcutaneously; repeat in ½ hour if necessary.
  3. Prescribe tripelennamine hydrochloride (Pyribenzamine) by mouth, 25 mg., every 4 hours.
  4. Refer to an ophthalmologist if the condition persists.

37–2.   Blepharitis
Treatment
  1. Examine for, and remove, ingrowing or turned under eyelashes.
  2. Cleanse the lids and remove scales from eyelashes. Chewing gum can be removed from the lids and lashes with ordinary cooking oil or by chilling with an ice cube.
  3. Prescribe an antibiotic ointment.
  4. Refer to an ophthalmologist if marked irritation is present.

37–3.   Chalazion. No emergency treatment is necessary. Refer to an ophthalmologist.

37–4.   Choroiditis. This condition causes no pain and is not the immediate result of trauma; therefore, it is for practical purposes never encountered as an emergency.

37–5.   Conjunctivitis. See also 37–40, below (*Differential Diagnosis Chart*).
Treatment
  1. Irrigate thoroughly and frequently.
  2. Instill sodium sulfacetamide drops (30%) every 4 to 6 hours during the day; apply an antibiotic ointment at night.
  3. Prescribe iced compresses two to three times a day.
  4. If condition persists for more than 48 hours, instruct the patient to consult an ophthalmologist.

37–6.   Corneal ulcers. (For traumatic, see 37–32, below.)
Treatment
  1. Determine the extent of the ulceration by staining with 1% fluorescein solution.

2. Give emergency treatment as outlined for *Keratitis* (37–20, below).

3. Instruct every patient with a corneal ulcer to report to an ophthalmologist within 48 hours.

37–7. **Dacrocystitis**
Treatment

1. ACUTE. Apply frequent hot compresses, with reference to an ophthalmologist within 24 hours.

2. CHRONIC. No emergency treatment is necessary. Evaluation by an ophthalmologist should be recommended.

37–8. **Ectropion** (Eversion of Lid). No emergency treatment is needed. The patient should be advised to consult an ophthalmologist.

37–9. **Edema of the eyelids**
A. *Inflammatory* (from styes, dacrocystitis, sinusitis, etc.)
Treatment

1. Apply hot compresses.

2. Give sedation and control pain as necessary.

3. Refer for determination and treatment of the underlying cause.

B. *Systemic* (renal or cardiac). No emergency treatment is needed. The importance of complete investigation of the cause should be stressed to the patient.

C. *Allergic.* Usually due to some type of local application or medication (mascara, eye shadow, lash curlers and dyes, eye drops, ophthalmic ointments, etc.). Recovery usually is rapid after stopping use of the offending substance.

37–10. **Emphysema of the lids.** Crepitus from air in the soft tissues generally means a fracture of the sinus wall.
Treatment

1. Apply a firm pressure bandage.

2. Warn the patient against blowing his nose.

3. Hospitalize immediately for head injury care.

37–11. **Entropion** (Inversion of Lid).
Treatment

1. Hold the lid in proper position if possible by Scotch tape.

2. Refer to an ophthalmologist for definitive treatment.

37–12. **Eversion of eyelids.** See *Ectropion* (37–8, above).

37–13.   Glaucoma. See also 37–40, below (*Differential Diagnosis Chart*).

>   *Treatment*
>   1. Whenever examination indicates the possibility of increased intraocular tension, referral AT ONCE to an ophthalmologist is indicated.
>   2. Rapid failure of sight, violent headache and severe ophthalmic pain—sometimes associated with nausea, vomiting and general depression—should suggest the possibility of a "glaucomatous attack" and call for immediate hospitalization.

37–14.   Herpes

>   **A. *Herpes Simplex.*** Immediate referral to an ophthalmologist. Treatment with 5-iodo-2-deoxyuride (IDU) may result in complete healing without vision loss.
>
>   **B. *Herpes Zoster Ophthalmicus***
>   1. Control severe pain by codeine sulfate, morphine sulfate or dihydromorphinone hydrochloride (Dilaudid).
>   2. Apply a protective bandage.
>   3. Refer to an ophthalmologist for treatment at once.

37–15.   Hordeolum. See *Stye* (37–24, below).

37–16.   Inversion of eyelashes. See *Trichiasis* (37–27, below).

37–17.   Inversion of eyelids. See *Entropion* (37–11, above).

37–18.   Iridocyclitis. See *Iritis* (37–19, below).

37–19.   Iritis (Iridocyclitis, Uveitis). See also 37–40, below (*Differential Diagnosis Chart*).

>   *Treatment*
>   1. Apply hot compresses—not over 38° C. (100.4° F.).
>   2. Apply eye patch.
>   3. Arrange for treatment at once by an ophthalmologist.

37–20.   Keratitis

>   *Treatment*
>   1. Examine thoroughly for, and remove, any foreign bodies.
>   2. If pain is very severe, phenacaine (Holocaine), dibucaine (Nupercaine), or ethylmorphine (Dionin) ophthalmic ointments may be applied—once only. COCAINE IN ANY FORM SHOULD NOT BE USED.
>   3. Apply an eye patch.

    4. Impress on the patient the need for immediate care
        by an ophthalmologist.
37–21. **Panophthalmitis.** Relieve the pain by anodynes or
opiates and hospitalize at once.
37–22. **Pterygium.** No emergency treatment is needed. Refer
to an ophthalmologist.
37–23. **Scleritis**
    Treatment
    1. Apply hot compresses.
    2. Arrange for immediate care by an ophthalmologist.
37–24. **Stye** (Hordeolum)
    Treatment
    1. Apply hot compresses.
    2. Incise and drain if the condition is localized.
    3. Prescribe 1% chlortetracycline (Aureomycin) or
        5% sulfathiazole ointment for home application.
37–25. **Symblepharon.** Refer to an ophthalmologist.
37–26. **Trachoma.** This infectious conjunctivitis is due to a
virus which is spread by personal contact. It may cause severe
scarring, occasionally blindness.
    Treatment
    1. Instruction regarding disposition of infected hand-
        kerchiefs, towels, etc.
    2. Sulfadiazine, 0.5 to 1.0 gm., by mouth three times
        a day.
    3. Penicillin, 600,000 units, intramuscularly.
    4. Sulfathiazole ophthalmic ointment.
    5. Reference to an ophthalmologist.
37–27. **Trichiasis** (Inversion of Lashes). If only a few lashes
are inverted, they may be removed with cilia forceps. If multiple or if severe pain, lacrimation, photophobia or ulceration is
present, the case should be referred to an ophthalmologist.
37–28. **Uveitis.** See *Iritis* (37–19, above).

TRAUMATIC CONDITIONS
    Vision of each eye should be tested by the Jaeger or Snellen
method or by reading tests or finger visualization before examination and recorded in the patient's chart in all cases of suspected eye injury.
37–29. **Injuries to the choroid**
    A. Rupture of the choroid can be caused by a severe con-
        tusion of the eyeball. The diagnosis as a rule cannot

be made on emergency examination, but suspicion of its presence requires immediate transference to an ophthalmologist.

B. Penetrating wounds may cause suppurative iridochoroiditis with exquisite pain requiring morphine sulfate or dihydromorphinone hydrochloride (Dilaudid) for relief. Hospitalization should be arranged as soon as possible.

37–30. **Injuries to the ciliary body.** Injuries to this area are in the so-called "danger zone" of the eye and not infrequently result in sympathetic ophthalmia (37–38, below). Immediate reference to an ophthalmologist is indicated if an injury to the ciliary body is suspected.

37–31. **Injuries to the conjunctiva**

A. *Foreign Bodies.* Usually foreign bodies are found lying on the inner surface of the upper lid and can be removed with or without 1% tetracaine hydrochloride (Pontocaine) anesthesia by brushing with a cotton applicator dampened with saline. If acute conjunctivitis or corneal irritation is present, an antibiotic ointment should be prescribed and an eye patch applied. If an abrasion is present, recheck examination by an ophthalmologist within 2 days should be arranged.

B. *Lacerations.* No attempt should be made to suture cuts in the surface of the conjunctiva. A sterile eye patch should be applied and the patient referred at once to an ophthalmologist.

C. *Burns.* (Also see Topic 28–14.) Thorough irrigation with tap water is the only treatment needed in mild cases. Moderately severe cases require cold or iced compresses and application of an antibiotic ointment. An eye patch should be applied and arrangements made for the patient to consult an ophthalmologist within 48 hours. Severe cases, especially electrical, acid or alkali burns, require immediate referral to an ophthalmologist.

D. *Injuries Caused by Intense Light* (Welder's Flash, Photophthalmia). Patients' stories are often inaccurate; therefore, a thorough search should be made for foreign bodies in the conjunctival sac, under the lids and on the cornea before a diagnosis of photophthalmia is made. If none is found and the history is indicative of a "flash," the following routine should be used:

1. Instill 2 drops of 1% tetracaine hydrochloride (Pontocaine) solution.
2. Cover with cold (preferably iced) compresses for 5 minutes.
3. Instill 2 drops of the following solution:

Phenylephrine (Neo-Synephrine) hydrochloride (1% sol.)	12.5 ml.
Tetracaine hydrochloride (Pontocaine)	0.25 ml.
Isotonic solution (buffered) q.s. ad	100.00 ml.

4. Cover with cold compresses for 5 minutes.
5. Instill 2 drops of castor oil.
6. Instruct the patient to apply cold or iced compresses and castor oil drops at home and to arrange for further medical care in 24 hours if acute discomfort persists.

37–32. **Injuries to the cornea**
  A. Foreign Bodies
   1. A history of any object striking the eye makes a thorough search for foreign bodies mandatory. Fluorescein (1 or 2%) is harmless and may be used to demonstrate breaks in the external layers of the cornea. The eye must be irrigated thoroughly after examination. A fresh solution of fluorescein should always be used. Exact localization of embedded or intraocular radiopaque foreign bodies can often be obtained by special radiologic techniques.
   2. Foreign bodies on, or embedded superficially in, the cornea may be removed under 1% tetracaine hydrochloride (Pontocaine) anesthesia, using a damp cotton applicator or a blunt eye spud. Removal of any residual rust ring requires reference to an ophthalmologist and should not be attempted as emergency treatment.
   3. NO ATTEMPT SHOULD BE MADE TO REMOVE DEEPLY EMBEDDED FOREIGN BODIES as an emergency measure. An eye patch should be applied unless the pressure of the pad might cause further penetration and the patient referred at once to an ophthalmologist.

4. AN ELECTROMAGNET SHOULD NEVER BE USED except under the direction of an ophthalmologist.

5. Defects (ulcers) of the cornea following removal of foreign bodies require application of a small amount of 5% sulfathiazole or 1% chlortetracycline (Aureomycin) ointment, protection of the eye with a patch, and reference to an ophthalmologist within 48 hours.

B. Contusions. Usually caused by some blunt object, contusions as a rule clear spontaneously (and slowly) without treatment. Internal bleeding and dislocation of the lens require immediate care by an ophthalmologist.

C. Burns. If corneal burns are small and superficial, treatment is the same as for conjunctival burns (37–31,C, above; and Topic 28–14); if extensive or deep, immediate care by an ophthalmologist is essential.

D. Wounds

1. SUPERFICIAL. These generally heal without complications, provided they are kept clean.

TREATMENT

   a. Irrigation followed by an antibiotic ointment.

   b. Application of an eye patch.

2. PENETRATING. Immediate care by an ophthalmologist is mandatory. X-rays should be taken to rule out, or localize, buried radiopaque foreign bodies.

37–33. **Injuries to the eyelids**

A. Ecchymosis ("Black Eye"). Direct trauma in the region of the eyes severe enough to cause ecchymosis may also cause severe underlying injuries. The following conditions which require immediate care by an ophthalmologist should be ruled out:

1. Lacerations of the cornea (37–32,D, above).

2. Fracture of the orbital wall (see 37–10, above; and 37–35, below).

3. Detachment of the retina, partial or complete (see 37–36, below).

Treatment. Cold compresses for 24 hours, followed by hot compresses and gentle massage. Injection of hyaluronidase in 1% procaine hydrochloride often is very effective. If a fracture is suspected from clinical and/or x-ray examinations, the patient should be hospitalized for observation and treatment.

B. Insect Bites. [Also see Topic 24 (*Allergic Reactions*); Topic 27 (*Bites*); and Topic 62 (*Venoms*).]

Cold compresses are indicated for control of swelling, which may be very marked. Antihistaminics may be of value.

C. Lacerations. Because loss of tissues of the eyelids may result in ectropion (37–8, above) or entropion (37–11, above) lacerations in this area should be thoroughly irrigated, but NOT DEBRIDED, before suturing. Antibiotics and tetanus antitoxin or toxoid (Topic 19) should be given if gross contamination is present.

Especially in vertical lacerations, suturing should be done with great care in order to prevent contractures. If the laceration extends through the eyelid, careful examination for damage to the eye should be done before suturing. If a through-and-through laceration is jagged or extensive, or if there is avulsion or loss of tissue, a sterile bandage should be applied and the patient hospitalized at once for operative repair and possible skin grafting to prevent marked cosmetic disfigurement.

37–34. Injuries to the iris

A. Nonpenetrating. Concussion with subsequent traumatic mydriasis is the most frequent cause. After instillation of 1 or 2 drops of 1% pilocarpine hydrochloride and application of an eye patch, the patient should be referred to an ophthalmologist.

B. Penetrating. This condition calls for application of an eye patch and immediate reference to an ophthalmologist for care.

37–35. Injuries to the orbit. If injury to the orbit is suspected from clinical and/or x-ray examination, immediate hospitalization for head injury care (Topic 43) is indicated. Fractures of the thin floor of the orbit require immediate surgical repair to avoid impaired binocular vision.

37–36. Injuries to the retina. Suspected or proved incomplete or complete detachment of the retina requires immediate reference to an ophthalmologist.

37–37. Injuries to the sclera. If injury to the sclera is suspected, the patient should be referred to an ophthalmologist WITHOUT DELAY for examination and treatment. X-rays should be taken to rule out embedded radiopaque foreign bodies if the history is suggestive (see 37–32, above).

37–38. Sympathetic ophthalmia. This very serious condition practically never occurs unless there has been a penetrating lesion of the opposite eye at some time in the past. RECOGNITION IN THE STAGE OF SYMPATHETIC IRRITATION MAY RESULT IN PREVENTING TOTAL BLINDNESS. The usual signs and symptoms of this stage are as follows:

1. Marked photophobia and lacrimation, with dimness of close vision.
2. Bizarre bright and colored sensations.
3. Neuralgic pain in and around the eye.

Any person with a history of a perforating injury to an eye AT ANY TIME IN THE PAST who complains of any of the signs and symptoms listed above in the uninjured eye should be referred immediately to an ophthalmologist.

37–39. Removal of contact lenses

A. Original Type. Marked irritation of the conjunctiva, intense lacrimation and cloudiness of vision may occur if contact lenses are not removed at frequent intervals. This problem was much more acute with the original contact lenses which were relatively large and depended on suction for fixation in functional position. A suction cup was the usual method of removal but breaking of the suction seal was sometimes required. Two methods were effective:

1. Prying up an edge of the lens with a small scalpel or eye spud. Local anesthesia was generally required.
2. Breaking the suction seal by a sudden jet of air injected under the edge of the lens, using a small syringe and a blunt needle.

B. Modern Type

1. Apply 1% tetracaine hydrochloride (Pontocaine).
2. Stain with fluorescein to make certain that the lens is still in place and to detect any breaks in the cornea.
3. Lift lens with a spatula and remove with suction cup.
4. Treat corneal ulcers as outlined in 37–6 and 37–32,D, above.

37–40. Differential diagnosis of conjunctivitis, glaucoma and iritis

	CONJUNCTIVITIS	GLAUCOMA	IRITIS
Aqueous humor	normal	cloudy	cloudy
Cornea	normal	steamy	clear
Eyeball	normal	hard	soft
Headache	never	frequent	frequent
Iris	normal	muddy	muddy
Nausea	never	frequent	occasional
Pain	slight	very severe	severe
Pupil	normal	dilated	small
Redness	marked	variable	circumcorneal
Vision	normal	marked to complete loss	some loss

38. FOREIGN BODIES

See also Topic 48–25 (*Foreign Bodies in Children*).
38–1. In the ears
Examine with an otoscope. Children frightened from previous attempts at removal often require sedation by a pentobarbital sodium (Nembutal) suppository before examination. If superficial, and if swelling of the wall of the external auditory meatus has not resulted from previous attempts at removal (usually at home), most foreign bodies can be removed with forceps or by carefully inserting a curved probe behind the object and gently working it outward. Gravity may help.

    A. Substances which will not absorb moisture can sometimes be removed by syringing. DO NOT ATTEMPT IRRIGATION for beans, peas, candy, etc.; absorption of moisture and subsequent swelling can cause serious and permanent damage. DO NOT IRRIGATE if there is suspicion or evidence of drum perforation.

B. *Foxtails* can usually be removed with forceps without difficulty. A few drops of any glycerin or petrolatum base ear drops instilled in the ear will result in immediate relief of discomfort and spontaneous evacuation if the patient will sleep with the affected ear against the pillow.

C. *Hot Slag* particles usually are loose in the canal and can be removed with a cotton applicator. If firmly adherent to the drum or if there is evidence of severe drum damage, treatment by an otolaryngologist should be arranged.

D. *Burns* (Topic 28–11), usually from hot slag, involving any part of the external auditory canal can be treated with any oily ear drops (provided the drum is not perforated), but severe burns of the drum require reference to an otolaryngologist.

E. *Insects* alive and buzzing in the external auditory canal will often fly or crawl out toward a flashlight held close to the external auditory meatus. If this maneuver is unsuccessful, removal by syringing may be necessary.

F. Referral to an otolaryngologist generally is required in the following instances:
  1. When there is damage to, or perforation of, the drum.
  2. When the foreign body cannot be removed on one or two gentle attempts.
  3. When the cooperation of the patient cannot be obtained.

38–2. **In the eyes.** See Topic 37–31,A, 32,A, and 38.

38–3. **In the nose.**

Foreign bodies in the nose are frequently encountered in small children; often, sufficient cooperation to permit removal of the object with forceps or a small wire probe cannot be obtained. Sedation by means of a pentobarbital sodium (Nembutal) suppository may be tried. However, if the child struggles or resists examination, hospitalization for use of a general anesthetic should be considered. If the parents take a reasonable attitude, postponement until care by an otolaryngologist can be arranged will result in no danger to the patient.

In some instances, foreign bodies will be expelled from the nares in infants and small children by sneezing. Many small children will sneeze if a puff of cigarette smoke is blown suddenly against the child's nose while his mouth is kept covered.

38–4. In the trachea, bronchi or esophagus. Also see Topic 48–25; and *Localization Chart* (Topic 48–40,B).

A. Cyanosis, air hunger and dyspnea, with a history of swallowing a foreign body, may require immediate action on the part of the physician as a lifesaving measure. If the patient is markedly cyanotic or moribund, mouth-to-mouth respiration (Topic 17–1) should be started (unless prevented by obstruction) and the following procedures done without hesitation:

1. Have the parents, relatives or friends leave the room unless their assistance will be needed.

2. Attempt dislodgement of the foreign body by concussion, utilizing the pull of gravity. A child can be held by his feet and his head tapped forcibly against the examining table or floor.

3. Perform a tracheotomy if necessary (for technique see Topic 17–11).

4. Give oxygen inhalations under positive pressure by face mask and rebreathing bag.

B. If signs and symptoms of irritation or obstruction are less severe, x-rays (anteroposterior and lateral) of the chest should be taken after examination of the posterior pharynx. If the radiopaque foreign body is in the trachea, its greater surface will appear in the lateral film; if in the esophagus the anteroposterior film will show the greater width. Small pointed or irregularly-shaped foreign bodies can sometimes be demonstrated by x-rays taken after the patient has swallowed a small cotton pledget saturated with barium.

C. Foreign bodies lodged in the trachea or bronchi which cannot be located with a laryngoscope and removed with long forceps require that the patient be transferred to a hospital as soon as his condition will permit; those in the upper gastrointestinal tract

generally require no treatment except reassurance
(especially of parents), a normal diet and observation, unless there is a chance of perforation.

D. If careful screening of all stool specimens for 3 days
indicates that the foreign body has not passed
through the gastrointestinal tract, further x-ray
studies should be made.

38–5. In the stomach and gastrointestinal tract. (Also see
Topic 48–25,G and H.)

A. If the object is small enough to pass through the
esophagus into the stomach and does not have any
extremely sharp points (C, below), it will generally
pass through the small and large bowel without
difficulty.

B. Nonradiopaque foreign bodies in the stomach can sometimes be visualized by x-rays taken immediately
after a few swallows of a cold carbonated beverage.
Any space-consuming object will cause a defect in
the gas shadow caused by the released carbon
dioxide.

C. Sharp-pointed objects should be watched carefully,
clinically and by x-ray. If any signs suggestive of
perforation or obstruction develop, immediate hospitalization for possible operative intervention must
be arranged.

38–6. In the musculoskeletal structures.
Whether the foreign bodies are wood (splinters, etc.), steel
or other metals (industrial accidents, household and auto accidents, bullets, needles, etc.), or dirt, gravel, rock (explosions,
falls, auto accidents, etc.), or semisolid (graphite, grease), the
general principles of treatment are the same.

A. Careful cleansing and irrigation.

B. Exploration (puncture wounds, bullet wounds, etc.) to
determine the extent of penetration. This should
be done with great care under direct vision if possible and with extension of the entrance tract under local anesthetic if necessary.

C. X-rays (AP and lateral). Skin markers should be placed
for reference before the films are taken if the
presence of a small, easily overlooked radiopaque
foreign body is suspected.

D. If the foreign body is superficial and easily accessible it should be removed by sharp dissection and debridement, followed by thorough irrigation. If there is any gaping or separation, primary closure should be done if within 6 hours of injury; after a longer period the wound should be debrided but should not, as a general rule, be sutured. [See Topic 55–20 (*Lacerations*).]

E. Deeply Embedded Foreign Bodies should be treated conservatively [tetanus antitoxin or toxoid (Topic 19), local treatment of point of entry (B, above), and observation]. Antibiotic therapy may be indicated, particularly if several hours have elapsed between the injury and the first treatment.

F. Musculoskeletal Foreign Bodies require hospitalization:
1. When there is evidence of severe or persistent bleeding which cannot be controlled by pressure.
2. If the location of the foreign body or its point of entry or course, together with clinical examination, indicates perforation of the pleura, pericardium, peritoneum or viscera.
3. If the foreign body lies within the skull.
4. If there is evidence of severe or extensive bone damage.
5. When evidence of nerve severance, injury or pressure is present.
6. If x-ray or clinical examination indicates that the foreign body lies within a joint.

38–7. **In the urethra.** See Topic 40–9,D; and Topic 48–25 (*Foreign Bodies in Children*).

38–8. **In the vagina**
1. Retained pessaries, tampons, etc., may require use of a speculum for localization and removal.
2. A variety of metallic or other objects inserted into the vagina or cervix in attempts to induce an abortion or by mentally deranged persons may require removal. A thorough examination to rule out perforation should be made.

39. GASTROINTESTINAL EMERGENCIES

39–1. **Neonatal conditions,** often associated with severe feeding problems, respiratory distress, abnormal elimination and signs of obstruction may require emergency care.

    A. Diaphragmatic Hernia (Topic 48–34).

    B. Imperforate Anus (Topic 48–34).

    C. Intestinal Atresia.

    D. Megacolon (Topic 48–34).

    E. Tracheo-esophageal Fistula.

All require immediate hospitalization for surgical evaluation and repair.

39–2. **Obstruction**

    A. Mechanical

        1. INTRALUMINAL

            a. Fecal impaction. If the patient is in acute discomfort from partial or complete obstruction, and rectal examination demonstrates a mass of hard-packed feces, an attempt may be made to remove the mass with the gloved finger. In elderly women, posterior and downward digital pressure through the vagina may cause sufficient dilation of the sphincter ani to allow the impacted mass to pass. These procedures are usually very painful and often unsuccessful. Premedication with rapid-acting barbiturates or meperidine hydrochloride (Demerol) is essential. Morphine sulfate and/or other opiates contract the sphincter ani and should not be used. Hospitalization for general anesthesia may be necessary if an attempt at digital removal is unsuccessful or is too painful to be tolerated. In less severe cases in which obstruction is not complete, the patient can be sent home with instructions regarding warm oil enemas and diet.

            b. Foreign bodies. See Topic 38–5.

            c. Gallstones (39–8, below).

2. EXTRALUMINAL
   a. Adhesions, usually postoperative.
   b. Hernia, incarcerated (39–5,B,3, below).
   c. Malignancies (39–4,C, below).
   d. Pyloric stenosis (Topic 48–34).
   e. Volvulus (Topic 48–57).

B. Nonmechanical
1. Inflammation, caused by enzymes, organisms and poisons.
2. Ischemia (mesenteric vascular occlusion).
3. Reflex following surgery or trauma.

C. Signs and Symptoms
1. Repetitious vomiting—may be fecal.
2. Abdominal distention and diffuse tenderness.
3. High-pitched bowel sounds.
4. Decreased elimination.
5. Progressive dehydration.

D. Treatment
1. No food by mouth.
2. Antiemetics parenterally.
3. Hydration parenterally and rectally (Topic 7).
4. Shock therapy (Topic 15–7).
5. Referral for hospital care.

39–3. **Perforation**

A. Esophageal. From corrosives, foreign bodies or instrumentation. May cause shock (Topic 15) and mediastinitis.

B. Intraperitoneal (gallbladder, intestines, spleen, stomach).
1. CAUSES
   a. Foreign bodies (Topic 38–5).
   b. Medications such as phenylbutazone (Butazolidin), reserpine and steroids.
   c. Trauma.
   d. Ulcerative processes.
2. SIGNS AND SYMPTOMS
   a. Abdominal pain and rigidity.
   b. Shock (Topic 15).
   c. Tenderness, local or generalized.
   d. Free air in the abdomen by x-rays.
3. TREATMENT
   a. Nothing by mouth.

    b. Shock therapy (Topic 15–7).

    c. Analgesics after the diagnosis has been established.

    d. Hospitalization for definitive care, usually surgical.

39–4. Hemorrhage

A. Severe bleeding from any point along the enteric tract can present a serious life-threatening situation. Gastrointestinal bleeding may be frankly evident from blood in the emesis or rectal discharge or may be occult with the patient initially presenting in a state of shock.

B. Treatment

1. Shock therapy (Topic 15–7).
2. Hospitalization for thorough clinical and laboratory investigation, treatment and observation, even when bleeding and anemia appear to be mild.
3. Rapid history from patient and relatives to determine causes contributing to hemorrhage that should also receive immediate treatment (i.e., use of anticoagulants or steroids, familial conditions such as hemophilia, improper diet, etc.).
4. Ice water lavage of stomach immediately for severe upper gastrointestinal hemorrhage.

C. Rectal Bleeding. All cases of rectal bleeding of undetermined cause, especially in persons over 50, should be considered as possible malignancies until proved otherwise.

1. HEMORRHOIDS. Loss of blood may be enough to cause shock (Topic 15).
2. CRYPTITIS. Inflammation of the crypts of Morgagni may cause anal spasm and pain, pruritus and frequent bowel movements in addition to bleeding.

    TREATMENT

    a. Sitz baths.

    b. Dilation of the sphincter.

    c. Antibiotic therapy.

D. Specific Poisons may cause severe gastrointestinal and rectal bleeding. See under Topic 49.

E. Ulceration, Infection and Inflammation. This group of pathologic conditions may be manifested clinically by anorexia, fever, nausea, vomiting, abdominal pain and tenderness and compounded by alteration of normal evacuation and fluid and electrolyte imbalance as well as hemorrhage.

SPECIFIC CONDITIONS
39–5. Anatomic defects

A. Achalasia. Persons with an atonic esophagus may develop sudden distress with dysphagia or respiratory difficulty from aspiration of gastric overflow or regurgitated food.

Treatment

1. Evacuation of the esophagus with an Ewald tube.
2. Referral to a gastroenterologist for evaluation and treatment.
3. Bronchoscopy if necessary for removal of aspirated food.

B. Hernia

1. AT THE FIRST VISIT a thorough and complete history MUST be taken on every case of claimed inguinal, femoral or ventral hernia when the condition is alleged to have arisen out of, or to have been caused by, the patient's work. This history should include the following points:

   a. Details regarding the exact effort which the patient was performing when he first felt subjective symptoms. This history should include the position of the patient while lifting or straining, weight of the object lifted, type of pain, presence or absence of nausea and/or vomiting, and general malaise.

   b. A statement regarding the type of work usually performed, and regarding any variation from the normal routine at the time of the alleged injury.

   c. A detailed interval history covering the period between the time of the alleged injury and medical examination.

   d. A specific statement from the patient regarding previous symptoms such as pain, swelling or bulging in the affected area. If the patient has had previous operative repairs on either side, full details of the onset of symptoms of the

original condition, with operative findings and
industrial status, should be obtained.

2. PHYSICAL EXAMINATION

    a. Presence or absence of a defect in support or a
bulge on inspection and palpation, especially
while coughing or straining.

    b. Size of the inguinal rings ON BOTH SIDES by
digital examination.

    c. Presence or absence of an impulse in the inguinal
canal, or at the site of the palpable defect, on
coughing or straining.

    d. Comparative tenderness on digital examination if
inguinal.

    e. If scrotal, ease of reduction by taxis.

3. TREATMENT

    INDUSTRIAL CASES (arising out of, or caused
by, employment and covered by state or federal
compensation laws). All strangulated hernias,
and some incarcerated hernias, are acute surgical emergencies and should be hospitalized for
immediate care. All other cases should be examined in detail and a First Report of Injury
(Topic 76) made out BUT NO TREATMENT OF
ANY KIND GIVEN. This includes recommendations for any type of home therapy and/or the
purchase of an athletic supporter or truss. Instead, the patient should be referred to the compensation insurance carrier or employer for disposition. He should be warned to report immediately for medical care if severe discomfort,
marked enlargement or irreducibility should
develop.

NONINDUSTRIAL CASES should be advised regarding operation, application of support, or other treatment;
or referred for surgical consultation.

C. Prolapse of the Rectum

1. IN INFANTS AND CHILDREN this condition is fairly
common. It is probably the result of congenital
defects in the firmness of the connective tissue
between the layers of the rectum.

TREATMENT

    a. Preliminary sedation.

      b. REDUCTION AT ONCE by manual replacement. The sooner this is accomplished, the easier the procedure. Delay results in shutting off the blood supply by sphincter spasm with resultant extreme edema.

      c. Elevation of the foot of the bed.

      d. Application of cold packs to decrease edema.

      e. Tight strapping of the buttocks.

      f. Immediate hospitalization for reduction under general anesthesia if the measures given above are unsuccessful.

    2. IN ADULTS, prolapse generally results from lesions (hemorrhoids, proctitis, polyps) which cause excessive straining at stool. Reduction by the methods outlined above is generally much more difficult than in children and recurrence more common.

      The patient should be hospitalized if:

      a. Replacement cannot be obtained on one or two attempts.

      b. There is discoloration of the prolapsed structures indicative of circulatory embarrassment.

      c. Marked edema is present.

      d. The prolapse recurs spontaneously after reduction.

39–6. Anorectal conditions

This area of the body is particularly prone to develop inflammatory conditions which are very painful and likely to be accompanied by bleeding.

    A. Cryptitis (39–4,C,2, above).

    B. Fissures. A small break in the continuity of the mucous membrane of the rectum or skin around the anus may cause itching, pain and bleeding on defecation. See *Pruritus Ani* (Topic 54–12).

  Treatment

    1. Sitz baths.

    2. Fecal softeners.

    3. Low residue diet.

    4. Sedation as necessary.

    5. Referral to a proctologist if symptoms are severe or persistent.

  C. Hemorrhoids (Piles)

    1. IF NOT THROMBOSED, but prolapsed or protruding, re-

placement with a lubricated gloved finger should be attempted. If this cannot be done because of acute pain or strangulation, inject 100 TRU (turbidity reducing units) of hyaluronidase in 2 ml. of 0.5% procaine into the swollen tissues at three or four different points. After a short wait, painless and complete replacement can usually be accomplished. Ethyl aminobenzoate (Benzocaine) suppositories and sitz baths at home should be prescribed and the patient instructed to arrange for further care if the symptoms persist or recur.

2. IF THROMBOSED, severe pain can be relieved by injection of a small amount of 1% procaine or lidocaine (Xylocaine) into the mucous membrane and evacuation of the clots through a small incision. Suturing is not necessary. The patient should be advised to take sitz baths until the acute inflammation subsides and to obtain further medical care if not completely relieved.

D. Prolapse. See 39–5,C, above.

E. Pruritus Ani. See Topic 54–12.

F. Stricture of the Rectum may occur following rectal surgery; more often, it results from infections such as lymphogranuloma venereum (Topic 61–4). No emergency treatment is indicated unless acute infection is present or complete obstruction has occurred. In the former, antibiotics and hot sitz baths may give relief; in the latter instance, the patient should be hospitalized for relief.

39–7. Appendicitis, acute
Surgical intervention is indicated as soon as the diagnosis has been established.

39–8. Cholecystitis, acute
Frequently a history of prior gallbladder complaints will be obtained. Obstruction of the biliary tracts from choleliths (or from inflammation following passage of a stone) or from infection may precede involvement of the gallbladder. Generally, pain is present in the right upper quadrant of the abdomen; the gallbladder itself may or may not be palpable.

Treatment. Referral for hospitalization and immediate surgical evaluation.

39–9.   **Diarrhea.** [See also Topic 48–17 (*Diarrhea in Children*).]
Diarrhea may present as an emergency situation with moderate or marked dehydration, incipient or frank shock, watery and bloody stools, high fever, tenesmus and "toxic state." Specific bacteria (Shigella and Salmonella), amebae, exogenous toxins, or acute fulminant ulcerative colitis may be the cause. Emergency treatment is, initially, massive general supportive measures; diagnostic procedures and specific therapy follow.

Determination of the specific cause of the diarrhea is indicated even in mild cases.

39–10.   **Diverticulitis**
In adults acute inflammation of diverticuli may cause signs and symptoms difficult to differentiate from an acute surgical abdomen. If perforation should occur, the treatment is emergency surgery. However, subacute inflammatory conditions characterized by pain, mild fever and bleeding are more common. Diverticulitis is one of the common causes of rectal bleeding in children.

> *Treatment*
> 1. In mild cases, control of the infection by antibiotics may give marked relief.
> 2. Start bland, low residue diet and fecal softeners.
> 3. Acute cases require immediate hospitalization.

39–11.   **Esophagitis and gastritis**
> *Treatment*
> 1. Treat as under peptic ulceration [*Hemorrhage* (39–4, A and B, above)].
> 2. Topical Xylocaine, 15 to 30 ml. orally, may give dramatic relief of symptoms.

39–12.   **Fecal impaction.** See 39–2, A, 1, a, above.

39–13.   **Fissure-in-ano.** See 39–6, B, above.

39–14.   **Hemorrhoids.** See 39–6, C, above.

39–15.   **Hernia.** See 39–5, B, above.

39–16.   **Impaction, fecal.** See 39–2, A, 1, a, above.

39–17.   **Intussusception.** See Topic 48–34.

39–18.   **Ischiorectal abscess.** (See also Topic 23–18.)
Complete disability from severe local pain and tenderness may be present, together with generalized abdominal distress and distention.

> *Treatment*
> 1. Administration of antibiotics.
> 2. Application of local heat by sitz baths.

3. Analgesics or sedation.

4. Referral to surgeon or proctologist for hospitalization and drainage under general anesthesia when the abscess has localized.

39-19. Pancreatitis, acute

This condition may come on suddenly although it is frequently preceded by symptoms of gallbladder disease, peptic ulcer or high intake of alcohol. Pain in the midabdomen with penetration to the back or flanks may be severe. Vomiting and paralytic ileus are common. Shock may develop and is an ominous early sign.

Treatment

1. Shock therapy (Topic 15-7).

2. Hospitalization for definitive care. General treatment is similar to that for acute cholecystitis except that surgical intervention need not be considered.

39-20. Piles. See 39-6, C, above (*Hemorrhoids*).

39-21. Polyps (ulcerative) may be mistaken for internal hemorrhoids if located near the anus; if in the rectum, they may cause recurrent rectal prolapse.

Treatment

1. Control of infection and edema by sitz baths, ethyl aminobenzoate (Benzocaine) suppositories and antibiotics.

2. Referral to a surgeon or proctologist for examination and treatment. These lesions may be premalignant.

39-22. Prolapse of rectum. See 39-5, C. above.

39-23. Ulcerative colitis. See under *Diarrhea* (39-9, above).

39-24. Vascular problems

Either arterial or venous pathology may be responsible for several types of gastrointestinal emergencies.

A. Esophageal Varices. See 39-4, above.

B. Mesenteric Artery Occlusion from thrombosis or embolism causes acute severe midabdominal pain with minimal or no abdominal tenderness and hyperactive bowel sounds. Ileus, shock and blood in the peritoneal space and stool are later manifestations.

Treatment

1. Treatment of shock if present (Topic 15-7).

2. Referral for surgical resection of the involved bowel.

C. Rectal Bleeding. See 39-6, above.

40. GENITOURINARY TRACT EMERGENCIES

40–1. Traumatic conditions

If injury to the urogenital tract is suspected, the attending physician should first perform a thorough physical examination of the abdomen, lower back, flanks and scrotum or perineum, followed by gross and microscopic examination of the urine for blood cells. Catheterization may be necessary but should be avoided whenever possible—a "clean-catch" or second glass specimen is usually satisfactory. If there is blood in the urine or if there is any reasonable doubt as to the nature or extent of the injury, the patient should be hospitalized at once for urologic examination and treatment.

40–2. Bladder injuries

Ruptures of the bladder may vary in degree from tears of a few fibers of the muscular wall with microscopic hematuria to large rents with extensive extravasation of urine, hemorrhage, peritonitis and shock. The most common causes are:

1. Fracture of the pelvis with perforation or laceration of the bladder wall by sharp bone ends.
2. Direct trauma over a distended bladder. Gross and microscopic examination of a "clean-catch" or second glass specimen of urine should be done at once if the type of injury suggests possible bladder damage. Cystograms may be indicated to confirm the diagnosis, but only under exceptional circumstances should these be done as an emergency procedure.

Treatment. All cases of proved or suspected bladder damage should be transferred at once for hospitalization. Shock, if present, must be treated (Topic 15–7) before transfer.

40–3. Kidney injuries

A severe blow over the flank or paralumbar muscles may cause a contusion or rupture of a kidney. Suspected cases should be hospitalized for observation, diagnosis and treatment.

Severe shock is common and must be treated (Topic 15–7) before the patient is hospitalized.

40–4. Orchitis

Direct blows to the scrotum, as well as straddling injuries, may cause traumatic orchitis with extreme pain, rapid swelling, nausea and vomiting, and complete temporary prostration. Hospitalization is rarely indicated, although it may be several hours before the acute discomfort and reflex nausea and vomiting decrease enough to allow any type of physical activity.

Treatment
1. Control of pain and anxiety by sedatives, anodynes and narcotics. Chlorpromazine hydrochloride (Thorazine) will often help to control reflex nausea and vomiting.
2. Application of cold compresses.
3. Support by a T binder or athletic supporter until swelling subsides.

40–5. Penis injuries

A. Abrasions. Cleanliness will promote rapid healing.

B. Contusions. No special care is required; the profuse blood supply will cause rapid recovery.

C. "Dislocation" from external trauma may result in displacement of the base of the corpus beneath the symphysis pubis or into the abdominal wall or scrotum.

Treatment
1. Replacement by manipulation and traction as soon as possible. A general anesthetic often is necessary.
2. Hospitalization if there is evidence of urethral damage.

D. "Fracture" of the shaft of the penis may be caused by direct trauma or (occasionally) may occur during coitus. Treatment consists of sedation and cold packs, followed by hospitalization if pressure from a deep hematoma interferes with urination, or if a hematoma beneath Buck's fascia does not absorb spontaneously.

E. Frenum Injuries may cause severe bleeding requiring suturing under local anesthetic for control.

F. Lacerations. Because of the redundant loose skin and abundant blood supply of the penis, surgical repair of lacerations usually can be performed without difficulty. Debridement should be minimal. If a large amount of skin or soft tissue has been lost, hospitalization for grafting is indicated. The patient should be informed in advance of repair that scarring may result in irreparable contractures and deformity—especially curvature during erections (chordee).

G. **Necrosis** of the portion of the penis distal to a constricting band (usually applied in an attempt to control urinary incontinence or improve sexual performance) may occur. If swelling (sometimes tremendous) will not allow removal of the round-and-round constriction with the aid of a lubricant, a general anesthetic is necessary. Extreme distal urethral edema may require use of a retention catheter. Because of the profuse blood supply, complete and rapid recovery is the general rule unless actual gangrene is present.

H. **Zipper Injuries.** See Topic 48–62.

40–6. Postcircumcision bleeding

Improper operative technique, especially in the use of the Gomco clamp, may result in bleeding, sometimes coming on several days after circumcision.

Treatment. Mild bleeding or oozing generally can be controlled by pressure. Gelfoam or Oxycel held snugly over the bleeding area may be necessary. Severe bleeding requires immediate surgical control by properly placed mattress sutures.

40–7. Scrotal injuries

Direct blows or straddling injuries may cause extensive bleeding into the areolar tissue of the scrotum, as well as injury to the penis and scrotal contents. Rupture of the membranous urethra must be ruled out by careful examination since even a suspicion of this condition requires immediate hospitalization before extensive extravasation of urine has occurred.

Treatment

1. Bed rest until the swelling subsides.
2. Sedatives and anodynes.
3. Support by means of a T binder, suspensory or athletic supporter.
4. Reference to a surgeon or urologist—evacuation of the hematoma or extravasated urine may be necessary.

   5. Hospitalization in severe cases. However, most pa-
      tients do very well on home care, provided the
      urethra is intact.

40–8. Testicular torsion usually occurs in children and requires immediate hospitalization if correction cannot be obtained by gentle manipulation. Differentiation from inguinal
hernia, epididymitis, hydrocele and hematocele may be very
difficult.

40–9. Urethral injuries

Characterized by urethral bleeding, pain and difficulty in
urination, injury to the urethra may be caused by:

   A. Severe scrotal injuries (40–7, above), especially those
        caused by straddling some hard object, with com-
        pression of the membranous urethra against the
        symphysis pubis.
   B. Displaced or comminuted fractures of the pelvis near
        the symphysis pubis.
   C. "Dislocation" (40–5,C, above) or "fracture" of the penis
        (40–5,D, above) by direct trauma.
   D. Introduction of foreign bodies into the urethra by chil-
        dren (Topic 48–27) and mentally deranged persons.
   E. Attempts at catheterization.

   Treatment
      1. Sedation by intravenous barbiturates. Pain may be
         severe enough to require a narcotic.
      2. Treatment of shock (Topic 15–7).
      3. Immediate hospitalization for urologic care.

40–10. Vaginal and vulval injuries

Marked swelling and profuse bleeding may result from tears
at delivery, blows, straddling injuries, forcible intercourse, attempted rape (Topic 11), insertion of foreign bodies or instruments and from caustic burns. Thorough examination after
cleansing and hemostasis is always indicated.

   Treatment
      1. Repair of small lacerations under local anesthetic.
      2. Hospitalization if:
         a. Large hematomas are present.
         b. Lacerations enter or closely approximate the blad-
            der or rectum.
         c. Blood loss has been excessive.

40–11. Nontraumatic conditions

40–12. Cystitis

Characterized by dysuria and bladder tenderness, cystitis rarely causes severe systemic reactions except in children (especially girls). It is one of the common causes of sudden temperature rise in small children. If suspected, a "clean-catch" or second glass urine specimen should be examined microscopically for pus and blood.

Treatment

1. Force fluids orally and, if necessary, intravenously.
2. Give appropriate antibiotics or sulfonamides as indicated by cultures and sensitivity tests.
3. Recommend bed rest until afebrile.
4. Prescribe bladder sedation.
    a. IN ADULTS. A mixture of tincture hyoscyamus and potassium citrate may give subjective relief from the burning and scalding sensation.
    b. IN CHILDREN. Mandelic acid preparations often give relief, provided fluids are restricted for at least 12 hours.
5. Refer to a urologist for further care. Severe cases may require hospitalization.

40–13. Epididymitis

The discomfort of an acute epididymitis is often severe enough to bring the patient for emergency care with the story that the pain developed following a lift or a strain. Investigation will generally disclose a nontraumatic etiology, although straddling injuries with contusion of the scrotum and traumatic orchitis (40–7, above) occasionally will cause an associated traumatic epididymitis. In boys, testicular torsion (40–8, above) must always be ruled out.

Treatment

1. Bed rest until the acute signs and symptoms subside.
2. Cold compresses.
3. Support by an athletic supporter or T binder.
4. Analgesics. Morphine sulfate in small doses may be required to control severe pain.
5. Reference for urologic care if afebrile; if afebrile, hospitalization as soon as possible.

40–14. Hydrocele

Even though the patient may insist that the excess fluid in the scrotal sac is very uncomfortable, drainage as a rule is not an emergency procedure. The patient should be advised to consult a urologist. In children, testicular torsion (40–8, above) must always be ruled out by careful examination, even if the transillumination test is positive.

40–15. Hydronephrosis

Diagnosis of this condition cannot be made from an emergency examination. All that can be done is to attempt to give symptomatic relief and to combat infection as outlined under *Cystitis* (40–12, above).

40–16. Nephritis (Bright's Disease)

If glomerular, degenerative or arteriosclerotic kidney disease is present or suspected, the only emergency measures required are:

1. Treatment of convulsions [Topic 33; and *Coma* (Topic 3)].
2. Treatment of congestive heart failure (Topic 29).
3. Arrangement for hospitalization for medical work-up and care.

40–17. Paraphimosis

Retraction of the foreskin can usually be reduced by application of cold compresses and steady constant manual compression of the glans penis for 10 to 15 minutes, followed by gentle traction on the prepuce. If this is unsuccessful, infiltration around the constricting ring of 150 turbidity reducing units (TRU) of hyaluronidase dissolved in 2 ml. of normal saline may make reduction possible. In rare instances hospitalization for use of a general anesthetic may be necessary.

40–18. Perirenal (perinephric) abscess

If this condition is suspected, immediate hospitalization for care by a urologist is indicated.

40–19. Periurethral abscesses. See Topic 23–26.

40–20. Phimosis

Basically due to chronically tight structures covering the glans penis, acute symptoms are usually brought on by trauma but occasionally may develop without known precipitating cause. If the acute swelling of the glans cannot be controlled by sedation and cold compresses and the constriction released by gentle manipulation, the patient should be hospitalized for surgical relief. Dorsal slits or other surgical procedures should NOT be done as emergency measures unless there has been prolonged constriction and delay in surgical treatment is anticipated.

40–21. **Retention of urine**

This very uncomfortable condition is a common and legitimate emergency. If any difficulty is encountered during catheterization (Topic 17–3), the patient should be given an anodyne and referred at once to a urologist. In any case, acute urinary retention is a sign of serious underlying pathology requiring urologic investigation.

Passage of sounds, filiform catheters or stylet-stiffened catheters should not be attempted unless the attending physician is familiar with, and skilled in, their use. Nonbreakable catheters (never glass!) should be used in females. For technique of catheterization, see Topic 17–3.

40–22. **Stone in the urinary tract**

The severe, radiating, often agonizing, pain caused by passage of a stone down a ureter is a legitimate emergency requiring immediate relief. However, because the clinical picture is chiefly subjective, it can be simulated convincingly by narcotic addicts. A careful history supplemented by review of any available previous records and examination of a urine specimen (obtained in the presence of an attendant) for red blood cells is essential before narcotics are administered or prescribed. In questionable cases x-rays of the abdomen may be necessary. A negative x-ray, however, does not rule out the presence of calculi—many are not radiopaque.

Treatment

1. Bed rest, with application of hot stupes to the abdomen.
2. Morphine sulfate, 15 mg., with atropine sulfate, 0.4 mg., subcutaneously or, if the pain is very severe, intravenously. Meperidine hydrochloride (Demerol), 50 to 100 mg., may be substituted if the pain is of moderate intensity.
3. Methantheline bromide (Banthine), 25 mg., intravenously.
4. Nitroglycerin in tablet form, 0.4 to 0.6 mg., sublingually.
5. Papaverine hydrochloride, 30 to 60 mg., intravenously.
6. Adiphenine hydrochloride (Trasentine), 0.25 gm. by mouth, or 0.12 gm. subcutaneously.

Sudden and complete subsiding of the acute pain indicates that the stone has passed through the ureter into the bladder;

when this occurs, reference to a urologist on a nonurgent basis is all that is indicated. If the pain persists, or if there is any question regarding the validity of subjective complaints and objective findings, hospitalization for observation, evaluation and treatment should be suggested. Narcotic addicts will usually suddenly remember a number of apparently good reasons for refusing hospitalization, particularly if it has been suggested, directly or indirectly, that a method of hospital treatment without use of narcotics is planned.

40–23.   **Urethritis**

   A. Specific (gonorrheal). See Topic 61–3.

   B. Nonspecific. Acute urethritis is a very common condition, especially in young females, and is often overlooked as a cause for urinary complaints. Prescription of a mild sedative for symptomatic relief is all that is required. Thorough pediatric or medical investigation should be recommended.

41.   GYNECOLOGIC CONDITIONS

41–1.   **Abortions.** See Topic 50–1.

41–2.   **Amenorrhea** (Absence of Menses). No emergency treatment is required.

41–3.   **Bartholin gland abscesses** may require incision and drainage if acute or fluctuant, but whenever possible the patient should be referred to a gynecologist for this procedure.

41–4.   **Dysmenorrhea** (Painful Menstruation)

   Treatment

   1. Application of hot stupes to the abdomen.
   2. Antispasmodics:
      a. Phenobarbital sodium, 0.06 gm., intramuscularly.
      b. Atropine sulfate, 0.4 mg., subcutaneously or intravenously.
      c. Adiphenine hydrochloride (Trasentine), 75 mg., or adiphenine hydrochloride, 50 mg., combined with phenobarbital, 20 mg., by mouth every 4 to 6 hours.

41–5.   **Ectopic pregnancy.** See Topic 50–3.

41–6.   **Menorrhagia** (Abnormally Profuse Menstruation)
   Treatment
       1. Severe cases require plasma volume expanders intravenously followed by hospitalization.
       2. Mild cases may be sent home for bed rest and given a prescription for ergonovine maleate (Ergotrate), 0.2 mg., orally every 4 hours. Gynecologic examination in 1 or 2 days should be recommended.

41–7.   **Metrorrhagia** (Bleeding between Periods)
   Treatment
       1. If excessive, hospitalize at once.
       2. If mild:
           a. Ergonovine maleate (Ergotrate), 0.2 mg., orally every 4 hours.
           b. Limited activity; preferably bed rest.
           c. Examination by a gynecologist as soon as possible.

41–8.   **Mittelschmerz** (Pain Midway between Periods)
   Differential diagnosis from an acute surgical condition may require hospitalization for laboratory studies and observation. Sedation and analgesics will control milder cases.

41–9.   **Pelvic inflammatory disease** (Salpingitis, Tubo-ovarian Abscess)
   If febrile, hospitalize at once; if afebrile, prescribe sedation, antibiotics in large doses and bed rest. The patient should be referred to a gynecologist for examination and care.

41–10.   **Postpartum bleeding**
   A. Mild Cases
       1. Limited activity; preferably bed rest.
       2. Ergonovine maleate (Ergotrate), 0.2 mg., by mouth three times a day for 3 days.
       3. Antibiotics for prevention of secondary infection.
       4. Gynecologic examination if bleeding persists.
   B. Severe Cases, especially those with fever, require immediate hospitalization. Shock therapy (Topic 15–7) may be necessary before transfer to the hospital. Intravenous injection of 1 ml. of oxytocin (Pitocin) in 500 ml. of 5% dextrose solution will control hemorrhage in some instances.

41–11.   **Pruritus vulvae**
   Topical anesthetics such as dibucaine (Nupercaine) ointment, with sedation, will usually control symptoms until the

patient can be seen by a gynecologist. Cellulitis of the external genitalia from fingernail excoriations may be severe enough to warrant hospitalization.

41–12. **Salpingitis.** See 41–9, above.

41–13. **Torsion of the pedicle of an ovarian cyst**

This condition requires surgical intervention at once. The diagnosis is often made at exploratory laparotomy for acute abdominal pain.

42. HAND INJURIES

Adequate treatment of injuries to the hand requires specialized knowledge, skill and experience—not only in the proper care of soft tissue injuries but also in traumatic orthopedics, peripheral nerve repair and plastic surgery, especially skin grafting. If the emergency physician is not sure of the proper procedures, even though the injuries appear to be minor, he should arrange for treatment as soon as possible by an experienced surgeon. Nerve and tendon function should always be determined on initial examination and recorded in detail in the emergency chart before any debridement or repair is begun. Except in very minor injuries involving other parts of the hand than the digit upon which the ring is worn, rings should always be removed, using a ring cutter if necessary.

42–1. **Abrasions of the hand**

    A. Cleanse thoroughly with a mild detergent, such as pHisoHex or with nonmedicated soap and water. Remove any superficially embedded foreign materials by sharp dissection under local anesthesia.

    B. Inspect carefully, using magnification such as an eye loupe if necessary. Remove any firmly adherent or deeply imbedded foreign bodies by sharp dissection under local anesthesia.

    C. Irrigate thoroughly; repeat B (above) if necessary.

    D. Apply a petrolatum gauze dressing. Bacitracin (Parentracin) gauze may be used in place of petrolatum gauze if infection is apparent or suspected. Dressings should be snug and securely anchored but not tight enough to interfere with circulation. Allowance should be made for the inevitable posttraumatic swelling.

E. Give tetanus antitoxin or toxoid (Topic 19) and broad spectrum antibiotics if warranted by the circumstances of the injury, if gross contamination has been present, or if more than 6 hours have elapsed since injury.

F. Impress on the patient the fact that the original dressing MUST be checked by a physician within 36 hours.

42–2. **Cellulitis of the hand**

Any evidence of infection of any part of the hand calls for immediate treatment to preserve maximal function and minimize permanent damage.

A. Elevation and partial immobilization by a splint and sling.

B. Control of pain. Narcotics may be required.

C. Administration of antibiotics in large amounts, preferably after cultures and sensitivity tests.

D. Administration of tetanus antitoxin or toxoid (Topic 19). If tetanus antitoxin is necessary, adequate amounts (3000 to 10,000 units) should be given.

E. Incision and drainage of small superficial abscesses with insertion of a small rubber dam drain if necessary. Spraying with ethyl chloride is usually adequate for anesthesia. The necessity of redressing in 24 hours should be stressed to the patient.

Incisions should always be made in the "safe areas" of the palm and digits to avoid severance of essential structures and function-limiting scarring.

F. Hospitalization is usually indicated under the following circumstances:

1. If a general anesthetic or forearm, brachial or axillary block will be required.

2. If the deep palmar spaces or flexor tendon sheaths are involved.

3. If the patient is not making satisfactory progress under conservative ambulatory treatment.

42–3. **Contusions of the hand**

A. Mild contusions require no emergency treatment. Cold

compresses for the first 12 hours, followed by hot soaks at home, will accelerate recovery.

B. If extensive hematomas are present, the hand or digit should be immobilized on a padded splint, elevated, anodynes given, and surgical or orthopedic follow-up care arranged. Severe crushing injuries may require hospitalization. Traumatic aneurysm of the palmar arteries has been reported following localized contusions.

C. *Subungual Hematomas*

1. Small hematomas should be evacuated only if severe throbbing is present. Painless removal of the blood beneath the nail by burning a small hole through the nail with a red-hot paper clip gives complete relief. As a rule, no return visit is necessary.

2. Hematomas with associated external wounds are potentially infected and require free drainage. A section of the nail should be removed with sharp-pointed scissors after a preliminary drill hole has been made, the blood evacuated, and a dressing applied and protected by an aluminum fingertip guard. Recheck in 24 hours is essential.

3. Incomplete avulsion of the proximal end of the nail may require completion of the avulsion under digital block anesthesia. Using sterile technique, the proximal portion, usually about one third of the nail, should be excised, blood removed from beneath the nail and soft tissue folds by irrigation, and a stay suture of No. 40 cotton inserted through the nail and soft tissue on each side. A Telfa dressing and protective guard should be applied, tetanus antitoxin or toxoid given (Topic 19) and follow-up care in 24 hours arranged.

D. Contusions of the joints of the fingers usually require splinting to minimize permanent limitation of motion from fibrosis of the joint capsule. IF THERE IS PAIN ON MOTION, SPLINT! Persistent gentle massage (inunction) of the bruised area with an ointment of hydrocortisone acetate (2½%) in neomycin sulfate (Neo-Cortef) will often decrease swelling and pain.

42–4. **Fractures of the hand**
   A. *Simple (Closed) Fractures*
   1. SCAPHOID (NAVICULAR) FRACTURES (Topic 45–8,C,9)
      require immobilization in a short arm plaster
      cast with the wrist in slight cock-up (grasping)
      position and the thumb in extreme abduction.
      The cast should extend to the metacarpophalan-
      geal joints of the fingers and include the distal
      joint of the thumb. Small chip or avulsion frac-
      tures of the carpal bones require splinting in
      plaster in a position which will relax ligamen-
      tous or tendon pull.
   2. SEMILUNAR (LUNATE) FRACTURES are often associ-
      ated with partial or complete dislocation which
      may be difficult to recognize on routine x-rays
      (see Topic 45–5,B, 9 to 12). If dislocation is
      present, hospitalization is indicated; if not, a
      short arm cast (elbow to metacarpophalangeal
      joints) should be applied.
   3. METACARPALS. (Also see Topic 45–8,C,11.)
      a. All undisplaced metacarpal fractures should be
         immobilized in plaster.
      b. Displaced fractures with angulation, overriding or
         comminution usually require hospitalization.
         An exception is the so-called "boxer's fracture"
         of the distal ends of the second to fifth meta-
         carpals (usually the fifth).
            After injection of a local anesthetic into the
         hematoma, correction of the volar angulation
         can usually be obtained by firm pressure dor-
         sally, using the proximal phalanx flexed to 90
         degrees as a lever. If x-ray or fluoroscopic ex-
         amination shows satisfactory reduction, the
         hand should be flexed over a roller bandage
         and immobilized with tape or plaster of Paris.
         Again the position should be confirmed by
         x-rays. Recheck examination in 24 hours, pref-
         erably by an orthopedist, should be arranged.
      c. Fractures of the medial angle of the proximal end
         of the metacarpal of the thumb (Bennett's
         fracture) usually require special orthopedic

care to prevent a large permanent disability from instability and loss of grip.

4. PROXIMAL AND MIDDLE PHALANGES

   a. If multiple, hospitalization is advisable. Single fractures, even though considerably displaced, usually can be manipulated into satisfactory position without difficulty under local anesthesia. A pulp pin inserted through the pulp of the ball of the injured digit on the volar side of the distal phalanx, with traction by rubber bands attached to a banjo splint, may be necessary to maintain satisfactory position and alignment. The attachments and pull of the flexor tendons should be kept in mind when splinting and applying traction; acute flexion at the proximal interphalangeal joint is required if the fracture is distal to the attachment of the flexor digitorum sublimus tendon.

   b. All phalangeal fractures should be immobilized in plaster or on aluminum splints extending well up on the palm. Recheck in 24 hours, preferably by an orthopedist, should be arranged.

5. DISTAL PHALANGES

   a. Fractures of the tuft require no treatment except protection with an aluminum splint.

   b. Fractures of the proximal lip of the dorsal aspect at the attachment of the extensor tendon (baseball finger, mallet finger) should be splinted in plaster, or an individually fitted aluminum splint applied as soon as possible. The proximal interphalangeal joint should be in 70 to 80 degrees flexion and the distal joint in hyperextension to obtain maximum relaxation of the extensor tendon.

B. **Compound (Open)** *Fractures* of any portion of the hand should be referred for hospital care with the following exceptions:

1. SHATTERING FRACTURES OF THE TUFT should be irrigated, debrided and closed, saving as much length as possible and avoiding suture lines on the tactile surface of the ball. Small loose frag-

ments of bone should be removed but larger pieces left in situ.

2. FRACTURES OF THE DIGITS ASSOCIATED WITH LOSS OR MACERATION OF THE SOFT TISSUES. A plastic amputation should be performed, SAVING AS MUCH LENGTH AS POSSIBLE, especially of a thumb. Amputated portions can sometimes be filleted and used as full thickness grafts (42–5,A, 8,C, below). Every precaution should be taken to insure satisfactory shape and thickness of the tactile surface of the stump, with minimal scarring. Digital nerves should be identified, clipped off, and allowed to retract to prevent the formation of neuromas. If the amputation is through the base of the nail, all nail matrix cells should be removed by sharp dissection and curetting.

42–5. **Lacerations of the hand**

In order to prevent limitation of function, every possible measure to prevent infection must be taken.

A. Principles of Treatment

1. Repair within 6 hours if possible. This limit may be extended to 12 hours if the wound is not deep or extensive and if there is no evidence of gross contamination or infection. Lacerations more than 12 hours old should be irrigated and debrided (42–5,A,8, below) but NOT SUTURED.

2. Preliminary washing and irrigation before debridement, using copious amounts of bland nonmedicated soap and water, followed by normal salt solution. If very painful, this preliminary washing may be done under a local anesthetic.

3. Application of sterile drapes after preliminary irrigation and cleansing of the wound and surrounding skin.

4. OBSERVANCE OF STERILE OPERATING ROOM TECHNIQUE. All persons, including the patient, if practical, should be masked. Cap, mask and sterile gloves should be worn by the surgeon, with a sterile gown as well if an extensive or lengthy procedure is contemplated.

5. Application of a tourniquet to obtain a relatively bloodless field. A rubber band around the base

of the digit is adequate in most finger cases. (Also see Topic 55–20.)

6. ANESTHESIA
   a. Local infiltration or digital block with 1 or 2% procaine or lidocaine (Xylocaine) is usually sufficient. Nerve blocks (forearm, elbow, brachial, axillary) give excellent results but require special techniques.
   b. Local anesthesia (infiltration or local nerve block) should be used unless:
      (1) The patient is comatose or in such a condition that pain perception is markedly decreased.
      (2) A very short procedure (for instance, one or two stitches) is planned.
      (3) There is reason to believe that the patient is sensitive to procaine or other local anesthetics.
   c. Administration of a general anesthetic should be postponed until AT LEAST 6 HOURS after the last intake of food or liquids.

7. EXAMINATION OF THE WOUND UNDER LOCAL ANESTHESIA FOR:
   a. Severance of large blood vessels, muscles, nerves or tendons.
   b. Fractures, dislocations or epiphysial displacements.
   c. Foreign bodies.
   d. Hematomas.
   e. Any openings into, or contamination of, joints, tendon sheaths or fascial spaces. If unexpectedly severe damage is encountered, the tourniquet should be removed (or loosened and re-applied if indicated), a sterile pressure bandage applied and the patient transferred AT ONCE to an adequately equipped hospital. Administration of a sedative may be advisable. The physician to whom the patient is being sent should be advised by telephone of all details and a written transfer sheet sent with the patient.

8. DEBRIDEMENT
   a. The object of debridement is to convert a wound lined with traumatized and potentially infected

tissue into a surgically clean wound. With a small toothed forceps, sharp scalpel and small curved scissors, sharp dissection should be used to remove any damaged structures to a depth of 1 to 2 mm., starting with the skin and working toward the depths of the wound. If necessary for adequate exposure the surface laceration should be extended, bearing in mind the areas of safe incisions in the hand. Nerves, tendons, blood vessels and articular surfaces should be preserved.

b. All dead spaces should be eliminated by mattress sutures after careful evacuation of blood clots. Bleeding not controllable by pressure should be stopped by clamping and tying with No. 000 plain catgut. Buried suture material, however, should be kept to an absolute minimum.

c. Completely severed small sections of soft tissue (for instance, fingertips) which are not badly macerated, in some instances (especially in small children) can be carefully cleaned, placed in sterile saline solution, and sutured back in place as full thickness grafts. The quicker this suturing is done, the better the chance of a "take." Intact skin from amputated parts which are to be discarded can be used for grafting denuded areas.

d. No antibiotics, antiseptics, disinfectants, sulfonamides or other substances of any type should be painted, sprayed, insufflated or sprinkled into the wound.

9. Closure

a. Bony surfaces, joints, nerves and tendons must be completely covered. If necessary, a pedicle graft with the base proximally can be transferred from the immediate neighborhood and the resultant defect covered with split thickness grafts.

b. Careful approximation of skin edges without inversion or undue tension is essential, using nonabsorbable sutures. Cotton (No. 40 or 50) and Dermalin are satisfactory. Interlocking adhesive "butterflies" often result in an excellent closure but must be inspected frequently to detect slippage.

B. Dressings. A small strip of sterile petrolatum gauze or a nonadherent dressing such as Telfa should be placed over the sutures and a pressure bandage applied to control oozing. Collodion dressings should never be placed directly over a wound because of the possibility of promoting growth of anaerobic organisms, and because of the difficulty in removal. Collodion, however, can be used very satisfactorily to hold the edges of the outer dressings in place, especially on persons sensitive to adhesive tape.

Except in very small lacerations, the following measures should be routine:

1. Splinting to limit motion and prevent tension on repaired structures.
2. Application of a sling; elevation.
3. Administration of large doses of penicillin or other antibiotics as indicated by sensitivity tests if the wound was grossly contaminated or surgical repair was delayed beyond the safe limit (42–5,A,1, above).
4. Protection against tetanus by antitoxin or toxoid (Topic 19).
5. Control of apprehension, anxiety and pain by acetylsalicylic acid (aspirin), barbiturates or narcotics.

C. Postoperative Care. Small superficial lacerations as well as more serious wounds require REMOVAL OF THE ORIGINAL BANDAGE IN 24 HOURS for inspection and to allow for swelling. Failure to stress to the patient the need for this recheck examination constitutes negligence (Topic 69–1).

42–6. **Nerve injuries in the hand**

A. Primary versus Secondary (Delayed) Nerve Suturing. Unless the emergency physician has had neurosurgical training, he should not attempt a primary nerve suture. If immediate referral for care by a neurosurgeon is not possible, careful debridement (42–5,A,8, above) should be performed and the ends of the severed nerve identified and "tagged" with a small knot of black silk or very fine stainless steel wire. Closure should then be done in the usual manner. The procedure should be explained to the patient (or parents, spouse or legal guardian) and secondary nerve suture by a neurosurgeon recommended. The optimum wait is generally accepted to be 21 days. Whenever possible, a basal electromyogram should be made since, as a rule, denervation potentials do not develop until about 21 days after injury.

B. Evaluation of Motor and Sensory Deficits. Localized pressure from crushing injuries, or from a too tight tourniquet, may result in motor and/or sensory loss distal to the point of pressure. Before any treatment is given, motor function and sensation should be carefully evaluated and noted in detail on the emergency chart. Slow recovery of complete function usually occurs if pressure is the only causative factor in the motor or sensory deficit.

42–7. Puncture wounds of the hand

The treatment of puncture wounds requires the exercising of good judgment and common sense by the attending physician. The method of injury, chance of infection, and possibility of buried foreign bodies must be considered. All puncture wounds should receive tetanus antitoxin or toxoid (Topic 19).

Enlargement of the wound tract, thorough irrigation, careful debridement and suturing are indicated for:

A. Gross contamination.

B. Possible foreign bodies embedded in the soft tissues (Topic 38–6).

If presence of an intra-articular foreign body is known or suspected, reference for specialized care is indicated.

C. Human bites (Topic 27–13).

D. Indelible pencil wounds, whether or not the lead is still present. These require extensive excision of all discolored tissue as soon as possible. [See Topic 49–54 (*Aniline Dyes*).]

42–8. Tendon injuries in the hand

A. In the Palm or Dorsum of the Hand. If inspection or tests of function show evidence of complete severance of a flexor or extensor tendon proximal to

the metacarpophalangeal joints, immediate referral
for specialized care is indicated. Partial severance
without separation or loss of continuity can be repaired after irrigation and debridement, using fine
silk or cotton for suturing.

B. In the Digits

1. FLEXORS. Refer for specialist care.
2. THUMB TENDONS (ANY). Refer for specialist care.
3. EXTENSORS. Severed extensor tendons (except in the
   thumb) retract very little and no true pulleys are
   present; therefore, repair can usually be accomplished at the time of emergency debridement
   and closure. Fine cotton or silk should be used,
   employing the Bunnell double-right-angle stitch
   and splinting for 3 weeks in full extension. The
   specialized flexible pull-out wire technique recommended by Bunnell should not be attempted as
   an emergency procedure unless the emergency
   surgeon has had adequate training in this
   method.
4. Extensor tendon injuries requiring special handling:
   a. Avulsion of the extensor tendon attachment to the
      proximal lip of the dorsal aspect of the distal
      phalanx, usually associated with tearing off of
      a small flake of bone—the so-called "baseball"
      or "mallet" finger. For treatment see 42–4,A,-
      5,b, above.
   b. Buttonhole longitudinal splitting of an extensor
      tendon at the proximal interphalangeal joint,
      causing "paradoxical flexion." After debride-
      ment, the longitudinal split in the tendon can
      be repaired easily using interrupted sutures of
      fine cotton or silk. Splinting in full extension
      for 3 weeks followed by gradually increasing
      active (no passive) motion usually results in
      recovery of full function.

43. HEAD INJURIES

Also see Topic 36–4 (*Excitement States*); Topic 47–1 (*Coma of Undetermined Origin*); Topic 48–8 (*Brain Injuries in Children*); and Topic 48–28 (*Head Injuries in Children*).

43–1. **General principles of emergency care of head injuries**

43–2. **The general condition** of the patient is the primary consideration in all head injuries. Blood pressure, pulse, pulse pressure, respiration, color, and especially DEGREE OR STATE OF CONSCIOUSNESS are rapid and accurate indices of the patient's condition. All should be checked as soon as possible and at frequent intervals thereafter. CHANGES IN CONDITION are the most important factors in the evaluation of head injuries. Rapid or progressive deterioration may indicate a serious condition, such as an epidural hemorrhage from the middle meningeal artery (43–20, below), requiring immediate surgical intervention as a lifesaving measure (Topic 20).

43–3. **Initial examination** is all-important and should be done first with the patient clothed (Topic 47–1) and later completely undressed. The following points should be covered in detail and recorded in the patient's record, giving negative as well as positive findings:

A. Temperature, pulse, respiration and blood pressure.

B. General appearance—position, condition of clothing, etc., when first seen.

C. Evidence of severe or multiple injuries requiring immediate attention (Topic 20).

D. Examination of the head for evidence of trauma (wounds, hematomas, depressions, bleeding from the ears, nose or throat, etc.).

E. State of consciousness and mental status:

  1. CLEAR. Presence or absence of retrograde amnesia, disorientation as to time and place and aphasia (perceptive and expressive) should be determined.

  2. SEMICOMATOSE. Response to commands and painful stimuli, delirious, restless.

  3. COMATOSE. No response to painful stimuli.
F. **Eyes.** Size and equality of pupils, reaction to distance
    and light, nystagmus, diplopia, coordination of ex-
    traocular movements, funduscopic examination.
G. **Motor Power.** Ability to move the facial muscles equally
    on both sides; weakness or paralysis (flaccid, spas-
    tic) of an extremity.
H. **Rectal Sphincter Tone.**
I. **Sensation.** Variations in perception of pin prick and
    light touch on the face, arms, legs and trunk.
J. **Special Senses.** Vision, hearing, smell, taste; position
    and vibratory sense.
K. **Reflexes.** Superficial (corneal, gag, abdominal, cremas-
    teric); deep tendon (biceps, triceps, radial, knee
    jerks, ankle jerks).
L. **Pathologic Reflexes.** Babinski response on each side—
    positive (extensor) or negative (flexor); Hoffman;
    clonus.

43–4. **Shock** does not usually accompany head injuries in
adults but may be encountered in children (Topic 48–47). If
present, it must be controlled (Topic 15–7) before definitive
treatment. Injuries elsewhere should always be looked for and
treated in order of urgency (Topic 20). A gradually decreasing
pulse pressure may be the only evidence of increasing intracranial pressure.

43–5. **Adequacy of the airway** is essential. Removal of mucus
and blood by postural drainage and suction should be begun
at once and continued as needed. If the patient is vomiting, his
head should be lowered and turned to the side and frequent
suction utilized to minimize the danger of secondary lung infection from aspirated vomitus. Emergency tracheotomy (Topic
17–11) may be lifesaving.

43–6. **Prophylactic injections** (tetanus or other antitoxins,
toxoid, antibiotics) may contribute additional insult to an already critically embarrassed organism and, therefore, should
be postponed until the patient's condition has stabilized.

43–7. **Sedation** should be avoided unless extreme restlessness
or excitement (Topic 36–4) is present, but should be used
without hesitation if forcible manual or mechanical restraint
would otherwise be necessary. Parenteral administration of
rapid-acting drugs whose effect is of short duration is preferable, although rectal administration may be advisable in some

circumstances—for instance, if a properly signed treatment permit (Topic 70–18) cannot be obtained. The oral route should never be used; it may cause vomiting which, in turn, may cause increased intracranial pressure with extension of intracranial damage.

Effective Sedatives:

1. Chlorpromazine hydrochloride (Thorazine), 25 to 50 mg., intramuscularly.
2. Prochlorperazine dimaleate (Compazine), 10 to 25 mg., intramuscularly.
3. Paraldehyde, 5 to 10 ml., intramuscularly.
4. Phenobarbital sodium, 120 to 180 mg., intramuscularly.
5. Chloral hydrate, 1 to 2 gm., by retention enema.

43–8. **Control of pain.** Opiates and synthetic narcotics are definitely contraindicated in the presence of head injuries because of the possibility of:

A. Loss of pupillary signs.

B. Depression of respiration.

C. Masking of signs of developing intracranial pressure. If serious injuries elsewhere in the body cause severe pain, small doses of codeine sulfate or meperidine hydrochloride (Demerol) may be given subcutaneously as a calculated risk. Morphine sulfate and dihydromorphinone hydrochloride (Dilaudid) should never be used.

43–9. **Unrelated conditions.** The clinical picture of acute head injury can easily be confused with certain endocrine disorders (Topic 35); intoxication from alcohol [Topic 36–1 and Topic 49–227 (*Ethyl Alcohol*)] or drugs (Topic 3–13), air embolism (Topic 60–3,B,4); caisson disease (Topic 26–3); diabetes (Topic 3–3); and heat stroke (Topic 57–4). If the history or physical findings suggest the possibiltiy of head injury the patient should be kept under close observation and control until the picture has clarified.

43–10. **Concussion of the brain.** [Also see Topic 48–8,A (*Concussion in Children*).] If details of the history or neurologic findings suggest the possibility of even a slight concussion, the patient should be kept under close observation for at least 2 hours after his condition has stabilized before release from control. If unrelated conditions (43–9, above) which might confuse the picture are present, close observation until the possibility of brain damage can be ruled out is mandatory. Frequent examinations for changes in condition (43–2, above) should be made and recorded chronologically in the patient's record. X-rays may be indicated to rule out fracture, or for medico-legal purposes (Topic 21–1); but unless necessary for determination of emergency therapy, they should not be taken until the patient's condition has stabilized. If in the considered opinion of the attending physician it is safe to send the patient home, specific instructions regarding observation for posttraumatic symptoms and signs should be given by the physician personally to responsible members of the family. These instructions should be in simple nonmedical language and cover the following points:

A. Development of any difference in size of the pupils.
B. Increasing or recurring headaches.
C. Development of any facial asymmetry or of muscle weakness anywhere in the body.
D. Development of persistent vomiting.
E. Increasing sleepiness or stupor, or variations from the usual personality or behavior pattern.

43–11. **Acute excitement states** (Topic 36–4), sometimes even mania (Topic 51–1), can follow brain concussion. Rapid-acting barbiturates, chloral hydrate, chlorpromazine hydrochloride (Thorazine), paraldehyde or prochlorperazine dimaleate (Compazine) should be used for sedation in doses large enough to make physical restraint unnecessary.

43–12. **Fractures of the skull.** See also Topic 48–28 (*Head Injuries in Children*).

43–13. **Linear fractures without depression** are surprisingly well tolerated, especially by children, provided the middle meningeal artery or its branches are not damaged (see 43–20, below).

The location, not the extent, of the fracture and the condition of the patient are the most important factors to be considered in disposition. All patients with proved or suspected skull fracture should be kept under close observation for at least 2 hours; patients without neurologic signs can be allowed to go home with instructions to responsible members of the family as outlined under *Concussion* (43–10, above). If the general and neurologic pictures indicate that the patient's condition is deteriorating, immediate transfer by ambulance to a hospital should be arranged.

43–14. **Depressed fractures** can easily be confused with the edge of a scalp hematoma. Palpation may be misleading and tangential x-rays are necessary to establish the diagnosis. Conservative treatment is ordinarily carried out. Elevation of depressed fragments is not an emergency procedure unless signs of rapidly increasing intracranial pressure are present. All patients with proved or suspected depressed skull fractures should be hospitalized for close observation.

43–15. **Compound (open) depressed fractures**
Treatment
   1. Immediate hospitalization is indicated after application of a turban-type head dressing.
   2. If the condition is noted during or after debridement, the galea and scalp should not be closed. Instead, after control of gross hemorrhage, a sterile dressing should be applied and the patient transferred at once to a hospital by ambulance.

43–16. **Basal skull fractures** have a high mortality rate. Diagnosis usually depends upon the clinical picture since this type of fracture often cannot be demonstrated by x-rays.

43–17. **Anterior fossa**
Treatment
   1. Place in a position of maximal drainage, usually on the side or face down.
   2. Caution the patient against blowing his nose.
   3. Give sedation as needed but avoid opiates and synthetic narcotics (see 43–8, above).
   4. Hospitalize by ambulance as soon as possible. Do not attempt to control rhinorrhea or nasal hemorrhage by packing or intranasal medication of any type.

43–18. **Middle fossa.** Blood or a mixture of spinal fluid and blood from an undamaged ear canal may be diagnostic.
Treatment
   1. DO NOT attempt to cleanse the external auditory canal.
   2. Cover the ear with sterile gauze and apply a turban-type head dressing.
   3. Warn the patient against blowing his nose.
   4. Give sedatives as needed but avoid opiates and synthetic narcotics (see 43–8, above).
   5. Hospitalize by ambulance as soon as possible.

43–19. Posterior fossa. Unless the fracture is compound (open) the diagnosis of fractures in this area of the skull can be made only by x-rays. No emergency measures except supportive therapy and hospitalization for observation are indicated.

43–20. Extradural (epidural) hemorrhage. [Also see Topic 48–22 (*Extradural Hemorrhage in Children*).] Tearing of the middle meningeal artery or its branches may cause collection of blood between the dura mater and the skull. Direct trauma, sometimes very slight, is the usual cause; persons between 20 and 50 years of age represent the majority of cases.

   A. Signs and Symptoms
   1. Disturbances of consciousness of varying degrees and length following a head injury.
   2. An asymptomatic "lucid interval" lasting from one-half hour to several days (not always present).
   3. Rapid deterioration of condition with symptoms and signs of cerebral compression (headache, vomiting, increasing stupor, decreased respiration and pulse rate, deep coma, contralateral hemiplegia, terminal vasomotor collapse). Unilateral dilation of the pupil occurs in about 75% of cases but may be transient. Funduscopic examination is of no value.

   B. Treatment. If the patient's condition is deteriorating rapidly, IMMEDIATE evacuation of the hematoma may be a lifesaving measure [Topic 20 (*Urgency Evaluation*)]. This should be done if possible in a properly equipped hospital; but if a delay in hospitalization is unavoidable, it should be performed in an emergency setting. Delay will result in irreversible brain damage from pressure. As soon as the acute compression of the brain is released, the acute emergency is over. Hospitalization for postoperative care should, of course, be arranged as soon as possible.

43–21. Subdural hemorrhage. The bleeding in this condition usually comes from a tear in one of the cerebral veins entering the dural sinuses, the result of direct trauma to the frontal or occipital regions. This hemorrhage is venous, and its pressure less than in extradural hemorrhage (43–20, above); hence, signs of brain damage are much slower—sometimes weeks—in developing.

    Treatment. Hospitalization for localization and definitive care is indicated as soon as signs and symptoms suggestive of increased intracranial pressure are noted.

43–22. **Lacerations of the scalp**
    Treatment

1. After a careful history and thorough examination for evidence of intracranial damage, the area should be prepared by wide shaving and cleansing of the surrounding scalp. Under 1% procaine or lidocaine (Xylocaine) anesthesia the skull should be palpated with the gloved finger and, if possible, inspected. If a depression or defect can be felt or seen, a sterile nonradiopaque dressing should be applied and x-ray studies (including tangential views) made before closure of the laceration. Negative x-rays do not rule out the presence of a fracture; therefore, if an apparent defect or variation from normal has been noted, the patient should be kept under close observation for at least 8 hours. Palpation and direct observation are often more accurate than x-rays, especially if a nondepressed linear or stellate fracture is present. Neurologic findings suggestive of brain injury, with or without evidence of skull damage, call for hospitalization for close observation and frequent determination of vital signs (43–2 and 3, above). It should be remembered that thickening of scalp layers by blood or fluid may simulate a fracture (43–14, above) and that the location of the lesion (43–13, above) is of great value in prognosis.

2. After irrigation with sterile saline and careful debridement, closure should be done with a single row of interrupted sutures of No. 40 or 50 cotton using a large curved needle and including if possible the galea and full thickness of the scalp. Pressure usually will control bleeding, but mattress sutures may be necessary. After closure

a pressure bandage should be applied to control oozing.

3. Tetanus antitoxin or toxoid (Topic 19) and antibiotics should be administered if gross contamination is present or if treatment has been delayed.

4. Hospitalization is not necessary unless excessive blood loss has occurred or signs of increased intracranial pressure (43–10, above) have been noted or develop.

5. All patients should be told to report to a physician for recheck examination in not more than 3 days. The patient, or a responsible member of the family, should be instructed in detail BY THE ATTENDING PHYSICIAN regarding signs and symptoms of increased intracranial pressure (43–10, above).

43–23. Management of serious head injuries awaiting transfer for hospital care

Routine Therapy and Handling

1. Insistence on absolute rest in a position most suitable for adequate drainage. Visitors, even members of the family, should be discouraged.

2. Insurance of an adequate airway by support of the angles of the jaw, positional drainage and application of suction as needed.

3. Administration of oxygen under positive pressure by face mask and rebreathing bag as needed for dyspnea and cyanosis.

4. Avoidance of oral medications; they may induce vomiting.

5. Limitation of fluids.

6. Frequent checking of state of consciousness, pulse, blood pressure, respiration, temperature and neurologic findings. These findings should be recorded on the patient's emergency chart and a summary, together with any x-rays, sent with the patient on transfer.

7. Use of gentle restraint and sedation as needed. Forcible physical restraint should be kept to a minimum; IF IT IS NECESSARY, SEDATION IS NOT ADEQUATE. An able-bodied attendant should be present at all times.

8. Use of cooling measures (ice bags, cold compresses.

blower, etc.) if the temperature is higher than 39° C. (102.2° F.).

9. Careful consideration, supplemented by consultation if practical, regarding spinal puncture to decrease pressure in the presence of rapidly increasing stupor or deepening coma if delay in hospitalization is anticipated. As a general rule, however, this should be deferred until the patient has been hospitalized.

10. Tactful and sympathetic handling of the patient's family, friends or other interested persons, with avoidance of specific statements concerning extent of injuries, condition, type and duration of further treatment, possible complications and prognosis.

44. METABOLIC DISORDERS

See also Topic 35 (*Endocrine Emergencies*).

44–1. **Acidosis**

Formation or accumulation of acid products in the body more rapidly than removal or neutralization can take place results in a characteristic train of symptoms. This disturbance in metabolism may be caused by:

A. Interference with Respiration by:
1. Asthma, bronchitis, pneumonia, emphysema or other pulmonary conditions.
2. Cardiac decompensation.
3. High concentration of carbon dioxide in the air.
4. Deep narcosis.

B. Alkali Deficiency from:
1. Acid ingestion.
2. Anesthesia.
3. Anoxia.
4. Dehydration.
5. Diabetes mellitus.
6. Excessive exertion.
7. Kidney failure.
8. Toxemia.

C. *Signs and Symptoms* (all may be modified, masked or intensified by the causative condition)
1. Headache, drowsiness and generalized weakness.
2. Pain in the abdomen and extremities.
3. Tachycardia.
4. Rapid respiration at first, later becoming weak and shallow.
5. Fruity odor to the breath.
6. Acetone and diacetic acid in the urine.
7. Progressive stupor and coma.

D. *Treatment*
1. Application of heat by warmed blankets or a warm air circulator. Hot water bottles should not be used if other means of applying heat are available.
2. Caffeine sodiobenzoate, 0.5 gm., intramuscularly.
3. Normal salt solution, 1000 ml., intravenously.
4. Treatment of the underlying causative condition if identified.
5. Hospitalization for acid-base balance determinations and definitive therapy (Topic 7).

44–2. **Addisonian crises.** See Topic 35–1.

44–3. **Adrenal insufficiency, acute** (Addisonian Crisis). See Topic 35–1.

44–4. **Air sickness.** This is not due to changes in atmospheric pressure but to motion. See 44–18, below (*Motion Sickness*).

44–5. **Alkalosis.** Alkali excess in the blood may be due to:

A. *Hyperventilation* (Topic 36–6), caused by:
1. High temperature—body or external (Topic 57–2, 3 and 4).
2. Hysteria (Topic 51–5 and 9).
3. Encephalitis (Topic 63–5).
4. Hyperpnea due to high altitudes [Topic 26–1 (*Altitude Sickness*); and Topic 26–6 (*Mountain Sickness*)].
5. Anesthesia (second stage).

B. *Increased Formation or Oversupply of Alkali from:*
1. Prolonged vomiting or gastric lavage.
2. Therapy by x-ray or radioactive substances.
3. Overzealous administration of alkaline substances.
4. Congenital metabolic variations from normal.

C. Signs and Symptoms

1. Restlessness, irritability and excitability.
2. Slow deep respiration; the rate may be as low as 5 per minute.
3. Signs of neuromuscular irritability:
   a. *Erb's Sign*. Muscular response to a very weak galvanic current.
   b. *Chvostek's Sign*. Twitching of the facial muscles brought on by tapping the skin just anterior to the external auditory meatus.
   c. *Trousseau's Sign*. An "obstetrical position" of the hand and fingers brought on by constriction of the arm above the elbow.

D. Treatment

1. If due to *hyperventilation,* see Topic 36–6.
2. If due to excess alkali:
   a. Discontinue alkali therapy.
   b. Force fluids by mouth or give 500 to 1000 ml. of a 1% solution of sodium chloride intravenously.
   c. Give calcium gluconate, 10 ml. of 10% solution, intravenously.
   d. Hospitalize for laboratory studies and treatment.

44–6.　**Altitude sickness.** See Topic 26–1 and Topic 26–6 (*Mountain Sickness*).

44–7.　**Caisson disease** ("Bends," Compressed Air Sickness, Decompression Sickness). See Topic 26–3.

44–8.　**Car sickness.** See *Motion Sickness* (44–18, below).

44–9.　**Compressed air sickness.** See *Caisson Disease* (Topic 26–3).

44–10.　**Diabetic coma.** See Topic 3–3.

44–11.　**Gout.** Acute totally disabling swelling and pain in the joints, especially of the feet, may occur with gouty arthritis.

Treatment

1. Morphine sulfate, 10 to 15 mg., or codeine sulfate, 0.06 gm., subcutaneously—1 dose only.
2. Colchicine, 4 ml. (0.2 mg.), intravenously followed in 4 hours by 0.5 mg. by mouth every hour for eight doses or until nausea or diarrhea become troublesome.
3. Dextrose 5% in saline, 500 to 1000 ml., intravenously.

4. Magnesium sulfate (Epsom salts), 30 gm., by mouth.
5. Referral for complete medical check-up after relief of acute symptoms and signs. Hospitalization is rarely necessary.

44–12. Hypercalcemia

High serum calcium levels may occur from excessive prolonged intake of vitamin D and in conditions such as metastatic malignancy, sarcoidosis, multiple myeloma and hyperparathyroidism (Topic 35–3, B). Manifestations are usually headache, nausea, vomiting, dryness of the mucous membranes of the nose and mouth, pruritus and urinary distress.

Treatment
1. Antinauseants as required.
2. Correction of fluid imbalance (Topic 7).
3. Referral for corticosteroid therapy. Hospitalization may be required.

44–13.   Hyperinsulinism. See Topic 3–3.

44–14.   Hyperparathyrodism. See Topic 35–3,B.

44–15.   Hyperthyroid crises. (See also Topic 35–5,B.)

Two types which may require emergency therapy are recognized:

A. The Activated Type, characterized by restlessness increasing to delirium, tachycardia, vomiting, diarrhea, dehydration, occasional jaundice and high temperature, sometimes as high as 41° C. (105.8° F.).

Treatment
1. Physical restraint until adequate sedation can be accomplished.
2. Oxygen inhalations by face mask and rebreathing bag.
3. Cold packs and antipyretics.
4. Immediate hospitalization.

B. The Apathetic Type, characterized by extreme prostration with muscular hypotonia, mental apathy and a relatively low temperature rise—not above 38.3° C. (101° F.).

Treatment
1. Administration of oxygen under positive pressure, preferably by face mask and rebreathing bag if cyanosis is present.

2. Treatment of shock, which may be terminal (Topic 15–7).

3. Immediate hospitalization.

44–16. Hypoglycemia. Although often used synonymously with "hyperinsulinism" (Topic 3–3), hypoglycemia is a much broader term. Its causes are as follows:

1. Abnormal functioning of the islets of Langerhans (Topic 35–2, C).

2. Liver, pituitary and suprarenal disorders.

3. Severe head injuries (Topic 43).

4. "Dumping syndrome" after gastric resection (Topic 35–2, D).

5. Administration of excessive amounts of insulin, or inadequate food intake after the usual dose of insulin. Occasionally, oral hypoglycemic agents may cause an acute picture.

6. Extreme muscular fatigue.

7. Pregnancy.

8. Sympathetic nervous system disorders, often functional.

9. Renal glycosuria.

10. Idiopathic hypoglycemia of infancy.

Signs, Symptoms and Treatment are the same as outlined for *Hyperinsulinism* (Topic 3–3).

44–17. Hypoparathyroid crises are caused by atrophy, degeneration, fibrosis or surgical removal of the parathyroid glands. See Topic 35–3, A.

44–18. Motion sickness.

Certain individuals who are particularly prone to air, car, sea or train sickness do not follow the usual course of rapid complete recovery following cessation of the motion. Nausea, vomiting and dizziness may be severe or persistent enough to bring the patient for emergency treatment. Any normal human being can be made sick by motion. The exact causal mechanism is not as yet fully understood, although labyrinthine vestibular stimulation undoubtedly plays a part. Vertical (rise and fall—elevators, ships, planes, buses, cars), linear (forward and backward, stop and go—cars, buses, planes, playground and carnival swings, etc.), or angular acceleration (the normal rhythmic pitch and sway of moving vehicles) or any combination of all three may be the precipitating motion, which may be reinforced, facilitated and enhanced by special sense stimuli such as sound, sight, taste, smell and perception of vibration. Undoubtedly psychologic and emotional states contribute to, and exaggerate, motion sickness although they cannot cause it.

A. Signs and Symptoms

1. Restlessness, general malaise, hypersensitivity to sensory stimuli.
2. Lassitude, yawning, pallor, difficulty in breathing.
3. Waves of nausea and vomiting, followed by acute depression, apathy and generalized prostration.
4. Vague and inconstant objective signs—increased pulse and blood pressure (transient only).

B. Treatment (prophylactic, symptomatic and definitive)

1. Avoidance of eating or drinking just before starting a trip.
2. Proper selection of a vehicle and location therein:
   a. As large a vehicle as possible.
   b. A central seat or cabin to minimize roll (sideways motion) and pitch (end-to-end, up-and-down motion).
   c. Smoothly driven vehicles—a bus is more stable than a passenger car, a jet more stable than a propeller-driven aircraft.
   d. Focusing the eyes on a distant object—especially while traveling by air.
   e. Avoidance of a seat over the rear axle in a bus or passenger car—the site of maximum up-and-down motion.
3. Belladonna alkaloids prophylactically as preliminary tranquilizers, sometimes combined with barbiturates or chloral hydrate.
4. Antinauseants. Repeated tests conducted by the U.S. Armed Services have resulted in the conclusion that the following are the most effective drugs for prevention and treatment of motion sickness of any type (air sickness, car sickness, sea sickness, etc.):
   a. Meclezine hydrochloride (Bonine), 25 to 50 mg., orally once daily.
   b. Cyclizine hydrochloride (Marezine) orally, 50 mg., three or four times daily; intramuscularly, 50 mg., three times a day; by rectal suppository, 100 mg., every 4 to 6 hours. For children the

dosage *must* be adjusted according to age (Topic 5).

c. Prochlorperazine dimaleate (Compazine), 10 mg., orally three or four times daily; intramuscularly (deep in buttocks), 10 mg., three times a day.

Compazine dosage in children should be adjusted according to the following schedule (orally or by rectal suppository)

Under 9 kilograms of body weight—not to be used.

9 to 12 kilograms of body weight—2.5 mg., not more than twice a day.

13 to 18 kilograms of body weight—2.5 mg., not to exceed three times a day.

19 to 40 kilograms of body weight—3 mg., twice a day.

5. Amphetamine or dextroamphetamine to combat depression.

6. Replacement therapy (Topic 7).

C. Prognosis. Complete recovery without residual ill-effects always takes place within a few hours of cessation of motion.

44–19. Parathyroid crisis. See Topic 35–3, B (*Acute Parathyroid Intoxication*).

44–20. Porphyria

Acute intermittent porphyria may cause signs and symptoms requiring emergency care in adults of both sexes. Abdominal pain, often severe enough to be mistaken for an acute surgical abdomen, may be the presenting complaint, but a wide variety of neurologic complaints of extreme severity may be confused with poliomyelitis, encephalitis or acute poisoning. The characteristic laboratory finding is the change in color of the urine to dark red or even black on exposure to sunlight.

Treatment

1. Control of severe pain by meperidine hydrochloride (Demerol).

2. Assistance with respiration (Topic 17–1). In severe cases, tracheotomy (Topic 17–11) may be necessary.

3. Sedation by chloral hydrate, paraldehyde or chlorpromazine hydrochloride (Thorazine). BARBITURATES SHOULD NEVER BE USED.

　　　4. Hospitalization during the usually prolonged recovery
　　　　　from acute episodes.

44–21. **Radiation sickness.** See Topic 64–4, B.

44–22. **Sea sickness.** See 44–18, above (*Motion Sickness*).

44–23. **Tetany**

A. Active

Signs and Symptoms

　　　1. Carpopedal spasm.
　　　2. Convulsions of varying degrees of severity. These
　　　　　may be generalized or unilateral or confined to
　　　　　isolated muscle groups.
　　　3. Spasm resulting from involvement of the autonomic
　　　　　nerve supply of the iris, bronchi, diaphragm,
　　　　　heart, gastrointestinal tract and bladder.

Treatment

　　　1. Treatment of the underlying condition.
　　　2. Carbogen inhalations or paper bag rebreathing if
　　　　　tetany is due to hyperventilation (Topic 36–6)
　　　3. Calcium gluconate, 10 ml. of 10% solution, intra-
　　　　　venously.
　　　4. Hospitalization for blood studies unless hyperventila-
　　　　　tion (Topic 36–6) is the causative condition.

B. Latent.
Caused by hypocalcemia, alkalosis or, occasionally, hyperphosphatemia, and characterized by
neuromuscular excitability, this condition is rarely
encountered as an emergency. Erb's, Chvostek's
and Trousseau's signs (44–5, C, above) are pathognomonic. No emergency treatment is required.
The patient should be referred for medical examination and evaluation.

44–24. **Train sickness.** See 44–18, above (*Motion Sickness*).

45. MUSCULOSKELETAL DISORDERS

45–1. Arthritis

Although the numerous conditions grouped under this general heading usually cause chronic symptoms, acute discomfort
caused by fulminating infections or by traumatic aggravation

of the underlying condition may require emergency care or hospitalization. Use of a bed board, home application of cold or heat, local massage and large doses of salicylates by mouth may give relief in some types of arthritis. One to 2 ml. of d-tubocurarine chloride in a repository medium (Tubadil) intramuscularly will usually relieve acute muscle spasm but requires close observation because of its respiratory depressant effect [Topic 49–168 (*Curare*)]. Muscle relaxants such as carisoprodol (Rela, Soma), 350 mg., orally three times a day, chlorzoxazone (Paraflex), 250 mg., orally three times a day, and orphenadrine citrate (Norflex), 2 ml. (60 mg.) intramuscularly, or one tablet orally, two or three times a day may be effective. Corticosteroids and phenylbutazone (Butazolidin) are not suitable for emergency therapy since their safe use requires controlled follow-up care. For treatment of gout see Topic 44–11.

45–2. **Back injuries**

Back injuries vary markedly in intensity and type from slight muscular strains to fracture-dislocation with cord damage and partial or complete motor and sensory paralysis.

    A. Fractures of any portion of the spine except transverse processes (45–8,C,6, below) usually require hospitalization. Careful handling during transportation with the emphasis on smoothness, not speed, is mandatory.

    B. Soft Tissue Damage (contusions, sprains, strains) may cause acute symptoms which often can be relieved by one or more of the following means:

      1. For control of this type of pain acetylsalicylic acid (aspirin) with or without codeine sulfate by mouth is very effective. In extreme cases morphine sulfate or dihydromorphinone hydrochloride (Dilaudid) can be given subcutaneously in the smallest possible effective doses.

      2. To decrease muscle spasm, cold packs often are of value, as are skeletal muscle relaxants (45–1, above).

      3. Application of local heat and gentle massage.

      4. Infiltration of "trigger points" with 0.5 or 1.0% procaine or lidocaine (Xylocaine).

      5. To lessen skin sensitivity, spraying of the painful areas with ethyl chloride.

6. Limitation of movement and support in the cervical area may be accomplished to some extent by snug application of a Thomas collar if the patient is ambulatory; severe injuries require careful handling and transportation in the supine position, sometimes with sandbags and manual traction, preferably applied by the attending physician. A lumbosacral or sacroiliac support or tight adhesive strapping may give relief if the injury is to the soft tissues of the low back.

45–3. Bursitis.

[Also see 45–12, below (*Peritendinitis*).] Inflammation of any of the numerous bursae of the body is very painful and may be totally disabling. Anodynes, including narcotics, should be given as needed to control the acute pain until the patient can receive definitive treatment. If the bursa is hot, red and swollen, penicillin, 600,000 units intramuscularly, or tetracyclines in adequate doses orally, may be of benefit, as may immobilization and spraying the skin over the affected part with ethyl chloride. Infiltration of the painful area with 1% procaine or lidocaine (Xylocaine) may give spectacular relief. Slower relief may follow daily intramuscular injections of 1 ml. (1000 mcg.) of vitamin B_{12}. Hot compresses are contraindicated; cold sometimes decreases the acute discomfort.

Injection of 1 ml. (25 mg.) of hydrocortisone acetate preceded by a local anesthetic directly into the affected bursa sometimes is of benefit. All patients should be instructed to make arrangements for follow-up care.

45–4. Cervical injuries. See 45–11, below (*Neck Injuries*).

45–5. Dislocations. Also see 45–7, below.

A. General Principles of Emergency Care. X-rays should always be taken before reduction of a dislocation is attempted. If a fracture is present, especially in the region of the shoulder or hip, reduction should be postponed until the patient has been hospitalized. If no fracture is present, reduction may be attempted by any of the approved methods. Morphine sulfate should be given 20 minutes before manipulation except in small children. Dislocated small joints or epiphyses can sometimes be reduced under a local anesthetic injected directly into the joint or into the hematoma caused by the injury.

BEFORE AND AFTER REDUCTION the circulation and nerve supply should be checked carefully and x-rays taken to verify the correct position and alignment. If one or two attempts at reduction by any method are unsuccessful, no further manipulation should be attempted; instead, the patient should be hospitalized for possible general anesthesia.

B. Dislocations Requiring Special Handling

1. ACROMIOCLAVICULAR SEPARATIONS if marked or complete are clinically apparent, but more often lesser degrees of separation can be demonstrated only by comparative x-rays of the shoulder girdles taken with a heavy weight in each hand.

   TREATMENT
   a. Mild cases require only support for 2 to 3 weeks with a Velpeau bandage.
   b. Severe cases require hospitalization for operative repair.

2. ANKLE DISLOCATIONS of any degree usually do not occur without accompanying fractures, especially of the avulsion type, and gross ligamentous damage. To prevent subsequent instability, hospitalization for surgical repair of the damaged ligamentous structures is usually necessary even if reduction of the dislocation has been accomplished as an emergency measure.

3. CARPAL DISLOCATIONS. See Topic 42–6; and 45–5,B,5, 9 and 12, below.

4. CERVICAL SPINE DISLOCATIONS. Also see 45–11 below (*Neck Injuries*); and Topic 47–7 (*Spinal Injuries and Compression*). Immediate hospitalization with the head and neck immobilized by sandbags is imperative. Manual neck traction during transportation may be necessary.

5. ELBOW DISLOCATIONS. [Also see *Radial Head Subluxations* (45–5,B,14, below).] Provided no fractures are present, dislocations of the elbow can sometimes be reduced under heavy sedation but without anesthetic by the following method:
   a. Have the patient lie face down on a high narrow table with the injured arm hanging down.
   b. Make gentle downward traction on the wrist.

   c. When the olecranon slides distally on the humerus with wrist traction continued, lift the humerus laterally.

   d. Check for complete reduction by x-rays.

   e. Immobilize with a Velpeau bandage.

   f. Arrange for a check-up on circulation and sensation in 24 hours.

      If reduction cannot be obtained in two attempts the patient should be hospitalized for reduction under general anesthetic.

6. EPIPHYSIAL DISLOCATIONS. See 45–7, below.

7. FINGER DISLOCATIONS. See *Phalangeal Dislocations* (13, below).

8. HIP DISLOCATIONS. Hospitalization for reduction under general anesthetic is always required.

9. LUNATE DISLOCATIONS. [Also see *Perilunar Dislocations*) (12, below).] Severe direct trauma to the wrist may cause rupture of the ligamentous structures at the distal end of the lunate with subsequent partial or complete rotatory displacement. Hospitalization is usually indicated because reduction may be difficult and operative fixation of the distal end of the bone may be necessary.

10. NASAL BONE AND CARTILAGE DISLOCATIONS. See Topic 46–4.

11. PATELLAR DISLOCATIONS. Direct trauma or violent contraction of the quadriceps femoris can cause lateral dislocation of the patella, especially if the lateral parapatellar ridge is lower than normal or genu valgus is marked. Medial dislocations are very rare. Reduction can usually be obtained without anesthetic by a sudden forcible thrust medially with the palm of the hand.

      Recurrent dislocations may require operative transference of the tibial tuberosity medially or revision of quadriceps pull as an elective procedure.

12. PERILUNAR DISLOCATIONS OF THE CARPUS. In this type of dislocation the lunate remains in normal relationship to the radius and ulna while all of the other carpal bones are displaced. Routine x-rays may be misinterpreted, especially if as-

sociated fractures of the scaphoid or cuneiform are present. Reduction is usually difficult and requires regional block or general anesthesia, followed by immobilization for 6 to 8 weeks in a plaster of Paris short arm cast.

13. PHALANGEAL (CARPAL) DISLOCATIONS. Limited almost exclusively to the metacarpophalangeal joint of the thumb and the proximal interphalangeal joints of the other digits, these dislocations can usually be reduced easily by traction and manipulation, often without anesthesia. If necessary, 1% procaine or lidocaine (Xylocaine) can be injected into the joint before manipulation. After reduction a short aluminum splint or plaster cast should be applied.

Immobilization for 3 weeks, followed by institution of active motion, will usually result in regaining full function, although some permanent thickening of the capsule may result.

14. RADIAL HEAD SUBLUXATIONS. Partial subluxation of the proximal end of the radius from the sling formed by the orbicular ligament occurs almost exclusively in small children in the toddling age, although it may occur in injudiciously handled infants. The mechanism of injury is usually a sudden jerk on the outstretched arm by an adult leading or lifting the child by the hand.

SIGNS AND SYMPTOMS

    a. Severe pain which is very difficult to localize.

    b. Refusal to fully extend the forearm. The child usually holds the arm with the elbow slightly flexed and the forearm supinated and resists any attempts at examination or motion.

    c. X-rays are of no value in diagnosis except to rule out associated conditions, especially displacement of the epicondylar epiphyses (45–7,B,3, below).

TREATMENT

    a. *Gentle Manipulation.* If the injury is recent, this can usually be done without anesthetic by:

        (1) Traction on the forearm.

        (2) Pressure over the radial head with the thumb.

(3) Gradual extension and supination of the forearm. A palpable (sometimes audible) snap indicates reduction.

   b. *Application of a Sling.* The parents should be instructed to encourage use of the arm as soon as the pain subsides.

15. SHOULDER DISLOCATIONS. If x-rays show a fracture associated with the dislocation, hospitalization is indicated. If there is no fracture, reduction may be attempted by one of several methods (Topic 17–10). Pain and apprehension should be controlled by a preliminary subcutaneous injection of morphine sulfate or dihydromorphinone hydrochloride (Dilaudid).

16. SPINAL DISLOCATIONS. These usually occur in the cervical or upper dorsal regions. See *Cervical Spine Dislocations* (45–5,B,4, above) and *Neck Injuries* (45–11, below).

17. STERNOCLAVICULAR DISLOCATIONS. These injuries are uncommon and usually heal satisfactorily if partially immobilized by tight adhesive strapping over a pressure pad and use of a sling. Severe cases require operative repair as an elective procedure.

18. TARSAL DISLOCATIONS. Slipping between the tarsal bones is usually of small degree but can be very painful and cause complete disability. Careful comparative x-ray studies are essential for diagnosis.

    Treatment consists of manipulative or open reduction with plaster cast immobilization. Hospitalization is usually required.

19. TEMPOROMANDIBULAR DISLOCATIONS. These dislocations are usually unilateral and, because of spasm of the powerful muscles controlling the jaw, are very difficult to reduce. If heavy pressure downward and backward (with the operator's thumbs well padded) does not cause reduction, the patient should be referred for a general anesthetic.

20. TOE DISLOCATIONS are easily reducible by gentle trac-

tion followed by strapping to adjacent toes for 7 to 10 days.

21. ULNAR SHAFT FRACTURES with radial head dislocation require open reduction in adults, closed manipulation in children.

45–6. Epicondylitis

The acute pain from this condition (probably a localized viral fibrositis) can sometimes be relieved by spraying with ethyl chloride. Temporary (sometimes permanent) relief follows infiltration of the painful area with a local anesthetic. Local heat may be of benefit in some cases; others, it makes worse. Application of a splint or cast to control rotation of the forearm as well as elbow and wrist motion may be necessary. Since the discomfort is often acute, anodynes are indicated until the patient can receive definitive orthopedic care.

45–7. Epiphysial displacements

A. Many of these displacements or slips reduce spontaneously. Examination for localized tenderness or guarding muscle spasm, and fluoroscopic examination for excess mobility, in addition to comparative x-rays of the uninjured side, are often necessary to establish the diagnosis. With certain exceptions (see B, below), if a loose epiphysis is in satisfactory position, a well-padded plaster of Paris cast should be applied and the position confirmed by x-rays through the cast.

B. Application of a temporary splint, control of pain and immediate transfer for orthopedic care are indicated if:

1. Associated fractures are present.
2. There is marked displacement of the epiphysis.
3. Any of the epiphyses around the elbow joint are involved. Special orthopedic evaluation is indicated in all injuries of this type.
4. The capital epiphysis of the femur is loose or displaced even slightly; this condition practically always requires operative reduction and fixation.
5. Reduction is unstable.
6. Sufficient cooperation to allow proper application of a cast cannot be obtained.

45–8. Fractures

A. All severe bone injuries require control of pain and

shock (Topic 15–7) as soon as possible. If a case is too difficult or too lengthy for the attending physician to handle on an emergency basis, a splint, support or cast should be applied and arrangements made for care by an orthopedist at once. DO NOT SPLINT AND TELL THE PATIENT TO REPORT THE FOLLOWING DAY. In 24 hours swelling and spasm are maximal, use of local anesthesia unsatisfactory, and adequate reduction much more difficult.

B. Morphine sulfate, 8 to 15 mg., or dihydromorphinone hydrochloride (Dilaudid), 2 mg., should be given subcutaneously at least 15 minutes before any attempt at reduction. In children 2 years of age or younger a pentobarbital sodium (Nembutal) suppository, 30 to 60 mg., should be substituted. In older children the dose of narcotic should be adjusted carefully to the age (Topic 5). Head injuries —apparent or suspected (Topic 43)—and severe crushing or penetrating chest injuries (Topic 31) are contraindications to the use of any narcotic.

C. The following fractures can often be treated in an emergency setting, with follow-up orthopedic care in 24 hours:

1. FRACTURES OF THE NASAL BONES OR CARTILAGES. See Topic 46–4.

2. FRACTURES OF THE UPPER OR LOWER JAW WITHOUT DISPLACEMENT OR DISTURBANCE OF DENTAL OCCLUSION. These require only control of pain and application of a four-tailed bandage, with reference to a dental surgeon for definitive care. (Also see Topic 26–7,C.)

3. FRACTURES OF THE CLAVICLE. Reduction of closed transverse or diagonal fractures of the medial three-quarters, even with considerable displacement or overriding, can generally be obtained by proper application of a clavicular cross or figure-of-eight bandage of stockinette and adhesive, reinforced if necessary with plaster of Paris. Fractures of the distal quarter require only a Velpeau bandage or a snug sling. Check x-rays should be taken in 24 hours, and be fol-

lowed by any modifications necessary to improve the position. Compound (open) and comminuted clavicular fractures require hospitalization.

4. Avulsion fractures (nondisplaced) of the greater tuberosity of the humerus. A Velpeau bandage plus anodynes for control of pain is all that is necessary.

5. Greenstick fractures. In these cases misalignment can generally be corrected without difficulty by manipulation after injection of 1% procaine or lidocaine (Xylocaine) into the hematoma at the fracture site. Position after reduction and application of plaster should always be checked by x-rays. Circulation and sensation should always be rechecked in 24 hours.

6. Fractures of transverse processes of the lumbar vertebrae are always painful but rarely serious, although injury to underlying intra-abdominal organs (Topic 55–1) must always be ruled out. Partial immobilization by strapping or application of a lumbosacral belt may decrease the pain. The site of the fracture may be infiltrated with 1% procaine or lidocaine (Xylocaine). The patient should be instructed to sleep on a hard bed. Anodynes as needed are in order, since any motion of the back may be very painful for 7 to 10 days after injury. Excessive application of local heat should be avoided. Cold may be beneficial.

7. Fractures of the ribs and sternum.
   a. Linear fractures of the sternum or fractures of one or two ribs without displacement usually require nothing but heat and anodynes. Strapping of the chest is ineffective and may result in the development of a traumatic pneumonitis. Infiltration of the hematoma at the site of the fracture with 1% procaine or lidocaine (Xylocaine) will lessen discomfort on breathing, as will blocking of the intercostal nerves proximal to the fractures.
   b. Marked displacement, multiple fractures (Topic 31–2,B), very severe pain, or evidence of trau-

matic pneumothorax (Topic 31–4) requires
immediate hospital care.

8. FRACTURES INVOLVING THE WRIST JOINT [COLLES',
   REVERSED COLLES' (SMITH'S)]. If comminution,
   displacement, misalignment or distortion of the
   articular surface of the wrist is present, accurate
   reduction is essential for a satisfactory functional result. Injection of 1% procaine or lidocaine (Xylocaine) into the joint and into the
   hematoma usually gives satisfactory anesthesia.
   Restoration of the correct angle of the articular
   surface and of the length of the radius is necessary; if not obtained under local anesthesia, the
   patient should be hospitalized for general anesthesia. If a satisfactory reduction (checked by
   x-ray or fluoroscopy) is obtained, a plaster cast
   (with pressure points well padded) extending
   from the upper third of the humerus to the
   proximal interphalangeal joints (including the
   base of the proximal phalanx of the thumb)
   should be applied with the elbow at 90 degrees
   and the forearm in neutral position. If an adequate, stable reduction has been obtained, the
   wrist should be immobilized in optimum grasp-
   ing position (slight dorsiflexion and slight ulnar
   deviation). After the cast has set, sensation and
   circulation should be checked carefully and x-
   rays taken. Tests of sensation and circulation
   should be repeated in 24 hours. In all cases follow-up care should be arranged so that in adults
   the cast can be shortened in 7 to 10 days to
   allow active motion of the thumb and fingers
   after pain, spasm and swelling have subsided.
   Shortening the cast is not necessary in children.

9. FRACTURES OF THE CARPAL (NAVICULAR) SCAPHOID.
   If marked comminution or displacement is present, a temporary splint should be applied and
   the patient referred at once for orthopedic care.
   If the position is satisfactory, a padded plaster
   short arm cast extending from just below the
   elbow to the metacarpophalangeal joints of the
   fingers and to the distal joint of the thumb

should be applied with the wrist in slight cock-up position and the thumb fully abducted. Follow-up orthopedic care for a lengthy period is indicated because of the danger of aseptic necrosis and nonunion.

10. FRACTURES OF THE OTHER CARPAL BONES. Immobilization by a padded arm and hand cast is all that is necessary unless comminution or displacement of fragments or associated dislocations [see 45–5,B,9, above (*Lunate Dislocations*) and 45–5, B,12, above (*Perilunar Dislocations*)] and soft tissue damage make hospitalization for orthopedic care in order.

11. FRACTURE OF THE METACARPALS.

a. *Without Displacement.* Apply a padded plaster cast, take check x-rays, check for sensory and circulatory changes and refer for orthopedic care in 24 hours. EXCEPTION: Bennett's fracture (Topic 42–4,A,3,c).

b. *With Displacement.* Angulation, overriding or comminution generally requires orthopedic care for reduction. Fractures of the distal ends of the second to fifth metacarpals (usually the fifth) are the exception. These "boxer's" fractures can usually be reduced without difficulty under local anesthesia injected into the hematoma, with correction of the volar angulation of the distal fragment by firm dorsal pressure using the proximal phalanx flexed to 90 degrees as a lever (Topic 42–4,A,3,b). Direct traction in the long axis of the metacarpal is useless in fractures of this type.

12. FRACTURES OF THE CARPAL PHALANGES

a. *Proximal or Middle Phalanges.* Apply an aluminum splint in corrected position (after reduction under local anesthesia if necessary) and refer for orthopedic care in 24 hours. Acute flexion is required if a fracture of a middle phalanx is distal to the attachment of the tendon of the flexor sublimus.

b. *Distal Phalanges.* A protective aluminum guard is all that is necessary. A throbbing subungual hematoma may require evacuation (Topic 42–3,C). For treatment of avulsion of the extensor tendon attachment (baseball finger), see Topic 42–4,A,5,b.

13. FRACTURES AROUND THE KNEE

    a. *Avulsion Fractures* due to partial tearing loose of the attachments of the collateral ligaments should be casted in a position which will relax the injured ligament, using a padded cast from the groin to the toes, with the knee slightly flexed and the ankle at 90 degrees. Follow-up orthopedic care is essential.

    b. *Plateau Fractures* without displacement: same as avulsion fractures, above.

    c. *Patellar Fractures* without separation or displacement of fragments require a well-padded, skin-anchored walking cast (groin to 2 inches above the ankle), with the knee in full extension.

    d. *Tibial Tubercle Fragmentation* (Osgood-Schlatter disease) is characterized by pain over the tibial tubercle on local pressure or contraction of the quadriceps femoris. X-rays of this condition may show the characteristic "crow beak" deformity but more often epiphysial fragmentation only. The treatment is the same as given under avulsion fractures, above.

14. TIBIAL SHAFT FRACTURES. If the fracture is relatively transverse (not spiral or oblique) and there is no displacement or misalignment, a long leg cast —groin to toes—should be applied with the knee in slight flexion and the ankle and foot at 90 degrees. Check x-rays must be taken and the patient referred for orthopedic care in 24 hours.

15. FRACTURES AROUND THE ANKLE JOINT

    a. *Avulsion or Sprain Fractures* should be immobilized in a plaster short leg cast with felt pressure pads over the injured area and other pressure points and the foot in 7 to 10 degrees plantar flexion. The foot should be inverted or everted to relax the injured collateral ligament. Although injection of a local anesthetic and manipulation to demonstrate widening of the ankle mortise is a valuable diagnostic aid, it SHOULD NOT BE DONE AS A THERAPEUTIC MEASURE (45–13,A, below).

   b. *Malleolar Fractures* without displacement of fragments or distortion of the ankle mortise may be treated by a short leg cast. Bimalleolar or trimalleolar fractures require hospitalization for reduction, as do any fractures resulting in distortion of the normal shape or width of the ankle joint.

16. Os CALCIS FRACTURES. Incomplete or linear fractures without displacement should be placed in a padded, well-molded, short leg cast and referred for orthopedic care within 12 hours. Any comminution, subastragaloid involvement or change in Boehler's angle makes hospitalization for manipulation and reduction necessary.

17. TARSAL AND METATARSAL FRACTURES. If the bones are in good position with preservation of the normal arch, a padded plaster short leg cast with the foot plate molded to the arch should be applied. If there is overriding or malposition of the fragments, or if several fractures are present, referral for orthopedic care is in order.

18. FRACTURES OF THE GREAT TOE

   a. *Proximal Phalanx.* These fractures often require hospitalization, since rotation and displacement of the distal fragment, which is very difficult to reduce and control, may be present. If the fragments are stable and alignment is satisfactory, a short leg cast with a heavy platform sole may be applied and arrangements made for orthopedic care within 2 to 3 days.

   b. *Distal Phalanx.* A cut-out shoe and metatarsal bar are generally all that is necessary.

19. FRACTURES OF THE PHALANGES OF THE SECOND TO FIFTH DIGITS OF THE FOOT. Strapping of the injured digit to its neighbor, a cut-out shoe and a metatarsal bar will generally allow the patient to continue with normal activity.

20. SACRAL AND COCCYGEAL FRACTURES may require hospitalization for a few days for control of acute pain. Usually, however, strapping the buttocks together or prescription of a rubber chair ring will allow home care. Sitz baths may be of benefit.

D. Immediate Transfer to a Hospital for Care (after administration of shock therapy and application of a splint if necessary) is required in the following types of fractures:

1. All compound (open) fractures except those of the distal phalanges of the fingers (Topic 42–4,A,5) and toes.

2. All fractures with marked comminution, displacement or overriding.

3. All skull fractures, suspected from history or clinical findings or proved by x-rays, in adults (Topic 43–12). In children (Topic 48–28), home care of linear or nondepressed fractures may be feasible if neurologic signs are absent and if the parents can be depended upon to recognize and report at once any changes in condition.

4. All cervical spine fractures, with or without evidence of spinal cord damage, suspected or proved (Topic 47–7).

5. All fractures of the dorsal and lumbar spine except transverse processes (45–8,C,6, above).

6. Rib fractures if multiple, comminuted, or markedly displaced (Topic 31–2) or associated with signs of pleural perforation or lung damage (Topic 31–4).

7. Sternal fractures with depression of fragments or evidence of mediastinal bleeding (Topic 31–2).

8. All fractures involving the head, neck, shaft or distal end of the humerus except incomplete or nondisplaced avulsion fractures of the greater tuberosity (45–8,C,4, above) and greenstick fractures without misalignment (45,8,C,5, above).

9. All pelvic fractures, with or without comminution, displacement or signs of bladder, urethral or intra-abdominal damage.

10. Bennett's fracture of the thumb (Topic 42–4,A,3,c).

11. Multiple carpal or metacarpal fractures with comminution, displacement or overriding (Topic 42–4,A,1,2 and 3).

12. Fractures of the shafts of both the radius and ulna, with displacement or overriding.

13. Shattering fractures of the radial head with depression or loss of contour of the articular surface. Small chip fractures require only use of a sling for 2 to 3 weeks with active motion within painless limits.

14. Olecranon fractures with comminution or separation of the fragments.

15. All fractures in and around the hip joint or acetabulum.

16. All fractures of the shaft or condyles of the femur. These fractures have a tendency to cause severe, sometimes delayed, shock. Supportive measures (Topic 15–7) before and during the transportation are always indicated, whether or not signs and symptoms of shock are present.

17. All complete oblique, spiral or other unstable fractures of the shaft of the tibia even though there may be no displacement or overriding.

18. Plateau fractures of the tibia with depression or distortion of the articular surface.

19. All fractures around the ankle resulting in mortise widening or distortion [avulsion fractures ("sprain-fractures"), fracture dislocations, bimalleolar and trimalleolar fractures].

20. Multiple tarsal or metatarsal fractures with comminution, displacement or overriding.

21. Fractures of the great toe [except the distal phalanx (45–8,C,18, above)].

22. Comminuted or displaced fractures of the upper or lower jaws.

45–9. **Myalgia.**

Also see 45–1, above (*Arthritis*). Muscle pain severe enough to require emergency treatment may be the result of a large number of conditions, including direct or indirect trauma, metabolic disturbances, postural strain, acute infections and certain poisons.

A. Treatment

1. Treatment of poisoning, if a toxic substance is the causative agent (Topic 49). Slow intravenous injection of 10 ml. of 10% calcium gluconate solution is very effective in control of this type of myalgia.
2. Control of pain by salicylates and codeine sulfate orally.
3. Local application of heat or, if better tolerated, cold.
4. Spraying of the skin over the painful areas with ethyl chloride.
5. Infiltration of painful myofibrositic nodules with 1% procaine or lidocaine (Xylocaine).
6. d-Tubocurarine chloride in a repository medium (Tubadil) intramuscularly, 1 ml. (containing 25 mg. of d-tubocurarine chloride) per 70 kilograms (154 lbs.) of body weight, if muscle spasm is present. Heat and massage to the site of injection increases the rate of absorption and should be avoided.
7. Reference for investigation and treatment of the underlying cause.

B. Special Types of Myalgia

1. NOCTURNAL CRAMPS ("Jumpy Legs"). Cramping in the leg muscles severe enough to interfere with sleep may occur in any age group but is more common in children and persons beyond 50. Fatigue probably is a causative factor. Treatment of severe cases consists of slow intravenous administration of 10 ml. of 10% calcium gluconate. In milder cases the patient should be instructed to take calcium lactate, 0.6 gm., by mouth three times a day. Methoxyphenamine hydrochloride (Orthoxine), 100 mg., by mouth at bedtime, may give complete relief.
2. "SHIN SPLINTS" occur in athletes, especially sprinters and hurdlers, and may cause very severe pain—probably from a combination of tendinitis and myofascitis.

TREATMENT

   a. Anodynes and sedatives for severe pain.
   b. Limited activity—complete rest if practical.

     c. Application of an elastic bandage.

     d. Reference to an orthopedist for physical therapy and instructions concerning strapping during exercise.

  3. MAGNESIUM DEFICIENCY, usually in chronic alcoholics and asthenic persons, may cause leg cramps, tremors and acutely painful paresthesias, especially burning sensations in the feet.

TREATMENT

     Magnesium sulfate, 2 gm., intramuscularly three or four times a day usually gives rapid and complete relief.

45–10. Myofibrositis.

Also see 45–9, above (*Myalgia*). Both acute myofibrositis, characterized by spasm, limitation of motion and muscle tenderness, and chronic myofibrositis, characterized by loss of normal elasticity, a "doughy" feeling on palpation and "trigger nodules" in the substance of the muscle, can cause severe discomfort.

Treatment

  1. Immobilization if muscle spasm is acute. In the cervical area a Thomas collar is effective, in the low back a lumbosacral belt will relieve discomfort.

  2. Anodynes. Codeine sulfate may be required.

  3. Muscle relaxants orally or, in severe cases, intramuscularly.

  4. Local application of heat or cold, depending upon tolerance.

  5. Injection of "trigger nodules" with a local anesthetic.

  6. Reference for physical therapy. Ultrasonic therapy is very effective after the acute stage.

45–11. Neck injuries

Severe injury to the neck should always be suspected and ruled out by careful clinical and x-ray examination whenever:

  1. There is a history of direct trauma to the head or neck, especially when the neck was flexed at the time of injury.

  2. The patient was riding in a moving or stationary vehicle which was involved in a collision.

  3. Any story is obtained of pain or sensory disturbances, no matter how transient, in the back of the head

or in the neck, shoulders or arms following a sudden jerking strain.

A. Fractures and Dislocations must be ruled out by careful clinical and x-ray examination before the patient is allowed to move his head or neck or to sit up. All questionable cases should be hospitalized BY AMBULANCE if clinical examination suggests the possibility of cervical fracture or dislocation, even if x-rays are negative. The patient's head should be supported in a neutral position BY THE PHYSICIAN OR A TRAINED ATTENDANT when the patient is moved from or to a stretcher. Ambulance transportation with the patient flat on his back—the head immobilized by sandbags—is relatively safe. The ambulance crew should be told that smoothness, NOT SPEED, is essential.

B. Severe Strains ("Whiplash" Injuries). A sudden jerk to the neck may cause extensive soft tissue damage and acute symptoms, often deferred for 12 to 24 hours, which are apparently out of all proportion to the trauma alleged to have been sustained. Acute soft tissue injuries often cannot be differentiated from fracture or dislocation and may require hospitalization for observation and special x-ray studies. Mild cases can be treated by partial immobilization by a Thomas collar, with application of heat (or cold) and gentle massage at home. Traction by means of a Sayre sling may be beneficial. The pain is often severe enough to require codeine or morphine sulfate hypodermically for relief. d-Tubocurarine chloride in a repository medium (Tubadil), 1 to 2 ml. intramuscularly, usually will relieve acute muscle spasm.

Posttraumatic symptoms (neck pain, limitation of motion, headache, dizziness) persist for a lengthy time after posterior cervical strains and require prolonged treatment for relief.

45–12. Peritendinitis

Also see 45–3, above (*Bursitis*). Whether or not x-rays show amorphous calcification in the affected area (usually the shoulder or hip), palliative treatment is all that can be given as an emergency measure. When the pain is extremely acute hospitalization for treatment is indicated, but relief (or, at least, decrease in acute discomfort) can often be obtained by:

A. Hot or cold packs. Heat is beneficial in the majority of cases but occasionally is unbearable.

B. Spraying with ethyl chloride.

C. Codeine sulfate, 0.03 to 0.06 gm., and acetylsalicylic acid (aspirin), 0.6 gm., orally every 2 to 4 hours usually will control pain; occasionally morphine sulfate, 10 to 15 mg., or dihydromorphinone hydrochloride (Dilaudid), 2 mg., subcutaneously may be necessary.

D. Infiltration with 1% procaine or lidocaine (Xylocaine) with or without hydrocortisone acetate. The patient should be warned that this procedure may result in a temporary flare-up of symptoms after the local anesthetic effect has worn off.

E. Application of a Velpeau bandage (a sling is usually not enough) if the shoulder is involved. Crutches may be necessary if the structures around the hip are affected.

45–13. **Sprains**

A. *Mild Sprains.* Patients with injuries with relatively minor ligamentous and soft tissue damage often request treatment after 24 to 48 hours because increased edema and pain have developed. In many cases involving the extremities, instructions regarding limitation of activity, compresses or soaks at home (cold if within 24 hours, hot if later) and the application of an elastic bandage are all that is required. Adhesive strapping should be avoided as much as possible; if it is applied, it should not cover any part of any subcutaneous tendon such as the heel cord. Severe cases may require casting in a position which relaxes the damaged ligaments. Round-and-round strapping should never be applied.

Unless there is a specific indication for the procedure, ambulation after injection of the structures around a weight-bearing joint with a local anesthetic should be prohibited because of the danger of the development of an unstable joint from healing of the ligaments in a lax position with resultant recurrent sprains and strains.

B. Severe Sprains

1. Avulsion type fractures should be ruled out by x-rays, especially in industrial injuries (Topic 76) and potential public liability cases (Topic 68).

2. Splinting by bias-cut stockinette or elastic bandages, metallic trough splints or plaster of Paris may be indicated. The patient should be given crutches if a severe strain involves a lower extremity and weight bearing causes pain.

3. If a cast is applied, it should be done as soon as possible after the injury before posttraumatic swelling has developed.

45–14. Tendon injuries

All lacerations, stab wounds and puncture wounds should be checked carefully by tests of function for tendon damage. A severe contusion may cause severance by compression of a tendon against a bony prominence. Tendons (especially the biceps in the arm and the soleus in the calf) may rupture as a result of severe muscle strain.

Treatment

A. All Cases of Suspected or Proved Tendon Severance should be referred for hospitalization and surgical care with the exception of:

1. Incomplete severances—these can be easily repaired under local anesthesia.

2. Extensor tendons of the fingers without retraction (Topic 42–8,B,3).

3. Extensor tendons (dorsiflexors) of the second to fifth digits of the foot without retraction. These can easily be repaired under local anesthesia using the Koch or Bunnell technique.

4. Severance of the palmaris longus tendon. No repair is necessary because this tendon is vestigial and serves no useful function in the wrist or hand.

5. Severance of the flexor tendons of the second to fifth digits of the foot. These do not require repair.

6. Rupture of the soleus tendon. Application of a plaster cast from the knee to the toes with the ankle in moderate plantar flexion is usually required, with referral to an orthopedist for follow-up care.

B. Traumatic Tendinitis
Treatment
1. Application of cold compresses to decrease edema and lessen acute pain.
2. Limitation of motion by strapping, splinting or casting.
3. Anodynes.
4. Reference for follow-up care.

C. Acute Tenosynovitis. Ambulatory treatment consisting of splinting, anodynes and antibiotics may be tried. Hospitalization is indicated if:
1. The infection is extending in spite of conservative therapy.
2. The patient will not cooperate in limitation of activity.
3. Incision and drainage are indicated.

46. NASAL CONDITIONS

46–1. **Aerosinusitis (sinus squeeze)**
Common in sports divers (Topic 26), this painful condition characterized by collection of bloody exudate within the sinuses is due to the effect of increased barometric pressure on partially blocked ostia.
Treatment
1. Avoidance of diving until all evidence of infection and edema have disappeared—usually 4 to 6 weeks.
2. Insurance of adequate sinus drainage by frequent use of decongestant nose drops. Sinus washing or drainage should not be done; antibiotics are of little, if any, value.

46–2. **Contusions**
Treatment
1. Rule out fractures of the skull, nasal cartilages or nasal bones by thorough clinical and x-ray examination. Injection of 150 TRU of hyaluronidase in 1% procaine or lidocaine (Xylocaine)

into the swollen areas will decrease edema and
allow more accurate evaluation.

2. Instruct the patient to apply cold compresses or an
icebag at frequent intervals during the first 24
hours; after 24 hours local heat should be substituted.

3. Refer the patient to an otolaryngologist if the swelling persists or if crepitation in the soft tissues
is present.

46–3. Epistaxis (nosebleed)

A. Nontraumatic Epistaxis may be caused by varicosities,
telangiectasis, hypertension, nasal polyps, abrasions
from nose-picking, tuberculosis, malignant disease,
hemophilia, acute infectious diseases, etc. The
emergency treatment is the same for all conditions:

1. Upright position to allow drainage.
2. Pressure on the nostrils with the fingers.
3. Mouth breathing.
4. Avoidance of blowing the nose.
5. Wedging of a pad of gauze, cotton or paper tissue
between the upper teeth and the upper lip.
6. Insertion of a gauze strip saturated with 1:1000
epinephrine hydrochloride (Adrenalin) solution
into the bleeding nostril.
7. Packing of the anterior nares with a sterile gauze
strip or petrolatum gauze (Topic 17–6,A). DO
NOT use iodoform or other medicated gauze.
8. Insertion of a posterior nasal pack. For technique
see Topic 17–6,B.
9. Intravenous injection of 20 mg. of sodium estrone
sulfate (Premarin) if oozing is present. Repeat
in one hour if necessary.
10. Hospitalization if the bleeding cannot be controlled
by the measures given above. Blood loss may be
sufficient to require treatment of shock (Topic
15–7) before transportation.

B. Traumatic Epistaxis. If there is any possibility that the
drainage from the nose following injury is a mixture of blood and spinal fluid, no packing or medication of any type should be inserted into the
nostrils. The case should be treated as a SKULL
FRACTURE and the patient hospitalized AT ONCE.

The presence of rhinorrhea can sometimes be confirmed by placing a drop of the bloody fluid on a white blotter; the presence of a light pink area around a darkened center indicates the presence of spinal fluid. For treatment, see 46–3,A, above.

46–4. **Fractures of the nasal bones and cartilages**
Treatment

1. Simple displaced fractures can usually be restored to normal alignment by digital manipulation. If depression is present, the fragment can be elevated by pressure with a blunt padded instrument within the nostrils.

2. Comminuted, compound (open) or depressed fractures, especially those which result in marked septal deviation or distortion, should be referred to an otolaryngologist for reduction and follow-up care.

46–5. **Hematomas**

If untreated or if treatment is delayed, hematomas may result in permanent saddling of the bridge. The patient should be referred to an otolaryngologist as soon as presence of a hematoma (usually septal or between the lateral cartilages and the nasal bone) is recognized. If a delay in treatment is anticipated, prophylaxis against tetanus (Topic 19) and antibiotics are indicated.

46–6. **Lacerations**

See Topic 55–20,B, for general principles of treatment. Since the nose is in the "danger zone," prophylaxis against tetanus (Topic 19) and antibiotics should be given routinely.

46–7. **Septal injuries**

All cases with septal deviation or distortion require care by an otolaryngologist.

47. NEUROLOGIC DISORDERS

47–1. **Coma of undetermined origin**

The neurologic emergency which probably requires the most careful immediate thought for correct management, diagnosis and treatment is deep coma of undetermined origin. A preset schedule, such as that outlined below, is essential for handling cases of this type.

A. Check vital signs (heart rate, respiratory rate and type, blood pressure, rectal temperature).

B. Clear and maintain an adequate airway with the patient prone or semiprone.

C. Maintain adequate ventilation (Topic 17–1) and circulation (Topic 17–2).

D. If no one is available to give any accurate information, delegate some person (preferably with professional experience) to trace, if possible and as soon as possible, the patient's background. This should include:

  1. Location where patient was found, and the circumstances.

  2. State of consciousness when found.

  3. Presence of medications, or instruments for their use.

  4. History of prior episodes of coma.

  5. Condition and complaints before development of coma.

E. Observe the patient closely—first fully clothed, then completely undressed—covering the following points:

  1. Clothing—mud, blood, semen, grease, grass, corrosive agents or other stains; alcohol or other odors; holes or tears; burns.

  2. Identification data—"dog tags" around neck or on wrist.

  3. Skin (including scalp)—puncture wounds, ticks, thermal or electric burns, contusions, ecchymoses, pallor, sweating, cyanosis of lips or fingernails, swellings, effusions, laceration of the genitalia, evidence of pregnancy.

  4. Musculoskeletal misalignment.

  5. Breath—alcohol, acetone, uremia, carbon tetrachloride, gasoline, the "musty" odor of hepatic failure.

  6. Respiratory pattern—rate, rhythm, paradoxical respiration, use of accessory muscles.

  7. The patient as a whole—make-up, tattooing, type of clothing, body hygiene, expression.

F. Draw a specimen of blood for:

  1. Hematocrit.

2. White blood count and differential.
3. Typing and cross-matching.
4. Blood chemistry.
    a. Glucose
    b. Blood urea nitrogen (BUN)
    c. CO_2
    d. pH and serum acetone.
5. Save 5 ml. of blood serum.

G. Start an intravenous infusion of 5% dextrose in water or saline, preferably with a plastic radiopaque intravenous catheter.

H. Perform a complete physical and neurologic examination covering the following points:
1. Sensorium.
2. Cranial nerves.
3. Cerebellar and meningeal signs.
4. Motor and sensory responses.
5. Reflexes:
    a. Superficial—corneal, abdominal, cremasteric and rectal sphincter.
    b. Deep tendon reflexes—biceps, triceps, patellar, Achilles.
    c. Pathologic.

I. Catheterize (Topic 17–3); leave Foley catheter in place.
1. Note volume output in 15 minutes; save for 24-hour specimen.
2. Routine urinalysis (specific gravity, pH, color, proteins, sugar and acetone and microscopic examination).

J. Lavage the stomach; save a specimen of aspirate for later analysis if indicated.

K. Recheck the mouth, rectum and vagina as depositories for foreign bodies and toxic substances.

L. Perform a lumbar puncture unless contraindicated. Examine cerebrospinal fluid at once for:
1. Pressure.
2. Color and turbidity.
3. Protein and sugar content.
4. Cells (including Gram stain).
    Save a specimen of cerebrospinal fluid for culture if indicated.

M. Take x-rays as indicated, but only if necessary positioning will not be harmful to the patient.

1. Skull series. One lateral should be taken on a large enough film to show any gross misalignment of the cervical spine.

2. Chest films if signs of thoracic or pulmonary pathology have been noted.

3. Areas of suspected injury as based on physical examination.

N. Take electrocardiogram for evaluation of cardiac status and for information regarding electrolytic balance (Topic 7).

O. Continue observation and investigation until a definite reason for coma has been determined. MORE THAN ONE FACTOR MAY BE CONTRIBUTORY!

P. Institute specific therapy as indicated while continuing diligent supportive therapy.

47–2. **Coma due to specific causes.** See also Topic 3.

A. *Bacterial Infections.* See Topic 32–16; Topic 48–38 (*Meningococcemia in Children*); and Topic 48–59 (*Waterhouse-Friderichsen Syndrome in Children*).

B. *Cerebrovascular Emergencies.* See Topic 43, Topic 60–2 (*Intracranial Bleeding*); Topic 60–3 (*Embolism*); and Topic 60–6 (*Thrombosis*).

C. *Convulsive Seizures.* See Topic 3–7 (*Epilepsy*); and Topic 33.

D. *Hypertensive Encephalopathy*

1. SIGNS AND SYMPTOMS
   a. Convulsions.
   b. Coma.
   c. Visual changes.
   d. Acute rise in blood pressure.
   e. Disappearance of neurologic signs on reduction of blood pressure.

2. TREATMENT
   a. Begin reduction of blood pressure by intramuscular injection of 2 to 4 mg. of reserpine. Start with the smaller dose in moderate cases or if the presence of azotemia is suspected.
   b. Hospitalize as soon as possible for close monitoring of the patient's neurologic, cardiac and

renal status and possible administration of ganglionic blocking agents.

E. Injury

1. EPIDURAL (EXTRADURAL) HEMORRHAGE. See Topic 43–20 and Topic 48–22 (*Extradural Hemorrhage in Children*).

2. HEAD INJURIES. See Topic 43.

3. SUBDURAL HEMORRHAGE. See Topic 43–21 and Topic 48–8 (*Brain Injuries in Children*).

47–3. **Myasthenia gravis**

A. Signs and Symptoms

1. Paresis of pharyngeal, oculomotor, facial and respiratory muscles. Skeletal muscles are involved in advanced stages.

2. Marked fatigability.

3. Aggravation of symptoms by stress.

4. Emergency situations usually related to aspiration of food, respiratory failure or infection.

B. Treatment

1. Place the patient in the recumbent position.

2. Clear the airway and support ventilation (Topic 17–1).

3. Give neostigmine, 0.5 to 1.0 mg., intramuscularly (unless the patient is a known myosthenic or neostigmine overdosage is suspected).

4. Inject edrophonium chloride (Tensilon), 10 mg. intravenously or 25 mg. intramuscularly. As a diagnostic measure 3 mg. intravenously will cause improvement in a myasthenia gravis crisis but will cause no change in neostigmine overdosage.

47–4. **Neuritis (neuralgia)**

Although many conditions (infections, trauma, toxins, viruses, poisons, pressure, etc.) may cause irritation and pain along the course and distribution of various nerves, the discomfort in most cases is not severe enough to bring the patient for emergency treatment. The chief exceptions are as follows:

A. Alcoholic Neuritis. Occurring mostly in female chronic alcoholics, the extreme discomfort caused by toxic neuritis from alcohol often requires prolonged hospital therapy. Control and sedation as indicated under Topic 36–3 (*Delirium Tremens*) is all that is indicated as an emergency measure.

B. Arsenical Neuritis. See Topic 49–63 (*Arsenic*).

C. Bell's Palsy (Peripheral Facial Nerve Paralysis)

Signs and Symptoms

1. Inability to close the eye, wrinkle the forehead or elevate the corner of the mouth on the affected side.
2. Drooling of saliva from the mouth.
3. Development of clinical picture following chilling or injury of the involved side.

Treatment

1. Immediate administration of 60 mg. of prednisone daily in divided doses for 2 or 3 days, then gradual tapering off over a 7- to 10-day period.
2. Application of an eye patch with a bland ophthalmic ointment.
3. Protection of the involved side from wind and cold.
4. Instruction in measures to prevent loss of facial muscle tone (upward massage, taping, etc.). Electrical stimulation may be indicated.

D. Causalgia. Severe burning causalgia following trauma probably has a reflex neuritic component. Relief can sometimes be obtained by oral administration of tolazoline hydrochloride (Priscoline), 25 to 50 mg., every 4 hours. More severe cases usually require a series of sympathetic blocks.

E. Herpes Zoster. (For eye involvement see Topic 37–14,B.)

Treatment

1. Protection of lesions from infection by:
   a. Petrolatum gauze or dibucaine (Nupercaine) ointment dressings.
   b. Dusting with thymol iodide.
2. Control of pain, if moderate, by sedation and analgesics; if severe, by codeine or morphine sulfate subcutaneously.
3. Administration of antibiotic therapy if bacterial infection is a complicating factor.
4. Hospitalization if the pain is severe or the lesions extensive.

F. Meniere's Disease
Treatment

1. MILD CASES
   a. Sedation through barbiturates.
   b. Control of pain during attacks by analgesics and codeine sulfate. Addictive opiates and synthetic narcotics should be avoided.
   c. Administration of dimenhydrinate (Dramamine), 50 to 100 mg., by mouth three times a day.
   d. Low sodium diet and diuretics may be helpful.
   e. Reference to an otolaryngologist.

2. SEVERE CASES
   a. Control of severe pain by morphine sulfate or dihydromorphinone hydrochloride (Dilaudid) subcutaneously, provided the patient has none of the stigmata of addiction (Topic 2–4).
   b. Hospitalization at once.

G. Peripheral Neuritis during Pregnancy is usually associated with pernicious vomiting (Topic 50–11).

H. Retrobulbar Neuritis
Signs and Symptoms

1. Headache and ocular pain on the affected side. Increase of ocular pain with eye motion or pressure.
2. Rapid impairment of vision—blurring and central scotomata.
3. Normal external appearance of the affected eye. Disk normal early; later, injection and blurring of margins.
4. Slow temporary constriction of the affected pupil in response to light.

Treatment

1. Prednisone, 60 mg., orally in a loading dose and then daily in divided doses. Taper the dosage downward as soon as improvement begins.
2. Referral to an ophthalmologist.

I. Sciatica
Treatment

1. Local application of heat or cold as tolerated. Massage usually causes an increase in discomfort.
2. Application of a lumbosacral belt.
3. Muscle relaxants in large doses every 4 hours by mouth for relaxation of mild spasm. In severe

cases with acute spasm d-tubocurarine chloride in a repository medium (Tubadil), 1 to 2 ml., intramuscularly may be of value. Local heat and massage to the site of injection should not be applied if this drug is used; too rapid absorption can cause dangerous respiratory depression [Topic 49–168 (*Curare*)].

4. Salicylates and codeine sulfate by mouth for pain. In severe cases morphine sulfate, 10 to 15 mg. subcutaneously, may be required. Sciatic pain is a frequent complaint of addicts; therefore, the patient should be checked carefully for evidence of addiction (Topic 2–4) before any narcotic is given.

5. Spraying of the painful areas with ethyl chloride.

6. Hospitalization if the pain is intractable and severe.

J. Trigeminal Neuralgia (Tic Douloureux)

Treatment

1. Control of pain by morphine sulfate or dihydromorphinone hydrochloride (Dilaudid) in the smallest possible effective doses. Sedatives and hypnotics are of no value. Because of its extreme toxicity trichlorethylene therapy should not be attempted as an emergency procedure.

2. Referral to a neurologist.

K. "Whiplash" Injuries of the Neck. (See also Topic 45–11,B.) Severe neuritis of the cervical nerves supplying the neck, head, shoulders, arms and hands may follow sudden jerking motions of the neck. In addition, irritation of the nervi vasorum may cause apparently unrelated pain through reflex mechanisms. Development of neuritic pain is often delayed for several days after injury.

Treatment. See Topic 45–11,B.

47–5. Paralysis

Loss of muscle power, partial or complete, sudden or progressive, usually results in a situation requiring emergency management.

A. Acute involvement of the muscles of deglutition may be caused by:

1. Botulism (Topic 49–97).

2. Diphtheria (Topic 32–4).

    3. Myasthenia gravis (47–3, above).
    4. Poliomyelitis, bulbar (Topic 32–21 and Topic 48–45).
    5. Tetanus (Topic 32–31).
    6. Brain or high cervical injuries.

B. Involvement of the muscles of respiration may occur in:
    1. Anterior poliomyelitis (Topic 32–21 and Topic 48–45).
    2. Cervical fractures and dislocations (C,5, or above).
    3. Head injuries involving the respiratory center in the medulla.
    4. Guillain-Barré syndrome (Topic 27–20,C).
    5. Acute intermittent porphyria (Topic 44–20).
    6. Familial periodic paralysis (47–5,F, below).
    7. Tick bites (Topic 27–20,C).
    8. Electric shock (Topic 3–5).
    9. Acute poisoning (Topic 3–13 and Topic 49).

Treatment
    Expired air respiration (Topic 17–1,A,B,C and D) or mechanical ventilation (Topic 17–1,F), often followed by tracheotomy (Topic 17–11) may be necessary as lifesaving measures. Neck injuries must be immobilized.

C. Paralysis of central nervous system origin may result from:
    1. Brain infarction or increased intracranial pressure resulting from cerebrovascular accidents (Topic 60–2).
    2. Space-consuming intracranial or cord tumors.
    3. Head injuries (Topic 43 and Topic 48–8 and 28).
    4. Vertebral fractures (Topic 45–8,D,5).
    5. Partial or complete dislocation of any portion of the spine (Topic 45–5).

D. Paralysis due to peripheral neuropathy may be caused by:
    1. Herniated intervertebral disk or discogenic disease.
    2. Neuritis.
      a. Metabolic.
      b. Toxic.
      c. Traumatic.
    3. Cauda equina syndrome.

E. *Hysterical Paralysis* (Topic 51–5) must always be considered if the exact causative factor is not known.

F. *Familial Periodic Paralysis.* This rare condition is characterized by recurrent episodes of profound paralysis and weakness associated with low serum potassium levels.

Treatment
1. Supportive therapy particularly for ventilation if involvement present.
2. Potassium chloride, 5 to 10 gms., by mouth.
3. Correction of severe hypokalemia and paralysis by slow (not to exceed 5 ml./min.) intravenous infusion of 500 ml. of 5% dextrose in water containing 3 gms. of potassium chloride (40 mEq. of potassium). Intermittent electrocardiographic monitoring is desirable (Topic 7).

G. No matter what the etiology may be, persons showing evidence of recent, progressive or extensive paralysis (except those who respond to simple emergency measures) should be hospitalized as soon as possible and receive appropriate supportive therapy enroute.

47–6. Peripheral nerve injury in the extremities
An injured peripheral nerve is recognized by the loss of motor function or sensory perception in areas usually innervated by that nerve. The location of injury can usually be determined by the presence of overlying soft tissue trauma or adjacent bone fracture and displacement.

Treatment
1. Splint the involved extremity.
2. Treat soft tissue injuries.
3. Refer to a surgeon for end-to-end anastomosis of completely severed nerves or decompression of severely compressed nerves.
4. Control of pain by anodynes or narcotics.
5. If possible, obtain an electromyogram in all cases of peripheral nerve injury as soon as possible after injury to rule out pre-existent pathology. This is particularly important in compensation cases (Topic 76). Degenerative changes do not develop until about 21 days after injury.

47–7. Spinal injuries and compression
See also under Topic 45–5 (*Dislocations*); Topic 45–8 (*Fractures*); and Topic 45–11 (*Neck Injuries*).

A. *Diagnosis.* All cases of suspected head or back injury, with or without a history of severe direct trauma, should be considered as possible cord injuries until the condition has been ruled out by careful general and neurologic examination. The following points should be checked at first examination of the patient:

1. Determine if possible the type of trauma sustained. Although relatively minor accidents may cause contusion or edema of the cord without fracture or dislocations, acute flexion and hyperextension injuries are more likely to result in cord damage.

2. Ask the patient where he hurts. Radicular pain is common with cord injuries, and careful localization of pain is very important.

3. Carefully palpate the spine, working downwards from the base of the skull, for:
   a. Deformity, especially prominence of a spinous process.
   b. Muscle spasm, guarding or fibrillation.
   c. Tenderness on pressure or percussion over the spinous processes.

4. Test for motion of extremities.

5. Check for reflex changes, abnormal reflexes and the condition of the sphincters.

6. Examine for sensory changes—test light touch, pain and vibratory sense.

7. If possible, take portable x-ray films of suspected areas, moving the patient as little as possible. As a rule, compression fractures are less likely to result in severe cord damage than fracture-dislocations and breaks through the laminae or pedicles. Serious cord embarrassment can be caused by contusion and compression as well as by partial or complete severance; therefore, careless handling during examination or transportation may result in irreparable damage.

B. Treatment

1. Immobilize the spine as much as possible by means of sandbags on each side of the head and body. Manual cervical traction or traction by a head halter may be necessary.

2. Treat for shock (Topic 15–7).

3. Transfer for hospitalization with immobilizing meas-

ures (sandbags, traction, etc.) in place. THE
ATTENDING PHYSICIAN SHOULD PERSON-
ALLY SUPERVISE LIFTING THE PATIENT
ONTO THE AMBULANCE STRETCHER. The
ambulance crew should be instructed specifically
that smoothness, not speed, is essential.

C. Compression without Trauma. Evidence of acute spinal
cord compression may occur in the absence of any
trauma. Spontaneous compression in these cases
is most frequently related to: epidural abscess,
collapse of a pathologic vertebral disk due to a
malignant process and, occasionally, spontaneous
hemorrhage. Treatment is as outlined above with
transfer for hospitalization and evaluation for appropriate surgical intervention.

D. Prognosis. No estimate of the amount of damage, or
of the permanence thereof, should ever be given,
based on emergency examination alone.

47–8. **Vertigo**

Vertigo may be objective (the environment seems to spin)
or subjective (the body seems to float or revolve in space) and
may be caused by any disturbance in any of the structures
(brain or end organs) concerned with transmission of the im-
pulses. Vertigo should be distinguished from dizziness which
is merely an unsteadiness caused by a sensation of motion
within the head.

Treatment. Removal or treatment of the cause of the vertigo
is the most important therapeutic measure. Although in some instances hospitalization is required, in many cases the following symptomatic
measures will give relief:

1. Bed rest.
2. Sedation by barbiturates, paraldehyde or bromides.
3. Intravenous administration of hypertonic dextrose
   solution.
4. Dimenhydrinate (Dramamine), 50 to 100 mg., by
   mouth.
5. Atropine sulfate, 0.4 to 0.6 mg., subcutaneously.
6. Chlorpromazine hydrochloride (Thorazine), 25 to 50
   mg., or prochlorperazine dimaleate (Compazine),
   5 to 10 mg., orally or intramuscularly.
7. Vitamin B_6 (pyridoxine hydrochloride), 25 to 50 mg.,
   intravenously.

48.　PEDIATRIC EMERGENCIES

Infants and children represent a relatively large proportion of emergency cases. Under certain circumstances, in these age groups, some conditions require a change from, or modification in, emergency therapy suitable for adults. Treatment for these conditions, and for some emergencies peculiar to children, is outlined in the subheadings under this topic. If the emergency treatment for any condition is the same for children and adults, or if treatment in children has been covered elsewhere, the topic number only is given for reference.

In all cases, drug dosages MUST be modified according to age (Topic 5) unless dosages by weight, age or skin surface area (S.A.) are specified.

48–1. **Accidents**

The home, especially the kitchen, is the most dangerous place in the world for children in the preschool age group. The highest accident rate is in children who are under the parents' "direct supervision." During the first years of life absolute protection of the child by the parents is essential; from then on, progressive education is necessary regarding the pull of gravity, the effects of heat, the inedibility of certain substances, and the unpleasant effects of water in the breathing apparatus. In one year in the United States alone, 15,000 children are killed, 50,000 are permanently injured, and at least 1,000,000 receive medical treatment for the results of home accidents, in most instances resulting directly from parental ignorance, carelessness or neglect.

For treatment see under the type of injury sustained.

48–2.　**Acidosis**

　A. Causes

　　1. Prolonged vomiting with subsequent dehydration from any cause.

　　2. Starvation.

　　3. Metabolic upsets.

　B. Treatment

　　1. Control of vomiting as outlined under *Alkalosis* (48–3, below).

2. Insurance of adequate oxygenation if dyspnea or cyanosis is present.

3. Hypodermoclysis or intravenous fluids as given under *Alkalosis* (48–3, below).

4. Immediate hospitalization of severe cases for laboratory evaluation and replacement therapy (Topic 7).

48–3.   Alkalosis may result in severe convulsions in children. Causes may be listed as follows:

A. Alkali Excess in the Blood
Treatment. Hospitalization for laboratory tests essential for determination of the therapy needed to restore the normal fluid-electrolyte balance (Topic 7).

B. Chloride Loss Due to Persistent Vomiting
Treatment
1. Nothing by mouth except cracked ice, or repeated sips of a cold carbonated beverage.

2. Complete rest. Sedation by a pentobarbital sodium (Nembutal) suppository may be necessary.

3. Chlorpromazine hydrochloride (Thorazine) intramuscularly, dose 0.5 mg. per kilogram of body weight. The effects of Thorazine in accentuating and prolonging the effects of sedatives and analgesics should be given due consideration.

4. Dextrose (2½%) in water and normal salt solution (equal parts) intravenously or by hypodermoclysis, 30 ml. per kilogram of body weight.

5. Hospitalization for laboratory determinations and correction of fluid-electrolyte imbalance (Topic 7).

C. Hyperventilation. See Topic 36–6.
D. Metabolic Abnormalities. (Also see Topic 44.)
Treatment
1. Administration of oxygen under positive pressure by oxygen tent or face mask and rebreathing bag.

2. Immediate hospitalization. Complex disturbances of sodium, potassium and chloride ions requiring careful replacement therapy (Topic 7) are usually present.

48–4.   Angioedema. [Also see Topic 24 (*Allergic Reactions*).]
Treatment
1. Epinephrine hydrochloride (Adrenalin), 0.2 ml. of

1:1000 solution subcutaneously, repeated at ½ hour intervals if necessary.

2. Diphenhydramine hydrochloride (Benadryl), 1 to 2 mg. per kilogram of body weight, subcutaneously.

3. Insertion of an endotracheal tube or performance of an emergency tracheotomy (Topic 17–11) if the edema involves the upper respiratory tract and is sufficient to prevent adequate aeration. If either procedure is done, hospitalization for follow-up care is indicated.

48–5. **Asphyxial states.** [See also Topic 25 (*Asphyxiation*).]

A. Asphyxia Neonatorum

1. MILD ASPHYXIA

SIGNS AND SYMPTOMS

a. Embarrassment of respiration.

b. Normal or rapid heart rate.

c. Normal muscle tone.

TREATMENT

a. Insurance of a clear airway by postural drainage, suction of the pharynx and trachea, and support of the angle of the jaw after ruling out the presence of foreign bodies (Topic 38–4).

b. Mouth-to-mouth respiration (Topic 17–1,A) if necessary, followed by administration of oxygen by tent or face mask.

c. Hospitalization as soon as possible.

2. MODERATE OR SEVERE ASPHYXIA

SIGNS AND SYMPTOMS

a. Extreme embarrassment or absence of respiration.

b. Heart rapid at first, then slowing terminally.

c. Poor muscle tone.

d. Skin livid or pale.

e. Gag reflex diminished or lost.

TREATMENT

a. Insurance of a clear airway by postural drainage, suction of the pharynx and trachea, and support of the jaw after examination for obstructive foreign bodies (Topic 38–4).

b. Direct inspection of the larynx. If the pharyngeal reflex is present and the vocal cords move, oxygen under positive pressure by face mask and rebreathing bag is indicated; if the pharyngeal reflex is absent, immediate endotracheal intubation or tracheotomy (Topic 17–11) must be done, with administration of oxygen under positive pressure through the tube.

c. Immediate hospitalization.

48–6. Asthma

Treatment

1. Rule out mechanical blockage from foreign bodies (Topic 38–4).

2. Start intravenous administration of 5% dextrose in saline as soon as possible.

3. Relieve dyspnea by subcutaneous injection of 1:1000 aqueous solution of epinephrine hydrochloride (Adrenalin). The dosage should be as follows:

> Under 2 years, 0.1 ml.
> 2 to 3 years, 0.2 ml.
> 3 to 6 years, 0.3 ml.
> 6 to 12 years, 0.5 ml.
> 12 to 15 years, 0.75 ml.

If necessary these doses may be repeated every ½ hour for three doses; repeated small injections are more effective and less dangerous than a single massive dose. In older children occasional use of 1:100 epinephrine hydrochloride (Adrenalin) solution in a nebulizer may give relief. Frequent or excessive use, however, is dangerous.

4. Give oxygen inhalations under positive pressure by means of a face mask and rebreathing bag. In mild cases an oxygen tent may give relief.

5. Prescribe theophylline ethylenediamine (aminophylline) suppositories, provided vomiting is not present. Aminophylline may also be given intravenously VERY SLOWLY in 20 ml. of 10% dextrose solution, 4 mg. per kilogram of body weight. Oral and intramuscular methods of administration are not satisfactory.

6. Give ephedrine sulfate or phenylpropanolamine hydrochloride (Propadrine), 12 to 25 mg., by mouth in older children.

7. Refer all cases to a pediatrician. Severe cases must be hospitalized. Penicillin or other antibiotics, as a rule, should not be administered as an emer-

gency measure unless facilities allow obtaining cultures before the antibiotic is given.

48–7. **Bites.** See Topic 27 and Topic 62 (*Venoms*).

48–8. **Brain injuries in children.** [Also see 48–22, 28 and 51, below; and Topic 43 (*Head Injuries*).]

A. Concussion of the Brain (Topic 43–10) is characterized by complete loss of consciousness for a period which may be very brief and fleeting or prolonged. Children tolerate brain concussion much better than adults—the younger the child, the greater the chance of rapid and complete recovery. Unless definite localizing signs of increased intracranial pressure are present, hospitalization usually is not necessary, provided the parents can be made to understand the importance of limiting the child's activity and of keeping a close watch for changes in condition. These changes indicative of increased intracranial pressure (Topic 43–10) should be specified in detail in simple nontechnical language to the persons responsible for the child's care.

B. Congestion (Edema) of the Brain is caused by swelling of the brain substance within its nonelastic bony case and is characterized by slow development of signs and symptoms of pressure. Early physical and neurologic examination usually discloses no abnormalities.

Early Symptoms and Signs
1. Severe headache or persistent vomiting, or both.
2. Hypersensitivity and irritability; drowsiness, apathy and other variations from normal behavior pattern.

Late Signs
1. Papilledema.
2. Increased initial spinal fluid pressure.
3. Localizing neurologic signs (rare).

Treatment
1. Hospitalization for close observation and symptomatic treatment.
2. Removal of a small amount of fluid by spinal tap, but not until the possibility of a chronic pressure increase as the cause of the clinical picture has been ruled out.

C. Contusion of the Brain predicates brain substance damage. The clinical picture depends upon the location and extent of damage. A history of transient unconsciousness may or may not be obtained.

Common Signs and Symptoms
1. Retrograde amnesia.
2. Acute excitement—sometimes maniacal.
3. Heavy breathing—occasionally of Cheyne-Stokes type.
4. Rapidly shifting and changing focal signs.
5. Convulsions—usually generalized.
6. Stupor or coma.
7. Spinal puncture may or may not show red blood cells, but usually the total protein content is elevated.

Treatment
1. Provided the child's condition has stabilized and the parents are reasonably intelligent and sensible, mild cases can be sent home with specific, detailed and well-understood instructions to the parents, or persons responsible for the child, to report any changes in condition immediately (Topic 43–2).
2. Severe cases require immediate hospitalization. Sedation by phenobarbital sodium subcutaneously or a pentobarbital sodium (Nembutal) suppository [dosage according to age (Topic 5)] may be necessary before transfer but should be avoided whenever possible.

   NO OPIATES OR SYNTHETIC NARCOTICS SHOULD EVER BE ADMINISTERED OR PRESCRIBED because of their respiratory depressant effect and because of the possibility of masking important clinical signs (Topic 43–7 and 8).

D. Edema of the Brain. See *Congestion* (48–8,B, above).

E. Epidural (Extradural) Hemorrhage. See Topic 43–20.

F. Skull Fractures. See Topic 43–12.

G. Subdural Hemorrhage. See Topic 43–21.

48–9. **Bronchitis.** See *Respiratory Infections* (48–44, below); and Topic 53–1.

48–10. **Burns**

(Also see Topic 28.) Many common household articles are

hazards to children and may cause burns of varying extent and severity. Hot coffee, tea, foods and grease, stoves, fireplaces, steam kettles and unguarded electrical outlets all lie in wait for the unwary and curious toddler. Scalding bath water, burns from playing with matches, even sunburn (Topic 28–27), can be fatal.

The treatment and prognosis in burns in children depend upon the five factors outlined in Topic 28–1, with some modifications for age.

A. Per Cent of Body Surface Affected. This can be roughly calculated by a modification for age of the "Rule of Nines" (Topic 28–1,A).

PART OF BODY	PER CENT OF BODY SURFACE				
	At birth	1 year	5 years	10 years	Adults
Head, face and neck	21	19	15	13	9
Right arm, forearm and hand	9	9	9	9	9
Left arm, forearm and hand	9	9	9	9	9
Thorax—front	9	9	9	9	9
Thorax—back	9	9	9	9	9
Abdomen—ribs to inguinal creases.	9	9	9	9	9
Back—ribs to subgluteal creases ...	9	9	9	9	9
Right thigh, leg and foot—front ...	6	6½	7½	8	9
Right thigh, leg and foot—back ...	6	6½	7½	8	9
Left thigh, leg and foot—front	6	6½	7½	8	9
Left thigh, leg and foot—back	6	6½	7½	8	9
Genitalia	1	1	1	1	1
	100	100	100	100	100

B. Depth of Burn (Topic 28–1,B). Accurate estimation of the depth is impossible on first examination, even in superficial (first degree) burns with slight erythema.

C. Location of Burn (Topic 28–1,C). Involvement of the head, hands, genitalia and feet requires careful evaluation because of the tendency of burns in these areas to cause severe shock in 24 to 48 hours from "burn edema" or expansion of the extracellular fluid spaces.

D. Time Elapsed since the Burn (Topic 28–1,D).

E. Age and General Physical Condition (Topic 28–1,E). In children up to 5 years of age severe shock may be caused by a partial skin thickness burn involving

as little as 10% of the total skin surface. Older
children will usually tolerate damage of as much
as 20 to 25% of the total skin surface without serious complications. If the child is below normal in
nutrition, development or general resistance, even
smaller burned areas may have serious sequelae.

Treatment. (Also see Topic 28–2.)

1. MINOR BURNS (first degree or superficial, involving
   less than 25% of the body surface).
   a. Place infants and small children under sedation
      with a pentobarbital sodium (Nembutal) sup-
      pository, 0.03 to 0.06 gm. In children 6 years
      old or older, small doses of codeine sulfate or,
      if the pain is very great, morphine sulfate,
      subcutaneously [dosage according to age
      (Topic 5)] may be necessary.
   b. Remove all contamination—especially the numer-
      ous materials which may be applied as "first
      aid" by inexperienced persons—by gentle
      sponging with a mild detergent, followed by
      warm, sterile saline solution.
   c. Apply a petrolatum gauze dressing.
   d. Administer tetanus antitoxin or toxoid (Topic 19).
2. SEVERE BURNS (second or third degree, involving
   more than 25% of the total body surface).
   a. Cover the burned areas with sterile towels or clean
      sheets.
   b. Control severe pain by small doses of barbiturates
      or, in older children, narcotics, in the smallest
      possible effective doses (Topic 5).
   c. Institute supportive therapy at once by:
      (1) Intravenous plasma volume expanders and
          electrolyte solutions (Topic 7), avoiding ex-
          cessive chloride intake. (NOTE: Before in-
          travenous administration of synthetic
          plasma volume expanders, 20 ml. of blood
          should be collected so that typing, cross-
          matching and other necessary tests can be
          performed more easily and accurately.)
      (2) Force saline solution by mouth after vomiting
          has stopped. Tap water should not be given.
   d. Use aseptic technique while cleansing the burned

areas with a mild detergent and sterile saline solution. All surface contamination should be removed. Loose flaps of charred or devitalized tissues should be trimmed off with sterile scissors. Blebs should NOT be opened or extensive debridement attempted.

e. Apply an occlusive dressing of petrolatum gauze or fine mesh gauze, held in place by bias-cut stockinette.

f. Elevate burned extremities and splint damaged joints.

g. Hospitalize at once. A detailed summary of all treatment must accompany the patient to the hospital.

For treatment of burns requiring special management see Topic 28–3.

48–11. **Cardiac emergencies in children**

(Also see Topic 29.) Except for cardiac arrest (Topic 29–2), the common heart conditions requiring emergency handling which occur in adults (Topic 29) are relatively rare in infants and children. However, certain cardiac conditions in infants and children do require immediate recognition and treatment, sometimes as a lifesaving measure.

A. Anoxemia (Acute) in Cyanotic Congenital Heart Disease. There is no satisfactory explanation for this acute oxygen want, usually occurring in infants but occasionally in older children. The anoxemia may last for a few minutes or persist for several hours with complete spontaneous recovery, or death may occur from cardiac arrest (Topic 29–2).

Signs and Symptoms

1. Irritability; vigorous crying followed by progressively increasing dyspnea and cyanosis.

2. Loss of consciousness from lack of adequate oxygenation.

3. Cardiac failure.

Treatment

1. Mouth-to-mouth respiration (Topic 17–1) until administration of oxygen under positive pressure by face mask or endotracheal catheter and rebreathing bag can be substituted.

2. Morphine sulfate, 0.2 mg. per kilogram of body

weight subcutaneously; or in extreme cases, 0.1 mg. per kilogram of body weight intravenously. (Do not use in infants or children under 3 years of age.)

3. Knee-chest position.

B. Congestive Failure (Acute)

Signs and Symptoms

1. Restlessness and irritability.
2. Cough, dyspnea and cyanosis.
3. Vomiting.
4. Edema, especially of the face.
5. Enlargement of the liver.

Treatment

1. Oxygen under positive pressure by face mask or endotracheal catheter.
2. Short-acting barbiturates intramuscularly or by rectal suppository or retention enema [dosage according to age (Topic 5)].
3. Lanatoside C (Cedilanid) intravenously, 0.04 mg. per kilogram of body weight (one dose only).
4. Hospitalization at once.

C. Paroxysmal Tachycardia. The cause of this condition is unknown although congenital heart disease, drug sensitivity and acute infections seem to play a part.

Signs and Symptoms

1. Rapid breathing but grayish pallor.
2. Irritability and sleepiness.
3. Vomiting.
4. Very rapid, often uncountable, pulse. Electrocardiograms show a regular rapid rate with absence of normal P waves and P-R intervals.
5. Enlargement of the heart and liver.

Treatment

1. Digital pressure over the carotid sinus—ONE SIDE ONLY.
2. Induction of vomiting by oral administration of 4 to 8 ml. of syrup of ipecac.
3. .Administration of oxygen under positive pressure by face mask or endotracheal catheter and rebreathing bag.
4. Subcutaneous injection of morphine sulfate, 0.2 mg. per kilogram of body weight, for extreme rest-

lessness but not in infants or children under 3 years of age.

5. Immediate hospitalization if steps 1 and 2 (above) are not successful. Detailed studies may be required to distinguish between ventricular and supraventricular tachycardia.

D. Rare Cardiac Emergencies in Children

1. PERICARDIAL TAMPONADE may be due to acute pericardial effusion or bleeding (Topic 29–4). Any overwhelming infection or injury to the heart or pericardium may be responsible.

SIGNS AND SYMPTOMS

a. Dyspnea.

b. Pulsations of the veins of the neck; paradoxical pulse.

c. Marked enlargement of the heart and liver.

TREATMENT

a. Administration of oxygen by face mask if extreme dyspnea is present.

b. Immediate hospitalization for evacuation of the excess pericardial fluid unless rapid degeneration in condition requires immediate aspiration (Topic 17–7).

2. STOKES-ADAMS SYNDROME. Congenital heart disease, rheumatic fever and diphtheria may cause partial or complete heart block. It also may be caused by poisoning from certain drugs, especially methacholine (Mecholyl) (Topic 49–334) and potassium salts (Topic 49–475 and 476).

SIGNS AND SYMPTOMS

a. Sudden collapse.

b. Cyanosis.

c. Convulsions.

d. Very slow, or absent, pulse, with absence of any heart beat by auscultation. Death usually occurs in a few minutes unless the heart beat becomes re-established.

TREATMENT available under emergency conditions rarely influences the outcome, but the following measures may be tried:

a. Mouth-to-mouth respiration (Topic 17–1) and closed cardiac massage (Topic 17–2,A).

    b. Intravenous or intracardiac injection of 0.5 ml. of a 1:1000 solution of epinephrine hydrochloride (Adrenalin).

    c. Subcutaneous or intravenous injection of atropine sulfate, 0.25 to 0.6 mg.

    d. Immediate hospitalization with heart-lung resuscitation continued en route. If equipment is available, stimulation by an artificial pacemaker may result in lifesaving re-establishment of the normal heart beat.

48–12. **Concussion of the brain.** See 48–8, above.

48–13. **Contagious diseases.** See Topic 32.

48–14. **Convulsions.** [Also see Topic 33 (*Convulsive Seizures*).]

  A. Causes. Convulsions are much more frequent in children than in adults. Hyperpyrexia caused by acute infections is by far the most common etiologic factor. Among other causative conditions are:

1. Alkalosis (48–3), above) from prolonged vomiting or hyperventilation (Topic 36–6).
2. Allergic reactions (Topic 24).
3. Brain abnormalities (congenital, developmental or traumatic).
4. Breath holding (occasionally).
5. Cerebral degenerative diseases.
6. Drugs—overdosage and personal idiosyncrasy (Topics 49 and 59 and 48–14,A,21, below).
7. Encephalitis (48–20, below).
8. Epilepsy (Topic 3–7).
9. Extradural hemorrhage (Topic 43–20).
10. Head injuries (Topic 43 and Topic 48–8 and 28).
11. Hypocalcemia from tetany (Topic 44–23), rickets or hypothyroidism.
12. Hypoglycemia (Topic 44–16), with or without diabetes.
13. Hysteria (Topic 51–5 and 9).
14. Intracranial blood vessel abnormalities (Topic 60–2).
15. Kernicterus in erythroblastotic infants.
16. Lead encephalopathy (Topic 49–313).
17. Meningitis (48–37, below)—fever may or may not be present.
18. Otitis media (Topic 34–12,B).

19. Parasitic infection.
20. Pneumonia (48–41, below; Topic 53–14; and Topic 63–11).
21. Poisoning from ingestion, inhalation of fumes, or absorption through the skin or mucous membranes of many substances (see under Topic 49). Among the more common are:

Amphetamines (49–45)
Arsenic salts (49–63)
Aspirin (49–69)
Atropine (49–71)
Bromates (49–99)
Caffeine (49–107)
Camphor (49–112)
Carbon tetrachloride (49–120)
Castor beans (49–123)
Chokecherry (49–144)
Codeine (49–153)
Ephedrine (49–212)
Ethyl alcohol (49–227)
Fluorides (49–242)
Gasoline (49–254)
Kerosene (49–303)
Lead salts (49–313)
Metaldehyde (49–349)

Methyl salicylate (49–363)
Moth repellents (49–371)
Mushrooms (49–373)
Naphthol (49–382)
Nicotine (49–389)
Opiates (49–420)
Organic phosphates (49–421)
Phenol (49–450)
Picrotoxin (49–465)
Quinine (49–493)
Saccharin (49–507)
Salicylates (49–511)
Silver nitrate (49–530)
Snake venom (Topic 27–17 and Topic 62)
Tetrachloroethane (49–120)
Thiocyanates (49–600)
Tobacco (49–611)

22. Septicemia and bacteremia (48–37, below).
23. Subdural hemorrhage (Topic 43–21).
24. Temper tantrums.
25. Tetanus (Topic 32–31).
26. Tetany (Topic 44–23).

B. Treatment. Convulsions, as a general rule, are self-limiting and of short duration and do not require heroic measures for control. The causative factor should be determined as soon as possible. Any or all of the following measures may be indicated if the convulsions are prolonged or repeated, and as protection against injury:

1. Prevention of self-injury such as tongue-biting or injuries to the musculoskeletal structures (strains, dislocations, fractures).
2. Insurance of an adequate airway by positioning; removal of mucus and secretions by suction, and support of the jaw.

3. Administration of oxygen by face mask if cyanosis is present.
4. Reduction of high fever by sponging with alcohol or tepid water, application of cold compresses, or ice water enemas.
5. Sedation by:
    a. *Suppositories or Capsules of*:
        (1) Pentobarbital sodium (Nembutal), 0.03 gm. for children under 2 years of age; 0.06 gm. for children more than 2 years of age.
        (2) Secobarbital (Seconal) according to the following dosage table:
            Under 1 year, 50 mg.
            1 to 2 years, 50 to 100 mg.
            2 to 3 years, 100 to 200 mg.
            3 to 5 years, 200 to 250 mg.
            Over 5 years, 250 to 330 mg.
    b. *Subcutaneous Administration* of phenobarbital sodium, 4 to 5 mg. per kilogram of body weight. Above 5 years the doses should be adjusted according to age (Topic 5).
    c. *Intravenous Administration of:*
        (1) Phenobarbital sodium, 60 to 120 mg.
        (2) Amytal Sodium, 60 to 120 mg.
        (3) Pentothal sodium, GIVEN ONLY BY, OR UNDER THE DIRECT SUPERVISION OF, AN ANESTHESIOLOGIST.
    NOTE: The intravenous route should be used only in very severe or protracted convulsions.
    d. *Rectal Instillation* (by retention enema) of:
        (1) Pentothal sodium, 0.4 ml. of 10% solution per kilogram of body weight.
        (2) Paraldehyde in olive oil, 0.4 ml. of 10% solution per kilogram of body weight.
    e. *Inhalations of Ether* by the open drop method if the convulsions cannot be controlled within 30 to 45 minutes by other means.
6. DETERMINATION OF CAUSATIVE FACTORS. If symptoms and signs suggestive of meningitis (48–37, below) or intracranial hemorrhage (Topic 43–20 and 21) are present, or if the convulsions are very severe and no extracranial cause can be found, spinal puncture as an emergency diag-

nostic procedure is indicated provided preliminary examination of the fundi shows no evidence of choked disks. The spinal fluid pressure and appearance (clear, turbid, bloody or xanthochromic), together with the presence or absence of block, should be noted.

NORMAL SPINAL FLUID IN CHILDREN

Cell count	0 to 5 per cu. mm. (mostly lymphocytes) (more than an occasional polymorphonuclear leucocyte or red blood cell in an atraumatic tap is abnormal)
Chlorides	120 to 130 mEq. per L.
Glucose	50 to 70 mg. per 100 ml.
Protein	15 to 40 mg. per 100 ml.
Pandy test	negative

7. HOSPITALIZATION in all cases except uncomplicated, easily controlled, febrile convulsions.

C. Do Not

1. Allow the child to injure himself during a convulsion.
2. Delay anticonvulsive treatment. If the convulsion is exceedingly prolonged, death may occur from exhaustion, high fever or cerebral accident.
3. Give chloroform by the drop method for control of convulsions; the margin of safety between the effective and lethal doses is too small.
4. Administer opiates or synthetic narcotics of any type.
5. Send a child home when the cause of severe or protracted convulsive seizures has not been determined. Hospitalization for thorough study is a "must."

48–15. Croup

This is a symptom complex (not a disease entity) caused by narrowing of the epiglottic aperture by edema or swelling. It is characterized by stridulous cough usually preceded by, or associated with, mild respiratory infection, and has a notorious tendency to develop without warning during sleep and to become worse very suddenly. Usually there is very little temperature rise. As the child coughs, his voice becomes progressively hoarser.

A. Treatment in the Home may be tried.

1. Position of comfort; most children are more comfortable sitting up.
2. Increase of moisture content of the air by

    a. Hot steam devices, placed where they cannot be upset.

    b. Running a hot shower in a closed bathroom.

    c. Use of a steam kettle if other means are not available. Every precaution should be taken to prevent burning the patient or other children if a steam kettle must be used.

3. Antipyrine by mouth, 0.06 gm. per year of age up to 3, repeated if necessary every 4 hours for four doses.

4. Syrup of ipecac, 4 ml. by mouth every 15 minutes for not more than six doses. Stop as soon as vomiting occurs.

5. Sedation by a pentobarbital sodium (Nembutal) suppository, 0.03 to 0.06 gm., or by camphorated opium tincture (paregoric) in small doses by mouth, provided the child is over one year of age.

B. Hospital Treatment is definitely indicated if the measures given above do not result in a decrease in signs and symptoms or if there is any suspicion of loss of airway patency.

48–16. Diabetic coma

(See also Topic 3–3.) Coma may develop in diabetic children with astonishing rapidity. Vomiting, acute infections or refusal of food for any reason may be the precipitating factor. Whenever possible a blood sugar determination should be obtained before treatment is begun.

For signs, symptoms and differential diagnosis of diabetic coma see Topic 3–3,B.

    Treatment

1. Intravenous injection of 25 ml. of the following sterile hydration solution per kilogram of body weight (Topic 7):

0.9% sodium chloride	200 ml.
Molar lactate	20 ml.
Distilled water q.s. ad	500 ml.

2. Intravenous injection of plasma volume expanders, 10 ml. per kilogram of body weight.

3. Subcutaneous injection of regular insulin, 1 to 1½ units per kilogram of body weight.

4. Hospitalization for further care. A detailed summary of findings and treatment must accompany the patient to the hospital.

48–17. **Diarrhea**
   A. Acute Toxic Diarrhea
   Treatment
   1. MILD CASES
      a. Discontinue all food or liquids by mouth if vomiting is present. When vomiting has been controlled (48–58), start on sips of boiled water or weak tea, supplemented in 8 to 12 hours by barley or rice water and boiled skim milk; later, add gelatin preparations and crushed ripe bananas.
      b. Give tincture of opium (laudanum) or camphorated tincture of opium (paregoric) by mouth provided the child is over 6 months old [dosage according to age (Topic 5)], and provided there is not excessive mucus in the stool.
      c. If infection is present, and the offending organism and its sensitivity are known, give the appropriate antibiotic; otherwise, avoid antibiotic therapy which in itself may cause diarrhea.
      d. Refer to a pediatrician for follow-up care.
   2. SEVERE CASES
      a. Stop intake of all fluids and foods by mouth if vomiting is present.
      b. Combat shock and dehydration by intravenous electrolytes and/or dextrose (Topic 7).
      c. Give oxygen under positive pressure by face mask and rebreathing bag if cyanosis or air hunger is present.
      d. Arrange for transportation at once to a hospital equipped for blood chemistry determinations and replacement therapy (Topic 7). A detailed summary of all emergency treatment must go with the patient to the hospital.
   B. Acute Infectious Diarrhea may require immediate hospitalization for isolation and treatment.

48–18. **Drowning**
(See also Topic 13–2.) In children, the most efficient methods of resuscitation, after insurance of a clear airway by postural drainage and suction, are:
   A. Mouth-to-mouth or mouth-to-nose respiration, with or without alternating gentle chest compression (Topic 17–1,A).

    B. The prone tilting visceral shift teeter-board method (Rickard)—for infants only. For technique see Topic 17–1,E.

48–19. **Electric shock.** See Topic 3–5.

48–20. **Encephalitis, acute.** (See also Topic 63–5.)

    A. Causes. Acute encephalitis with high fever, restlessness, headache, delirium, convulsions and coma may be caused by many conditions in children. Among these are:

      1. Choriomeningitis, lymphatic.

      2. Contagious diseases, especially chickenpox (Topic 32–3), measles (Topic 32–15), Coxsackie and ECHO viruses, mumps (Topic 32–17) and poliomyelitis (Topic 32–21).

      3. Epidemic and equine encephalitis (Topic 63–5).

      4. Herpes simplex (Topic 63–9).

      5. Lymphopathia venereum (Topic 61–4).

      6. Poisoning (Topic 49) due to ingestion, inhalation of fumes or dust or absorption through the skin or mucous membranes of many substances. Notorious offenders are:

Alkyl mercury compounds (49–30)	Morphine and other opiates (49–370)
Arsenic compounds (49–63)	Sulfathiazole (49–569 and Topic 59–68)
Carbon monoxide (49–119)	
Iodoform (49–293)	Tetraethyl lead [49–229 (*Ethyl Gasoline*)]
Isopropyl alcohol (49–300)	
Lead and its salts (49–313)	Thallium (49–597)

      7. Polioencephalitis (Topic 32–21).

      8. Smallpox vaccination (very rare—practically never occurs in children under the age of 3).

      9. Toxoplasmosis (usually chronic but occasionally may be acute).

    B. Treatment

      1. SYMPTOMATIC

        a. Alcohol or tepid water sponges to reduce fever.

        b. Sedation as given under *Convulsions* (48–14, above).

        c. Acetylsalicylic acid (aspirin) to relieve headaches and to lower the temperature.

        d. Treatment for poisoning as given under Topic 49.

2. Immediate transfer to a hospital equipped for isolation, adequate investigation and definitive therapy.

48-21. **Excitement states.** (Also see Topic 36.)

A. Causes. Acute excitement states in children may be caused by fear, high fever, psychologic conflicts at home or elsewhere, or by trauma, especially chest injuries (Topic 31) and head injuries (Topic 43; Topic 48–8, above, and 28, below). Since there seems to be some relation between extreme excitement and cardiac arrest (Topic 29–2), children should be under sedation when they are taken to the operating room and should be watched carefully by an anesthesiologist during any surgical procedure.

B. Treatment

1. Restraint—gentle manual if possible, mechanical if necessary.
2. Sedation by:
   a. *Barbiturates.* A pentobarbital sodium (Nembutal) suppository, 0.03 to 0.06 gm., is generally adequate in small children. In older children phenobarbital sodium, 6.5 mg. per kilogram of body weight intramuscularly, may be required.
   b. *Chloral Hydrate* by mouth in orange juice or a carbonated beverage, 0.4 ml. of 10% solution per kilogram of body weight; total not over 10 ml.
   c. *Paraldehyde* by retention enema or intramuscularly, 0.15 ml. per kilogram of body weight.
   d. *Chlorpromazine Hydrochloride* (Thorazine) orally, rectally or intramuscularly in children over 2 years of age.

DOSAGE BY AGE
2 to 4 years, 5 mg.
4 to 6 years, 8 mg.
6 to 8 years, 10 mg.
8 to 15 years, 15 mg.

DOSAGE PER KILOGRAM OF BODY WEIGHT
Orally or intramuscularly, 0.5 mg.
Rectally, 1.0 mg.

NOTE: If Thorazine or allied drugs are used, the dosage of barbiturates or narcotics should always be reduced by at least one-half because of the potentiating effect of phenothiazines (Topic 59–53).

3. Hospitalization if a chest injury (Topic 31) or a head injury (Topic 43; Topic 48–8, above, 28, below) is present or suspected. Acute excitement may be the only indication of very severe intrathoracic or intracranial damage in children.

4. Reference to a pediatrician for investigation and treatment of the causative factors.

48–22. **Extradural (epidural) hemorrhage**

(Also see Topic 43–20.) This condition is relatively uncommon in infants and children.

Signs and Symptoms

1. A history of a fall or of a blow on the head, sometimes apparently very unimportant.

2. A period of unconsciousness of varying length followed by a lucid interval. This, however, is not always present; coma may persist from the time of injury, or coma may develop without previous impairment of consciousness.

3. Dilatation of the pupil on the injured side.

4. Twitching or progressive weakness of the muscles of the face or of the extremities on the side opposite the head injury, followed by a convulsive seizure.

5. Aphasia, with progressively increasing stupor; then coma, with slow pulse and labored respiration.

6. Terminal rapid pulse and temperature elevation.

Treatment

1. Sedation by intravenous or rectal barbiturates (see 48–14,B,5, above).

2. IMMEDIATE hospitalization. Surgical exploration and control of the bleeding vessel, usually the middle meningeal artery or one of its branches, must be performed as quickly as possible. This is one of the few instances where speed in transportation to a hospital equipped for brain surgery is essential.

48–23. **Eye injuries and infections.** See Topic 37.

48–24. **Falls**

Since children must learn about the effects of gravity by sad experience, it is not surprising that the incidence of injuries caused by falls is quite high, especially in the 6 months to 3 years age group. Carelessness of the parents is, of course, the most important factor. The distance the child falls may be of importance but a severe, even fatal, injury may occur from what is apparently a minor incident. Conversely, a fall of many feet may result in little, if any, injury, especially in very small children. Careful physical examination and close observation over at least 6 hours for changes in the state of consciousness and development of localizing neurologic signs is essential (Topic 43–2). Treatment of the different types of injuries resulting from falls is covered under their respective headings.

48–25. **Foreign bodies**

(See also Topic 38.) Contrary to general belief, unless actual obstruction or danger of perforation is present, foreign bodies in the respiratory and alimentary tracts do not represent urgent emergencies.

    A. In the Ear. See Topic 38–1.

    B. In the Eye. See Topic 37–29, 30, 31, 32 and 33.

    C. In the Nose. See Topic 38–3.

    D. In the Throat. [See also Topic 38–4 and *Localization Chart* (48–40,B, below)]. If the child is cooperative, removal of small sharp objects (fish bones, splinters, sucker sticks, toy arrows, etc.) imbedded in the gums, hard palate, posterior nasopharynx or tonsillar fossae may be possible. In many cases, particularly after attempts at removal at home, transference to a hospital where a general anesthetic can be given is necessary.

    E. In a Bronchus. (See also Topic 38–4.) Immediate hospitalization for bronchoscopic examination, localization and removal is indicated. Emphysema caused by the ball-valve action of the foreign body, and aspiration pneumonia, may develop if the obstruction is not removed. Peanuts are especially dangerous due to the action of an absorbable alkaloid, arachine.

    F. In the Esophagus. (See also Topic 38–4.) Hospitalization is required if x-rays at 6 to 8 hour intervals show no progress in 24 hours, if severe pain is present or if there is clinical evidence of obstruction.

    G. In the Stomach. (See also Topic 38–5.)

        1. Rounded objects under $1\frac{1}{2}$ inches in size will usually pass through without complications unless the child is very small. No changes in diet should be made or laxatives or cathartics given.

2. Sharp objects (straight pins, open safety pins, needles, large glass fragments, etc.) require close clinical and x-ray observation, preferably in a hospital. Lack of progression or shift in position, or clinical evidence suggestive of perforation are indications for gastroscopic or surgical exploration and removal.

H. In the Intestinal Tract. (See also Topic 38–5.) Close observation is usually all that is required. Any object which will enter and leave the stomach will almost always go the rest of the way. Severe pain, abdominal rigidity and clinical and x-rays signs of obstruction or perforation are indications for hospitalization for surgical removal (Topic 38–5).

I. In the Soft Tissues or Skeletal Structures. See Topic 38–6.

48–26.   **Gastrointestinal tract emergencies.** (See also Topic 39.)

A. Diarrhea. See 48–17, above.

1. INFECTIOUS. Immediate hospitalization for isolation and treatment is mandatory.

2. TOXIC. See 48–17, above.

B. Foreign Bodies. See Topic 38–5 and 48–25, above.

C. Hemorrhage. Persistent or recurrent bleeding of any degree from any part of the gastrointestinal tract in any child in any age group requires immediate thorough investigation and treatment, preferably in a hospital. In severe cases with extensive blood loss, intravenous plasma volume expanders and replacement fluids (Topic 7) and support of the circulation by vasopressor drugs (Topic 15–7) may be necessary before and during transfer to the hospital.

D. Poisoning. See 48–43, below, and under the appropriate heading under Topic 49.

E. Surgical Abdominal Conditions. (See also Topic 22.) In infants and children acute abdominal conditions requiring surgical intervention are most commonly due to:

1. Appendicitis (Topic 39–7).
2. Foreign bodies (Topic 38–4 and 5 and 48–25, above).
3. Hernia, strangulated or incarcerated (48–31, below).
4. Intussusception (48–34, below).

5. Malformation of the large or small bowel (48–34, below).
6. Meckel's diverticulum.
7. Peptic ulcer with perforation (Topic 39–3,B).
8. Pyloric stenosis (48–34, below).
9. Trauma—especially rupture of the spleen (Topic 55–30).

All require immediate hospitalization for careful differential diagnosis.

48–27. **Genitourinary tract emergencies.** (See also Topic 40.)

A. Anuria. Sudden decrease in output, or complete shutting off, of urine may be caused by:

1. OBSTRUCTION of the urethra with resultant distended bladder from:

a. Inflammation or edema
Treatment

(1) Hot compresses or baths.
(2) Gentle dilatation with a small catheter. Insertion of an in-dwelling catheter, using sterile technique (Topic 17–3), may be necessary but should not be attempted by a physician unfamiliar with the technique.
(3) Antibiotic therapy after determination of the offending organism and its sensitivities.
(4) Hospitalization in severe cases for care by a urologist.

b. Insertion of foreign bodies into the urethra.
Treatment

(1) Gentle "milking" of the male urethra from the base of the penis toward the glans sometimes allows removal through the meatus.
(2) Surgical removal with the aid of a urethroscope. This procedure requires hospitalization.

2. KIDNEY DISEASES

Acute and chronic glomerulonephritis are the conditions most frequently found in children.

TREATMENT

a. Catheterize (Topic 17–3) if the discomfort is acute.
b. Hospitalize for pediatric care.

3. EXTRARENAL CONDITIONS, especially cardiac decompensation.

TREATMENT. Hospitalize for pediatric care.

4. CENTRAL NERVOUS SYSTEM DISEASE OR INJURY

TREATMENT. Hospitalize for diagnosis and treatment, preferably under the care of a neurologist.

5. OVERDOSAGE OF SULFONAMIDES. (See also Topic 49–569.)

TREATMENT

    a. Check the urine for sulfa crystals; if present, stop the offending drug at once.

    b. Force fluids by mouth.

    c. Give sodium lactate, 250 to 500 ml. of M/6 solution, intravenously (Topic 7).

    d. Hospitalize for pediatric care if the anuria is complete or if the history indicates or suggests excessive intake of, or sensitivity to, sulfonamides (Topic 59–68).

B. Bladder Injuries. See Topic 40–2.

C. Cystitis. Infections of the bladder are very common in girls and should be ruled out by urinalysis in all cases of unexplained high fever or abdominal pain. See also Topic 40–12.

D. Kidney injuries. See Topic 40–3.

E. Paraphimosis. See Topic 40–17.

F. Renal Colic. See Topic 40–22.

G. Testicular Torsion. (See also Topic 40–8.) This condition must always be differentiated from incarcerated hernia (48–31, below), epididymitis (Topic 40–13) and orchitis (Topic 40–4). If gentle manipulation under sedation does not correct the torsion, IMMEDIATE referral for operative relief is indicated.

H. Urethral Injuries. See Topic 40–9.

48–28.   **Head injuries.** (See also Topic 43 and 48–8, above.)

    A. Head injuries are far better tolerated by children, especially infants, than by adults. Neurologic examination is not satisfactory or reliable in determining the extent of the injury, no matter what the age of the child. Neither is the history, as the severity of the accident often has little, if any, relation to the amount of intracranial damage. All children with known or suspected head injuries should be examined AT FREQUENT INTERVALS for signs and symptoms of increased intracranial pressure (Topic 43–2).

B. Changes in Condition are the most important factors in evaluation and prognosis.

1. STATE OF CONSCIOUSNESS. A prolonged acute excitement state (Topic 36 and 48–21, above) often indicates a poor prognosis.

2. SHOCK (Topic 15) is unusual following head injuries in adults, but severe, sometimes terminal, shock may occur in children following head injuries which appear to be comparatively mild.

3. PUPILLARY SIGNS
   a. Pinpoint pupils are usually considered to be indicative of severe brain stem damage.
   b. Dilated fixed pupils may indicate extensive brain damage.
   c. Unilateral dilation of the pupil usually is transient and of little importance; if persistent, it may indicate severe brain damage.

4. REFLEX CHANGES
   a. Hyperactive deep tendon reflexes in children may indicate severe contusion of the brain (48–8, above) with a poor prognosis for complete recovery.
   b. Complete loss of deep tendon reflexes may follow severe brain stem injury. The prognosis is poor.
   c. Hyperactivity of deep tendon reflexes on one side only suggests local brain damage on the opposite side of the head with a favorable prognosis following adequate therapy.
   d. Clonus. Same as c, above.
   e. Positive Babinski ("up-going toe"). Same as c, above.

Treatment. See Topic 43.

48–29. **Heat emergencies.** See Topic 57–2, 4, and 8.

48–30. **Hemorrhage.** See Topic 8; Topic 39–4 (*Gastrointestinal Hemorrhage*); Topic 43 (*Head Injuries*); 48–21 and 28, above; and Topic 60–1 and 2 (vascular emergencies).

48–31. **Hernia**

A. Diaphragmatic. Diagnostic symptoms and signs (progressive dyspnea, cyanosis, shift of the heart to the right) result from encroachment of the stomach and small bowel into the chest, the so-called "upside down stomach." This condition is usually the result of congenital weakness, but occasionally severe trauma is the precipitating factor.

Treatment. Immediate hospitalization for surgical exploration and repair. The sooner this is accomplished, the better the prognosis.

B. Femoral. Protrusion of a loop of bowel through a femoral ring is rare in infants and children, but does occur. Surgical repair as soon as possible is indicated if the hernia cannot be reduced by gentle manipulation; if reduction is possible, repair becomes an elective procedure.

C. Inguinal. In children, these hernias are almost always direct and represent a surgical emergency only if evidence of strangulation is present. Support by a tight-fitting binder is often all that is necessary until operative repair can be done as an elective procedure.

D. Umbilical. This is by far the commonest type of infantile hernia. Incarceration and strangulation practically never occur. Repeated reassurance of the parents is often the most important part of therapy. Spontaneous closure without treatment usually occurs.

48–32. **Hiccups.** See Topic 53–7. In infancy, gentle pressure over the upper abdomen after each feeding is usually all that is necessary.

48–33. **Hypoglycemia.**

[Also see Topic 3–3 (*Coma*) and Topic 44–16 (*Metabolic Disorders*).] Blood sugar levels below 40 mg. per 100 ml. from any cause may cause signs and symptoms requiring immediate therapy.

Signs and Symptoms
1. Restlessness and hunger.
2. Dilated pupils; increased pulse rate.
3. Convulsions followed by coma.

Treatment
1. Orange juice or sugar-containing carbonated beverages by mouth are usually all that is necessary in mild cases without unconsciousness or vomiting. If vomiting is present, 500 ml. of 5% dex-

trose in water should be given intravenously (Topic 7).

2. Severe cases should be hospitalized at once after intravenous administration of 10% dextrose in saline (Topic 7). Convulsions (48–14, above) should be controlled before transfer.

3. All cases should be under pediatric supervision as soon as possible.

48–34. Intestinal obstruction

(Also see Topic 39–2.) Early recognition of obstruction is essential for successful therapy. Among the many causes are:

1. Annular pancreas with compression of the duodenum.
2. Foreign bodies. See Topic 38–5 and 48–25,H, above.
3. Hernia with strangulation (usually inguinal). See 48–31,C, above.
4. Ileus—from meconium or following abdominal injury.
5. Pyloric stenosis.
6. Intussusception and volvulus.
7. Imperforate anus, intestinal atresia at any level, megacolon, and other congenital or developmental abnormalities.

Treatment. No matter what the cause, suggestive or conclusive evidence of intestinal obstruction in children requires immediate hospitalization for diagnosis and possible surgical treatment.

48–35. Ketosis

Children store a relatively small amount of glycogen in the liver; hence, in the absence of adequate insulin therapy, or in the presence of an acute infection, unconsciousness may develop very rapidly in diabetic children.

Treatment. See 48–16, above.

48–36. Lacerations. See Topic 55–20.

48–37. Meningitis

(See also Topic 32–16 and 48–59, below.) Among the many organisms which may cause meningitis are:

Arboviruses. (Topic 63–1)	Meningococcus
E. coli	Pneumococcus
Friedländer's bacillus	Staphylococcus
Hemophilus influenzae	*M. tuberculosis*

All may cause identical clinical pictures: stiff neck, high fever, convulsions and coma.

Treatment

1. Prevention of injury during convulsions (48–14,B, above).
2. Insurance of an adequate airway by postural drainage and suction.
3. Reduction of fever by sponging, ice packs and other available means.
4. Spinal puncture under isolation technique for determination of pressure, appearance and chemical findings, with identification of the causative organism. Disposition will depend upon the established diagnosis, since isolation precautions not available in many general hospitals may be required.

48–38. **Meningococcemia**

[Also see 48–59, below (*Waterhouse-Friderichsen Syndrome*).] Development of signs and symptoms suggestive of this very serious condition—especially rapid development of petechiae—requires IMMEDIATE massive antibiotic therapy, preferably intravenously, while transfer for hospitalization is being arranged.

48–39. **Migraine**

(See also Topic 30–21.) Migraine may occur in infancy but is more common in children between 5 and 10 years of age. Although there is a strong hereditary tendency toward the condition, attacks may be precipitated by allergic conditions, acute or chronic infections, errors in refraction, psychogenic disturbances, fatigue, lack of sleep or other breaks in the normal habit pattern.

A. *Signs and Symptoms*

1. Nausea and vomiting, with abdominal pain severe enough to be mistaken for an acute surgical condition, are the main symptoms in children under 12 years of age; over 12, headaches are predominant.
2. Vertigo, scintillation and scotomata are common; hemianopsia, rare.
3. Edema of the face and eyelids.
4. Cardiac symptoms—"precordial migraine."
5. Disturbances in smell.
6. Headaches which become more severe and more frequent as the child grows older (possibly because

it is difficult to determine whether or not a small child has a headache).

B. Treatment
1. Acetylsalicylic acid (aspirin) will control mild cases.
2. Ergotamine tartrate, 1 mg. by mouth for a child of 6, repeated in 1 hour, usually will give some relief.
3. Codeine sulfate may be necessary in severe cases [dosage according to age (Topic 5)], but should not be prescribed for children under 10 years of age. Morphine sulfate, meperidine hydrochloride (Demerol) and dihydromorphinone hydrochloride (Dilaudid) should never be used because of their addictive tendencies.
4. Antihistaminics, barbiturates, epinephrine hydrochloride, ephedrine sulfate and diphenylhydantoin (Dilantin) are of little, if any, permanent value although transient relief may be obtained. Methysergide maleate (Sansert) is of value as a preventive agent but not therapeutically.
5. Reference to a pediatrician for follow-up care is always indicated.

48–40. **Obstruction of the breathing apparatus**
A. Diagnosis. Dyspnea of varying degrees of severity is the one characteristic sign of obstruction of the respiratory tree. Obstruction may occur at any level; therefore, effective treatment depends upon accurate and rapid localization.

B. Localization Chart—Respiratory Obstruction

Symptom or Sign	LEVEL OF OBSTRUCTION				
	Larynx	Pharynx	Trachea	Bronchi	
Voice changes	Hoarse or absent	Blurred or thick	Normal	Normal	
Cough	Stridulous, "croupy"	Persistent, scratchy	Reflex irritative	Reflex irritative	
Swallowing	Difficult	Difficult	Usually normal, but occasionally painful	Normal	
Dyspnea	Inspiratory	Positional	Inspiratory	Often present with wheezing	
Cyanosis	Usually absent	May be present— relieved by position changes	Rare	Often present	
Intercostal retraction	Inspiratory	Usually absent	Inspiratory	If a large bronchus is blocked	
Breath sounds	Normal	Normal	Normal	Absent over collapsed lung	
Restlessness, excitement, apprehension	Often acute	Intermittent; acute during episodes of dysphagia and dyspnea	Rarely occur	Acute if a large bronchus is blocked	

C. Causes of Obstruction
1. ALLERGY
   a. Allergic edema associated with acute tracheobronchitis (48–44, below).
   b. Angioedema (48–4, above).
   c. Asthma (48–6, above).
2. DEVELOPMENTAL ABNORMALITIES such as tracheo-esophageal fistula.
3. INFECTIONS
   a. Croup (48–15, above).
   b. Diphtheria (Topic 32–4).
   c. Pneumonia (48–41, below and Topic 53–14).
   d. Poliomyelitis (48–45, below and Topic 32–21).
   e. Tracheobronchitis (48–44, below).
4. MECHANICAL
   a. Foreign bodies (Topic 38–4 and 48–25, above).
   b. Swallowing the tongue. This may occur following severe direct trauma to the head or face, during convulsions or while in coma.
      Treatment consists of pulling the tongue back into normal position by whatever instruments are available (it is almost impossible to do manually, even in a small child) and support of the angles of the jaw. If these measures are unsuccessful, tracheotomy (Topic 17–11) must be done immediately as a life-saving measure.
   c. Pressure from outside the respiratory tract.

D. Treatment consists of supportive and palliative measures awaiting determination and treatment of the cause.

48–41. Pneumonia. (Also see Topic 53–14 and Topic 63–11.)
Signs and Symptoms
1. Persistent cough with high fever.
2. Grunting respiration.
3. Dilation of alae nasi with each breath. Respiration rate increased to 50 or above per minute.
4. Dyspnea and cyanosis caused by reduced vital capacity and pain on breathing, not by obstruction.
5. Characteristic x-ray changes—involvement by lobes if due to pneumococcal infection; patchy infiltration if due to other organisms (including viruses).

Treatment
1. Insurance of an adequate airway.
2. Oxygen inhalations by face mask or tent.
3. Hospitalization for pediatric care.

48–42. **Pneumothorax.** (Also see Topic 53–16.)
   A. Causes. This condition is uncommon in children but
        may occur from:
   1. Birth injury.
   2. Pneumonia (48–41, above).
 •3. Injuries to the chest. Because of the elasticity of the
        chest wall in children, there may be no external
        evidence of trauma, but through the "accordion-
        action" of direct force, severe damage may occur.
   4. Spontaneous (nontraumatic) rupture of an emphy-
        sematous bleb, usually apical.
   B. Signs and Symptoms
   1. Dyspnea and cyanosis.
   2. Absent breath sounds.
   3. Mediastinal shift—demonstrable clinically and by
        x-rays.
   C. Treatment
   1. Insurance of an adequate airway by postural drain-
        age and suction.
   2. Oxygen inhalations by tent. A face mask and re-
        breathing bag may be necessary if dyspnea and
        cyanosis are severe.
   3. Aspiration of the air using a medium bore needle
        and gentle suction. [Also see Topic 31–5 (*Tension
        Pneumothorax*).]
   4. Bed rest at home under the care of a pediatrician
        is all that is required in mild cases; severe cases
        with massive collapse or signs of tension pneu-
        mothorax (Topic 31–5) require hospitalization
        until re-expansion of the lung has taken place,
        or until any infection has cleared.

48–43. **Poisoning**
More than 500,000 children receive medical treatment every
year for poisoning; more than 500 a year die.
   It is conceivable that any of the substances listed under
Topic 49, and many more, might cause acute toxic signs and
symptoms. Children are taught from earliest infancy that in
order to live and grow they must put substances into their

mouths. As a result of negligence, carelessness and ignorance of parents and other adults, children have access in and around their homes to an almost endless list of toxic substances.

For the general principles of treatment of acute poisoning refer to Topic 49–3. In all instances, the doses of medicines recommended in various treatments should be adjusted to the age of the child (Topic 5) unless doses based on age or weight are specified.

For signs and symptoms and treatment of toxicity from specific substances, see under alphabetical arrangement, Topic 49–11 to 673; for poisonous cultivated or garden plants, begin with Topic 49–674.

48–44. **Respiratory infections**

A. Bronchitis in children, especially infants, almost invariably involves the terminal bronchioles. It may be associated with acute laryngotracheobronchitis (D, below) and with a patchy pneumonia (48–41, above).

Signs and Symptoms

1. Toxic appearance.
2. Temperature of 38.8 to 40.6° C. (102 to 105° F.).
3. Persistent cough with coarse rales and rhonchi on auscultation.
4. Dyspnea, occasionally cyanosis.
5. Febrile convulsions.

Treatment

1. Insurance of an adequate airway by postural drainage and suction. Tracheotomy is almost never necessary.
2. Oxygen by face mask or tent if cyanosis is acute. Moisture often is beneficial.
3. Control of convulsions (48–14, above).
4. Strict pediatric supervision with administration of sulfanilamides and antibiotics as indicated. Hospitalization may be necessary in severe cases.

B. Croup. See 48–15, above.

C. Diphtheria. Infections from this specific organism are now fortunately relatively rare. Immediate treatment must be given if the condition is even suspected (Topic 32–4).

D. Laryngotracheobronchitis. Acute infections of these sections of the respiratory tract must be distinguished from croup (48–15, above), diphtheria (Topic 32–4) and mechanical obstruction. It is often associated with, and complicated by, capillary bronchitis (bronchiolitis) (Topic 53–2) and patchy pneumonia (48–41, above).

Signs and Symptoms

1. Croupy symptoms (48–15, above) often begin during the day and persist in spite of treatment.
2. Extreme toxicity with a high temperature.
3. Acute dyspnea and cyanosis.

Treatment

1. Insurance of an adequate airway. This includes performance of an emergency tracheotomy (Topic 17–11) if necessary.
2. Oxygen inhalations by tent or face mask if extreme dyspnea and/or cyanosis is present.
3. Warm, moist air inhalations. Many varieties of very efficient and safe patented devices are on the market, but the old-fashioned steam kettle (with precautions against burning the patient or other members of the family) is often the only means available in the home for producing warm moisture.
4. Antibiotic therapy based whenever possible upon cultures and sensitivity studies.
   a. Penicillin, 300,000 to 600,000 units, intramuscularly.
   b. Oxytetracycline (Terramycin) chlortetracycline (Aureomycin) or tetracycline (Achromycin) intramuscularly, 15 to 20 mg. per kilogram of body weight, repeated in 8 hours if necessary.
5. If there is evidence of allergic edema, epinephrine (Adrenalin) hydrochloride (1:1000 solution) may be given subcutaneously provided there is no tachycardia or evidence of impending heart failure.

> DOSAGE
> Under 2 years, 0.1 ml.
> 2 to 3 years, 0.2 ml.
> 3 to 6 years, 0.3 ml.
> 6 to 12 years, 0.5 ml.

6. Hospitalization for pediatric care in severe cases,

particularly if there is evidence of respiratory tract obstruction (48–40,B, above).

E. Nasopharyngitis. Aside from blocking of the nostrils of infants by crusts of thick secretion, nasopharyngitis rarely requires emergency care. Its chief importance is that it may simulate the prodromal picture of various more serious conditions such as poliomyelitis (Topic 32–21, and 48–45, below); otitis media (Topic 34–12,B); or (rarely) mastoiditis (Topic 34–10).

Treatment
1. Removal of crusts from the nostrils in infants.
2. Shrinking of the nasal mucous membranes with 0.25% phenylephrine hydrochloride (Neo-Synephrine) drops or spray.
3. Administration of antihistaminics if an allergic factor is suspected.
4. Sulfonamide or antibiotic therapy if indicated by cultures and sensitivity tests.
5. Home care, especially complete bed rest and copious fluids. Hospitalization is practically never necessary.

F. Otitis Media. See Topic 34–12,B.

G. Pneumonia. See 48–41, above; Topic 53; and Topic 63–11.

H. Tonsillitis. Acutely inflamed and swollen tonsils, sometimes sufficient to cause dysphagia and dyspnea, are very common in childhood.

Treatment
1. Soft or liquid diet.
2. Icebags or cold compresses to the throat.
3. Penicillin, 200,000 to 600,000 units, intramuscularly. Tetracycline (Achromycin) and/or oxytetracycline (Terramycin), 20 mg. per kilogram of body weight, may be of benefit.
4. Acute cases with extreme toxicity or edema require hospitalization and strict pediatric supervision.

I. Tracheobronchitis. See *Laryngotracheobronchitis* (D, above).

48–45. Respiratory paralysis in anterior poliomyelitis
(See also Topic 47–5.) Emergency tracheotomy (Topic 17–11) is an absolute necessity if symptoms and signs indicat-

ing airway obstruction cannot be cleared by postural drainage and suction. No patient in the acute stage of infantile paralysis should be transported until a tracheotomy has been performed if there is any possibility of the development or progression of respiratory paralysis requiring ventilation assistance.

48–46. **Serum reactions.** (Also see Topic 24, and Topic 59–66.)

> *Treatment*
> 1. Epinephrine hydrochloride (Adrenalin), 1:1000 solution, subcutaneously.
>
> > DOSAGE
> > Under 2 years, 0.1 ml.
> > 2 to 3 years, 0.2 ml.
> > 3 to 6 years, 0.3 ml.
> > 6 to 12 years, 0.5 ml.
>
> 2. Tripelennamine hydrochloride (Pyribenzamine) or diphenhydramine hydrochloride (Benadryl) subcutaneously, 5 to 7 mg. per kg. of body weight.
> 3. If the above methods are unsuccessful, hospitalization at once.

48–47. **Shock**

(See also Topic 15.) The chief difference between shock in children and that in adults is that in children the changes in condition described under Topic 15 may develop very rapidly and become irreversible before they are recognized. Identification of these early changes depends upon frequent and careful observation and examination. In children a slowly falling rectal temperature is often indicative of incipient shock. As a general rule, treatment of shock (Topic 15–7) takes precedence over all other emergency procedures except control of gross hemorrhage and restoration of respiration.

48–48. **Skull fractures.** See Topic 43–12; and 48–8 and 28, above.

48–49. **Smoke inhalation**

[See also Topic 25 (*Asphyxiation*).] The dangers of inhalation of smoke by infants and children are often unrecognized. The onset of secondary, serious signs and symptoms may be delayed for 1 to 5 hours after exposure.

> *Treatment*
> 1. Insurance of an adequate airway by postural drainage and suction.
> 2. Relief from dyspnea and anoxia by mouth-to-mouth, mouth-to-nose or mouth-to-adjunct respiration

(Topic 17–1), followed by oxygen inhalations under positive pressure by face mask and re-breathing bag when the equipment is available.

3. Control of pain and restlessness by barbiturates rectally or intramuscularly or, in severe cases in older children, by morphine sulfate subcutaneously or intravenously [dosage according to age (Topic 5)].

4. Hospitalization for at least 48 hours for treatment of the inevitable edema of the respiratory tract.

48–50. **Stings.** See Topic 27 (*Bites*); Topic 56; and Topic 62 (*Venoms*).

48–51. **Subarachnoid hemorrhage**

(See also Topic 60–2,C.) This condition is rare in infancy and childhood unless other severe head injuries are present. It can practically never be diagnosed except at operation.

48–52. **Subdural hemorrhage.** See Topic 43–21.

48–53. **Suffocation**

[See also Topic 25 (*Asphyxiation*).] In spite of popular belief to the contrary, very few infants and small children "smother" in bedclothes or from lying in unusual positions. In almost all cases, the apparent "accidental mechanical suffocation" is caused by an overwhelming acute respiratory infection. A few instances may be due to congenital heart defects. These facts should be kept in mind in the emergency handling of cases of alleged "suffocation."

48–54. **Sunstroke** (Heat Exhaustion). See Topic 57–8.

48–55. **Tetanus.** [Also see Topic 14 (*Serum Sensitivity and Desensitization*); Topic 19 (*Tetanus Immunization*); and Topic 32–31.]

A. Immunization. Of all reported cases of tetanus, 50 to 70% occur in children. Because immunity is not derived from the mother, active immunization of all children at an early age by a series of toxoid injections is very important. Fluid or aluminum hydroxide toxoid is preferable to alum-precipitated toxoid because it produces a faster rise in antitoxin titer. In badly contaminated wounds, tetanus antitoxin in adequate doses (Topic 19) should be given after testing for sensitivity to horse serum (Topic 14).

B. Treatment. See Topic 32–31.

48–56. **Tetany.** See Topic 44–23.

48–57. **Volvulus**

[Also see *Intestinal Obstruction in Children* (48–34, above).]
Twisting of the small bowel usually results from improper developmental rotation of the duodenum and may cause symptoms and signs of high intestinal obstruction developing during the first few hours of life or months or years later. The diagnosis cannot be made on symptoms and physical findings alone but requires thorough x-ray studies.

> **Treatment.** Hospitalization is indicated whenever volvulus is suspected. Operative untwisting of the distal portion of the duodenum may be lifesaving.

48–58. **Vomiting**

 A. Prolonged and Persistent Vomiting, no matter what its cause, will result in acute dehydration, acidosis or alkalosis, and complete collapse from exhaustion in children. Occasional regurgitation or vomiting in infants and children is of no clinical importance.

 B. Control of Prolonged Vomiting Depends on Four Factors:
  1. Physiologic rest of the stomach—nothing by mouth.
  2. Correction of any water-electrolyte imbalance by administration of appropriate fluids intravenously or by hypodermoclysis (Topic 7).
  3. Identification and treatment of the cause.
  4. Gradual resumption of a normal diet.

 C. Treatment
  1. Give nothing by mouth except ice chips.
  2. Insist on complete rest. Sedation by means of a pentobarbital sodium (Nembutal) suppository may be necessary.
  3. In children accustomed to chewing gum, meclizine (Bonine) gum, 25 mg., chewed for 5 or 10 minutes, often gives lasting relief.
  4. Administration of equal parts of 5% dextrose in water and normal salt solution intravenously (or, in less severe cases, by hypodermoclysis), 25 ml. per kilogram of body weight.
  5. Intramuscular injection of chlorpromazine hydrochloride (Thorazine), 0.6 mg. per kilogram of body weight.
  6. Hospitalization for supportive therapy, laboratory studies, correction of fluid-electrolyte imbalance

(Topic 7) and determination and treatment of the underlying cause is essential if the procedures outlined above do not result in cessation of vomiting.

48–59. Waterhouse-Friderichsen syndrome

[Also see 48–38, above (*Meningococcemia*).] Acute adrenal insufficiency and bacteremia (usually meningococcic) represent a true emergency. Early recognition of the clinical picture and immediate appropriate treatment may be lifesaving.

A. Signs and Symptoms
1. Sudden onset of acute malaise, chills and high fever, followed by dyspnea and cyanosis.
2. Gradually decreasing blood pressure with a gradually increasing pulse rate.
3. Rapid development of petechiae.
4. Acute respiratory and circulatory collapse—often terminal.

B. Treatment
1. Start oxygen under positive pressure immediately if cyanosis is acute or progressive.
2. Give plasma volume expanders or 5% dextrose in saline intravenously, 25 ml. per kilogram of body weight.
3. Support the blood pressure in older children by intravenous or intramuscular caffeine sodiobenzoate [dosage according to age (Topic 5)]. Caffeine is not well tolerated by infants and small children and should not be used if the patient is under 5 years of age.
4. Arrange for immediate hospitalization for isolation, laboratory studies, determination of the causative organism and specific therapy. If hospitalization is delayed for any reason, aqueous adrenal cortical extract therapy should be begun. As an emergency measure, 2.2 ml. of aqueous adrenal cortical extract per kilogram of body weight is safe.

48–60. Wheezing

[Also see 48–40, above (*Obstruction of the Breathing Apparatus*).] Development of acute wheezing in a child is an urgent medical emergency until the cause has been determined.

Causes

1. Bronchial asthma—allergic (most common) (48–6, above).
2. Foreign bodies (48–25, above).
3. Pulmonary or vascular tree abnormalities—congenital.
4. Congestive heart failure (48–11,B, above).
5. Bronchiolitis (48–44, above).
6. Pancreatic pathology—usually cystic fibrosis.
7. Mediastinal tumors.

Treatment. Depends upon the causative factors. Persistent acute wheezing for which the cause cannot be determined is an indication for hospitalization.

48–61. Wringer injuries

Confined almost exclusively to children of run-about age, wringer injuries can result in extensive permanent disability. Severe crushing and avulsion of soft tissues, abrasions, lacerations, friction burns, and nerve and blood vessel damage may occur. Fractures and epiphysial damage, usually of the hand, wrist or elbow, may be demonstrable by x-ray but are surprisingly rare.

Treatment

1. Control of panic and pain by pentobarbital sodium (Nembutal) suppositories in children under 4 years of age. Morphine sulfate subcutaneously may be indicated in older children [dosage according to age (Topic 5)].
2. Splinting, followed by x-rays.
3. Repair of soft tissue damage by:
   a. Cleansing of abrasions and superficial lacerations; application of petrolatum or bacitracin (Parentracin) gauze dressings.
   b. Debridement, evacuation of hematomas, obliteration of dead spaces, and suturing of gaping, deep or extensive lacerations (Topic 42–5 and Topic 55–20), under general anesthetic if necessary.
   c. Reduction of any fractures amenable to office or home care (Topic 42–4), followed by application of a removable type of splint or plaster shell.

       d. Administration of tetanus antitoxin or toxoid (Topic 19).

       e. Streptokinase-streptodornase (Varidase), 0.5 ml. (5000 units), intramuscularly twice a day, accompanied by a broad spectrum antibiotic.

       f. Arrangement for observation within 24 hours. Extreme edema, common following crushing injuries, often requires loosening of dressings, especially around the digits and elbow. Hospitalization is advisable in severe cases, especially those with suspected or known circulatory impairment.

       g. Explanation to the parents or legal guardian of the injured child of the potential seriousness of the injury and of the possible need for secondary skin grafting, tendon suture or nerve repair at a later date.

48–62. Zipper injuries. [Also see Topic 40–5,F (*Lacerations of the Penis*).]

    A. Although other redundant loose soft tissues may occasionally be involved, zipper injuries to the penis—especially the prepuce—are by far the most common. Proper removal under emergency conditions may prevent marked deformity.

    B. Removal is usually easy if the cooperation of the patient can be obtained. Small children should be quieted by a pentobarbital sodium (Nembutal) suppository; older children should receive a small subcutaneous injection of morphine sulfate, dosage according to age (Topic 5). The zipper—its supporting fabric cut from the clothing by scissors, if necessary, BUT NOT BENT OR CUT WITH WIRE CUTTERS—should be held firmly by both ends, and closed a short distance further, then gently disengaged. A short inhalation anesthesia sometimes must be used, but dibucaine (Nupercaine) ointment rubbed gently on the skin is generally adequate.

    C. After removal

      1. Apply an antiseptic ointment dressing.

      2. Suggest cold compresses for 12 hours; then hot sitz baths.

3. In older male patients recommend use of a suspensory.

D. DO NOT

1. Inject a local anesthetic. The resultant edema makes removal more difficult. In addition, acute toxic reactions (Topic 59–10,B) may occur because of extreme vascularity of the tissues and subsequent rapid absorption.

2. Cut through the zipper with a metal-cutting instrument; this may lock the teeth so that the slide cannot be pulled back.

3. Use sharp dissection. A gaping laceration requiring surgical closure may result in scar tissue and irreparable deformity (chordee).

49. POISONING, ACUTE

49–1. Definition (Sollmann) "A poison is any substance which, acting directly through its inherent chemical properties, and by its ordinary action, is capable of destroying life or of seriously endangering health, when it is applied to the body externally, or in moderate doses (to 50 gm.) internally." This definition specifically excludes injurious physical, mechanical and bacterial agents, and substances which are toxic only in very large doses.

49–2. Classification

A. Irritant Poisons

1. Simple irritants.
2. Corrosives—produce direct destruction of tissues.

B. Nerve Poisons (Neurotoxins)

1. Convulsants—cause spasms and convulsions.
2. Somnifacients—cause sleep and coma.
3. Cardiac poisons—embarrass, and eventually stop, the heart action.

C. Blood Poisons (Hematoxins). Alter the hemoglobin and/or blood corpuscles, especially the oxygen-carrying ability, with resultant cyanosis.

49–3.   **General principles of treatment**
49–4.   **Removal of the toxic substance as soon as possible**

A. From the Skin and Mucous Membranes. Wash with
   large amounts of water [for exception see *Titanium
   Tetrachloride* (49–608)] diluted with the appropriate chemical antidote, i.e., for acids, soap; for
   alkalies, acetic acid, lemon juice or vinegar.

B. From Wounds or Following Hypodermic Administration
   1. Limit activity.
   2. Apply a tourniquet if the wound is on, or the injec-
      tion has been made into, an extremity in order
      to limit diffusion of the poison by vascular and
      lymphatic channels.
   3. Apply suction, excise or cauterize.
   4. Induce hypothermia.

C. From the Lungs. After determining that the airway is
   patent, start artificial respiration by mouth-to-
   mouth, mouth-to-nose, manual or mechanical methods at once. Direct administration of air or oxygen
   under positive pressure is the most effective method
   and should be substituted for any of the other
   methods at the earliest possible opportunity. See
   Topic 13 (*Resuscitation*) and Topic 17–1,F.

D. From the Alimentary Canal and Gastrointestinal Tract.
   Swallowed poisons should be evacuated by emetics
   or lavage unless definite evidence of mucous membrane corrosion is present even though the patient
   has vomited and several hours have passed since
   ingestion. If it is known or suspected that the
   poison has been swallowed with suicidal intent
   (Topic 16), other body cavities should be examined
   and evacuated if necessary.
   1. LAVAGE. Washing of the stomach is indicated if the
      vomiting center is paralyzed (as in deep mor-
      phine or chloral hydrate poisoning) and in most
      cases of known or suspected ingestion of acutely
      toxic substances, provided that the danger from
      the toxic substance is considered to be greater
      than the risk of possible aspiration during lavage.
      It should not be used if a corrosive poison [see
      Acids (49–19), *Alkalies* (49–28) and *Lye* (49–
      323)] has been swallowed, in advanced strych-

nine poisoning (49–565), or if an acute excitement state (Topic 36) is present. For technique of *Lavage,* see Topic 17–4.

2. EMESIS. Measures to cause vomiting are indicated in
all cases, except when the vomiting center is
paralyzed or if a corrosive poison has been swallowed (see above). Vomiting will often result in
removal from the stomach of food or other large
particles which will not pass through a stomach
tube. If emetics are ineffective, lavage is indicated because most emetic drugs in themselves
have some toxicity.

   a. Household measures to induce vomiting
      (1) Insertion of a finger as far as possible into
          the throat, with a prop (preferably wood)
          between the teeth to prevent finger injury.
      (2) Gargling with soapsuds.
      (3) Swallowing of large amounts of table salt or
          household mustard in warm water.

   b. Subcutaneous injection of apomorphine hydro-
      chloride, 5 mg. This is the most effective em-
      etic because of its direct action on the vomiting
      center. DO NOT GIVE FOLLOWING COR-
      ROSIVE POISONS. Apomorphine is contra-
      indicated in children under 6 years of age
      because of its secondary depressant action.

   c. Administration of SYRUP (not the fluidextract) of
      ipecac, 15 ml. by mouth, followed by large
      amounts of warm water, repeated in ½ hour
      (once only) if necessary. Fluidextract of ipe-
      cac is 14 times stronger than the syrup and
      should never be used—deaths have been re-
      ported from confusion of the two preparations.
      Parents of children given syrup of ipecac
      should be informed of its deferred depressant
      side action which may last for 2 to 3 hours
      after an emetic dose. No treatment except
      forewarning and reassurance of the parents
      is required.

3. CATHARSIS. Because many toxic substances can be
   absorbed by, or cause irritation of, the small and
   large bowel, emptying is indicated. Saline cathar-

tics, especially magnesium sulfate (Epsom salts), are usually given by mouth or instilled through the stomach tube after lavage.

E. From the Peritoneal Cavity. Peritoneal dialysis is a relatively new method of removal of toxic doses of many substances from the body which is very effective in the treatment of severe cases of barbiturate, wood alcohol and other poisoning. For technique see Topic 17–9.

F. From the Circulating Blood. This may be accomplished by replacement or exchange transfusions of properly matched blood.

49–5. Destruction of the poison by antidotes

A. Acids. Give alkalies by mouth (magnesium, soap, chalk, baking soda).

B. Alkalies. Give weak acids by mouth (vinegar, lemon juice, orange juice).

C. Organic Poisons (alkaloids, glucosides, etc., and phosphorus). Give oxidizing agents such as one-half strength hydrogen peroxide, or potassium permanganate, 0.12 gm. to a glass (200 ml.) of water by mouth, followed by gastric lavage.

D. Hydrocyanic Acid. Give potassium permanganate, 0.12 gm. to a glass (200 ml.) of water; one-half strength hydrogen peroxide; or 5% sodium thiosulfate ("hypo") solution by mouth, followed by gastric lavage with 1:2000 potassium permanganate solution. For intravenous therapy (sodium thiosulfate, 5%, and methylene blue) see *Cyanides* (49–170).

E. Narcotics (natural or synthetic). Nalorphine hydrochloride (Nalline) intravenously. [See under *Morphine* (49–370).]

F. Heavy Metals. Dimercaprol (BAL). (49–74)

49–60. Precipitation of the poison

A. Tannic Acid, 4 ml. (one teaspoonful) in 100 ml. (½ glass) of water, or one cup of strong tea, is harmless and may be of benefit in poisoning from the following substances:

Aluminum (49–36)
Apomorphine (49–61)
Antipyrine [see *Acetanilid* (49–11)]
Digitalis (49–191)

Iron (49–296)
Lead (49–313)
Cinchona alkaloids [see *Cinchophen* (49–148)]
Cobalt (49–151)
Colchicine (49–154)
Copper (49–157)
Silver (49–530)
Strychnine (49–565)
Veratrine (49–639)
Zinc (49–666)

B. Alkaloids in General. Give tincture of iodine, 1 ml. (15 drops) in 100 ml. (½ glass) of water.

C. Arsenic. Ferric hydrate with magnesia has a questionably beneficial effect.

D. Barium. Magnesium sulfate (Epsom salts) by mouth forms a less toxic compound.

E. Mercuric Salts. Give sodium thiosulfate or sodium formaldehyde sulfoxylate by mouth.

F. Metals. Give raw eggs. Egg albumen is particularly effective against metallic mercury.

G. Opiate-containing Substances. [See *Codeine* (49–153), *Heroin* (49–268), and *Morphine* (49–370)]. Give calcium (lime water, chalk).

H. Phosphorus. Give cupric sulfate by mouth to form an insoluble coating of metallic copper.

49–7.   **Absorption of the poison by**

A. Charcoal (activated charcoal, animal charcoal or "bone black").

B. Demulcents—raw eggs, boiled starch, flour, milk.

49–8.   **Symptomatic treatment of**

A. Respiratory Failure

1. Insurance of an adequate airway.

2. Artificial respiration by mouth-to-mouth, mouth-to-nose, manual or mechanical methods, followed by administration of air or oxygen under positive pressure by face mask or endotracheal catheter and rebreathing bag. See Topic 13 (*Resuscitation*).

3. Temporary reflex respiratory stimulation by oral intake of 2 ml. (½ teaspoonful) of spirits of ammonia in a glass (200 ml.) of water.

B. Circulatory Failure. As outlined under *Shock* (Topic 15).

C. Pain. Control by codeine sulfate, morphine sulfate, di-hydromorphinone hydrochloride (Dilaudid), or meperidine hydrochloride (Demerol) intramuscularly or intravenously in the smallest possible effective doses, provided respiratory depression will not be harmful to the patient. Calcium gluconate (10% solution) injected slowly intravenously will usually relieve acute muscle pain.

D. Cooling or Chilling
1. Application of warmed blankets or clothing.
2. Use of a cast dryer or bed warmer if available. DO NOT USE HOT WATER BOTTLES if other means of keeping the patient warm are available.

E. Convulsions. See Topic 33 (*Convulsive Seizures*); and Topic 48–14 (*Convulsions in Children*).

F. Coma. See Topic 3.

49–9. **Treatment of specific poisons.** The alphabetic list (49–11 to 49–673) on the following pages includes substances which may give toxic signs and symptoms from inhalation of fumes or from skin absorption as well as by ingestion. Unless otherwise specified, ingestion is the mode of entry.

49–10. **The universal antidote,** referred to elsewhere in the text, is made up as follows:

CHEMICAL CONSTITUENTS	HOUSEHOLD EQUIVALENTS
2 parts activated charcoal	2 parts burned toast
1 part magnesium oxide	1 part milk of magnesia
1 part tannic acid	1 part strong tea

One tablespoonful (15 ml.) of the mixture should be given in a glass (200 ml.) of warm water whenever:
1. The exact nature of the poison has not been determined.
2. A delay in instituting lavage is anticipated.
3. An emetic is to be given.

POISONS

....A....

49–11. **ACETANILID** (Acetophenetidin, Aminopyrine, Antipyrine, Pyramidon. Also see Topic 59–4.)

A. Signs and Symptoms
1. Nausea and vomiting.
2. Cyanosis, especially of the face.
3. Cold, clammy skin.
4. Feeble pulse, slow respiration.

B. Treatment
1. Universal antidote (49–10), followed by emetics.
2. Gastric lavage with 500 ml. of 1:2000 potassium permanganate solution.
3. External heat.
4. Caffeine sodiobenzoate, 0.5 gm., intramuscularly.
5. Oxygen therapy by face mask and rebreathing bag.
6. Methylene blue (1% solution in 1.8% sodium sulfate solution), 50 ml., intravenously very slowly if evidence of acute methemoglobinemia is present.
7. Hospitalization if a large amount has been ingested or cyanosis is extreme.

49–12. **ACETIC ACID**

The most common cause of acute acetic acid poisoning is ingestion of "essence of vinegar," a common household flavoring agent.

A. Signs and Symptoms
1. Severe pain in the upper alimentary tract.
2. Grayish white ulcers in the mouth and throat.
3. Vomiting, sometimes bloody.
4. Cold, clammy skin; subnormal temperature.
5. Rapid, shallow respiration.
6. Acute dyspnea, sometimes pulmonary edema (Topic 52).
7. Collapse.

B. Treatment
1. Demulcents; milk is the most effective.
2. Gastric lavage with warm lime water.
3. Oxygen inhalations under positive pressure by face mask or intranasal catheter and rebreathing bag.
4. Caffeine sodiobenzoate, 0.5 gm., intramuscularly.
5. Metaraminol bitartrate (Aramine) intramuscularly or intra-

venously or 4 ml. of a 0.2% solution of arterenol bitartrate (Levophed) in 1000 ml. of 5% dextrose in saline, preferably through a plastic intravenous catheter to support the blood pressure for lengthy periods. The rate of injection must be regulated by frequent blood pressure determinations.
  6. Treatment of pulmonary edema (Topic 52–3).
  7. Hospitalization in severe cases.

49–13. ACETOARSENITES

These compounds are powerful pesticides and extremely toxic.
For treatment see *Arsenic* (49–63)

49–14. ACETONE (Dimethyl Ketone, Propanone)

Inhalation of fumes or ingestion may cause severe toxic manifestations.
  A. Signs and Symptoms
    1. Characteristic fruity odor on breath.
    2. Severe gastrointestinal symptoms—nausea, vomiting, abdominal pain.
    3. Rapid fall in temperature, pulse, respiration and blood pressure.
  B. Treatment
    1. Emetics or gastric lavage.
    2. Caffeine sodiobenzoate, 0.5 gm., intramuscularly.

49–15. ACETOPHENETIDIN (Phenacetin). See *Acetanilid* (49–11)

49–16. ACETYLCHOLINE

  A. Signs and Symptoms. Sweating, salivation, dyspnea, tightness in chest, excessive micturition, collapse.
  B. Treatment
    1. Atropine sulfate, 1 mg., intramuscularly.
    2. Oxygen therapy under positive pressure.
    3. Caffeine sodiobenzoate, 0.5 gm., intramuscularly. Arterenol bitartrate (Levophed) given intravenously in 1000 ml. of 5% dextrose in saline may be necessary if marked hypotension is present. Metaraminol bitartrate (Aramine) can be given subcutaneously, intramuscularly or intravenously for a similar vasopressor effect.

49–17. ACETYLENE

This commonly used commercial gas causes rapid onset of deep narcosis when inhaled in high concentrations. Lower concentrations cause slight intoxication characterized by dizziness and mental confusion.

Treatment
1. Stop exposure.
2. Give oxygen inhalations under positive pressure by face mask or intranasal catheter and rebreathing bag.

49–18. **ACETYLSALICYLIC ACID.** See *Aspirin* (49–69) and *Salicylates* (49–511).

49–19. **ACIDS** [Acetic, Acetic Anhydride, Carbolic (Phenol), Hydrochloric (Muriatic), Lactic, Nitric, Sulfuric (Oil of Vitriol), Trichloracetic, etc.]

For exceptions to the therapy outlined below see *Hydrofluoric Acid* (49–278), *Oxalic Acid* (49–425), *Pyrogallic Acid* (49–486), and *Tannic Acid* (49–576).

A. Treatment of External Contact
Repeated flooding with large amounts of water; application of a paste of sodium bicarbonate.

B. Treatment of Ingestion
1. DO NOT USE STOMACH TUBE OR EMETICS if concentrated acid has been swallowed.
2. Neutralize with aluminum hydroxide, magnesium oxide, milk of magnesia, milk, chalk, egg white or soap solution. DO NOT USE SODIUM BICARBONATE because of possible stomach distention.
3. Give olive oil, 200 ml. (1 glass) by mouth, for relief of gastric distress.
4. Apply external heat.
5. Inject morphine sulfate, 8 to 15 mg., intravenously for severe pain.
6. Administer caffeine sodiobenzoate, 0.5 gm., intramuscularly.
7. Perform a tracheotomy (Topic 17–11,B) if edema of the glottis is severe.
8. Hospitalize if there is any evidence of corrosion.

49–20. **ACONITE** (Aconitine)

Known as blue rocket, monkshood, wolfsbane, friar's cowl or mousebane, this flowering plant is common in gardens. Ingestion of the flowers, foliage or stems by children may cause severe toxic symptoms. Acute poisoning also may result from mistaking the aconite plant for horseradish, or from ingestion of medicinal compounds containing aconite.

A. Signs and Symptoms
1. Burning sensation in the mouth and throat; acute dysphagia; impairment of speech.
2. Vertigo.
3. Eye signs—lacrimation, muscle imbalance, diplopia.

    4. Paresthesias, generally starting with the fingers, sometimes involving the whole body.

    5. Nausea, vomiting and diarrhea.

    6. Hypotension.

    7. Tonic and clonic convulsions.

    8. Respiratory failure.

B. Treatment

    1. Emptying of the stomach by emetics and/or gastric lavage with 1:2000 potassium permanganate solution, provided convulsions have not developed.

    2. Application of external heat.

    3. Control of convulsions (Topic 33–2).

    4. Immediate institution of oxygen inhalations under positive pressure by face mask and rebreathing bag.

    5. Intramuscular injection of caffeine sodiobenzoate, 0.5 gm., in mild cases; or of arterenol bitartrate (Levophed), or metaraminol bitartrate (Aramine) in 1000 ml. of 5% dextrose in saline intravenously if the blood pressure is very low.

C. Prognosis. Poor in most cases. Fatalities have been reported from ingestion of 20 ml. of the tincture and from as little as 2 mg. of aconitine. Twice as much is rapidly and invariably fatal.

49–21. ACROLEIN

This commercial solvent, used in the resin industry, may cause acute toxic symptoms through inhalation of fumes as well as by ingestion.

A. Signs and Symptoms

    1. A feeling of tightness in the chest.

    2. Sleepiness.

    3. Vertigo, sometimes syncope.

    4. Nausea and vomiting.

    5. Diarrhea.

B. Treatment

    1. Removal from exposure.

    2. Oxygen inhalations under positive pressure, preferably by a face mask and rebreathing bag.

    3. Symptomatic.

C. Prognosis. Complete recovery in a short time unless severe irritation of the respiratory tract has occurred.

49–22. ALCOHOL. See *Ethyl Alcohol* (49–227), *Isopropyl Alcohol* (49–300), *Methyl Alcohol* (49–358) and *Alcohols (Higher)* (49–23).

49–23. ALCOHOLS (Higher)

The aliphatic liquid alcohols (amyl, butyl, ethylhexyl, isoamyl, etc.) are used extensively in industry as solvents. All are extremely toxic if ingested.

For signs and symptoms of toxicity and treatment, see *Amyl Alcohol* (49–48).

49–24. **ALDEHYDES.** See *Formaldehyde* (49–246) and *Formalin* (49–247).

49–25. **ALDRIN**

This complex insecticide is similar in actions and toxicity to *Dieldrin* (49–188).

49–26. **ALIPHATIC HYDROCARBONS**

These petroleum derivatives are used widely as cleaners, fuels and solvents. For toxic symptoms and treatment see *Kerosene* (49–303).

49–27. **ALIPHATIC THIOCYANATES** (Lethanes). See *Thiocyanates* (49–600).

49–28. **ALKALIES**

A. Treatment of External Contact
Flood with large amounts of water; then wash with vinegar or weak acetic acid. Use weak boric acid solution in the eyes after prolonged irrigation with tap water.

B. Treatment of Ingestion
1. Neutralize with vinegar or acetic acid in water.
2. Give demulcents—white of egg, olive oil.
3. Inject caffeine sodiobenzoate, 0.5 gm., intramuscularly.
4. Hospitalize if evidence of erosion or corrosion is present or if ingestion of a large amount of a strong alkali is known or suspected to have occurred.

DO NOT USE a stomach tube or give emetics if concentrated solutions have been swallowed or if marked erosion of the mucous membranes of the mouth or throat is present.

49–29. **ALKALOIDS IN GENERAL**

Treatment
1. Tincture of iodine, 1 ml. in 100 ml. (15 drops in ½ glass) of water by mouth.
2. Gastric lavage with large amounts of 1:2000 potassium permanganate solution.
3. Application of external heat.

4. Caffeine sodiobenzoate, 0.5 gm., intramuscularly.

49–30. ALKYL MERCURY COMPOUNDS

These compounds, especially the chlorides and phosphates, are widely used commercially as seed fungicides.

A. *Signs and Symptoms*
1. Fatigue and myalgia.
2. Headache and vertigo, sometimes associated with hyperactive reflexes and ataxia.
3. Decrease in visual fields.
4. Delirium and hallucinations.

B. *Treatment.* If symptoms follow ingestion, emetics and gastric lavage are indicated. If from fumes, oxygen inhalations after removal from exposure will result in rapid and complete recovery.

49–31. ALKYL SODIUM SULFATES

These complex compounds are the active agents in many household detergents (Drene, Dreft, Teel, etc.). Their toxicity is very slight. Emetics followed by a saline cathartic should be given if large amounts have been ingested.

49–32. ALLETHRIN (Allyl Cinerin) is similar in use and toxicity to *Pyrethrum* (49–483).

49–33. ALOIN

This irritant laxative acts only on the large bowel and has no serious systemic effects.

49–34. ALPHA NAPHTHYL THIOUREA. See *ANTU* (49–60).

49–35. ALUM. See *Aluminum and Its Salts* (49–36).

49–36. ALUMINUM AND ITS SALTS [Aluminum Ammonium Sulfate (Alum), Aluminum Acetate, Aluminum Chloride].

All of the soluble salts of aluminum may cause gastroenteritis if taken by mouth; the only treatment needed is demulcents. The oxide and hydroxide are insoluble and harmless.

49–37. **AMANITA POISONING.** See *Mushroom Poisoning* (49–373).

49–38. **AMINOAZOTOLUENE.** See *Scarlet Red* (49–517).

49–39. **AMINOPHYLLINE.** See Topic 59–3.

49–40. **AMINOPYRINE.** See *Acetanilid* (49–11) and Topic 59–4.

49–41. **AMIZOL (ATA)**

The toxicity of this herbicide used especially for control of poison oak and ivy is probably low, but following ingestion emetics should be given at once as a precautionary measure.

49–42. **AMMONIA** (Refrigerants, Household Cleansers, Medications). [Also see 49–503 (*Rocket Fuels*).]

A. Treatment of External Contact
Wash the skin, or irrigate the eyes, with copious amounts of water.
B. Treatment of Ingestion
1. Have the patient drink large quantities of dilute fruit juices or vinegar.
2. Start artificial respiration or oxygen inhalations at once if dyspnea or cyanosis is present. Tracheotomy (Topic 17–11) may be lifesaving and should be done without hesitation if any edema of the glottis is present.
3. Apply external heat by means of warm blankets, bed warmer or cast dryer.
4. Inject caffeine sodiobenzoate, 0.5 gm., intramuscularly.
DO NOT use a stomach tube, prescribe emetics or respiratory depressant narcotics, or use hot water bottles for external heat.

49–43. **AMMONIATED MERCURY**

This has about the same toxicity as bichloride of mercury if ingested. Systemic effects also may occur from absorption through the intact skin. For treatment see *Bichloride of Mercury* (49–87).

49–44. **AMMONIUM PICRATE** (Carbazotate)

This substance is used in explosives and fireworks. For treatment see *Picric Acid* (49–464).

49–45. **AMPHETAMINE SULFATE** (Dexedrine, Benzedrine)

Ingestion of more than 20 mg. a day, or too frequent use of inhalers, may cause toxic signs and symptoms. Following inhalation, the toxic picture usually develops within 5 to 10 minutes; after ingestion, a time lag of 30 to 45 minutes is common.

A. *Signs and Symptoms*
1. Acute restlessness, inability to relax.
2. Flushed face, later becoming pale.
3. Mydriasis.
4. Dryness of the mucous membranes of the nose, mouth and throat.
5. Rapid pulse. Blood pressure increased.
6. Shallow respiration.
7. Collapse.

B. *Treatment*
1. Empty the stomach by gastric lavage.
2. Inject rapid acting barbiturates intravenously.
3. Give oxygen by face mask or catheter and rebreathing bag.
4. Hospitalize for observation and treatment for 24 to 48 hours.

49–46. **AMYGDALIN**

Amygdalin occurs in peach and apricot pits and in bitter almonds. For treatment see *Cyanides* (49–170).

49–47. **AMYL ACETATE** (Banana Oil, Pear Oil). Also see *Plastic Cements and Glues* (49–469).

A. *Signs and Symptoms*
1. Headache; conjunctivitis, often acute.
2. Nausea and vomiting.
3. Muscular incoordination.
4. Laryngeal edema with or without dyspnea and cyanosis; sometimes pulmonary edema (Topic 52).
5. Severe central nervous system depression.

B. *Treatment*
1. If from inhalation, remove from exposure; if from skin contact, remove all clothing (including shoes and socks) and wash contaminated areas thoroughly with soap and water; if from

ingestion, institute gastric lavage immediately using large amounts of water unless profuse vomiting has occurred.

2. Give caffeine sodiobenzoate, 0.5 gm., intramuscularly or intravenously.

3. Combat dyspnea and cyanosis by administration of air or oxygen under positive pressure by face mask or intranasal catheter and rebreathing bag.

4. Hospitalize if signs of laryngeal edema, pulmonary edema or marked central nervous system involvement are present.

49–48. AMYL ALCOHOL

This alcohol is used extensively as a solvent for lacquer and explosives and is very dangerous if ingested or if fumes in high concentration are inhaled.

A. Signs and Symptoms
1. Sleepiness and headache.
2. Nausea and vomiting.
3. Irritation of the throat.
4. Anorexia.
5. Coma, twitching and death.

B. Treatment. As outlined under *Amyl Acetate* (49–47) and *Ethyl Alcohol* (49–227).

49–49. AMYL NITRITE

A. Signs and Symptoms
1. Cyanosis, at first of the lips, later spreading to the fingers, toes and remainder of the body.
2. Anoxemia from methemoglobinemia.
3. Coma and death from circulatory failure.

B. Treatment
1. Gastric lavage if ingested.
2. Oxygen inhalations under positive pressure, preferably by endotracheal catheter and rebreathing bag.
3. Caffeine sodiobenzoate, 0.5 gm., intramuscularly.
4. Ephedrine sulfate, 15 mg., intramuscularly.
5. Plasma volume expanders intravenously until whole blood transfusions can be arranged. Metaraminol bitartrate (Aramine), 50 to 200 mg., or arterenol bitartrate (Levophed), 4 ml. of 0.2% solution in 1000 ml. of 5% dextrose or saline (or added to the plasma volume expander), may be necessary if shock is severe.
6. Methylene blue (1% solution in 1.8% sodium sulfate solution), 50 ml., very slowly intravenously. This can be repeated every 45 minutes until 200 ml. have been given.

49–50. ANESTHETICS, INHALATION. See Topic 59–8.

49–51. **ANESTHETICS, INTRAVENOUS.** See *Pentothal Sodium* (49–444).

49–52. **ANESTHETICS, LOCAL.** (Also see Topic 59–10.)

A. *Injection, ingestion or absorption* of excessive amounts of any of the local anesthetics may cause:
1. Extreme excitement, euphoria and laughter; or acute depression and apprehension.
2. Pallor followed by dyspnea and cyanosis.
3. Tachycardia.
4. Convulsions.
5. Respiratory and/or cardiac collapse—especially cardiac arrest (Topic 29–2).

B. *Treatment*
1. If injected in an extremity apply a tourniquet if time will allow.
2. If ingested, give universal antidote (49–10) or tannic acid by mouth; follow with gastric lavage with large amounts of 1:2000 potassium permanganate solution.
3. In all cases, start oxygen under positive pressure by mask and rebreathing bag as soon as the condition is recognized or suspected. Sedatives and/or analeptics may be necessary but should be used with great caution and only if there is a specific indication for them. Phenobarbital sodium, 0.1 gm., and Amytal Sodium, 0.2 gm., intramuscularly, are the most effective sedatives. In extreme cases pentobarbital sodium may be given intravenously and cautiously.
4. Treat cardiac arrest (Topic 17–2 and Topic 29–2).

49–53. **ANILINE**

Aniline is a very powerful and dangerous liquid of wide commercial use which is also used as a rocket propellant (49–503). It may cause toxic symptoms and signs by ingestion or absorption through the intact skin.

A. *Signs and Symptoms*
1. Peculiar grayish pallor.
2. Amblyopia and decrease in visual fields, photophobia, scotomata.
3. Dyspnea, often acute.
4. Hypotension.
5. Generalized myalgia, sometimes very severe.

B. *Treatment*
1. Removal from exposure to fumes.
2. If ingested, immediate emetics and gastric lavage with any weak acid, followed by 30 ml. of magnesium sulfate (Epsom salts) by mouth.
3. Caffeine sodiobenzoate, ephedrine sulfate, and metaraminol bi-

tartrate (Aramine) or arterenol bitartrate (Levophed) parenterally for circulatory support.
4. Oxygen inhalations.
5. Calcium gluconate, 10 ml. of 10% solution, intravenously for
acute muscle pain.
6. To prevent toxic symptoms from absorption through the skin,
immediate and thorough washing with dilute vinegar (acetic
acid) followed by soap and water in large amounts.
C. **Prognosis.** Complete recovery after 6 to 8 hours. Never fatal.

49–54. **ANILINE DYES**

Poisoning from the many varieties of aniline dyes is most common in
children who have ingested colored crayons, sucked indelible pencils, or
drunk or eaten shoe polish. Absorption from colored diapers may cause
acute toxic symptoms in infants. The toxic picture (apathy, dyspnea, occasional gastrointestinal upsets and convulsions) is due to methemoglobinemia.

A. *Treatment*
1. Gastric lavage and/or emetics if the toxic material has been
swallowed.
2. Stimulants (analeptics).
3. Oxygen under positive pressure by face mask or endotracheal
catheter.
4. Plasma volume expanders intravenously until whole blood transfusions can be given. Exchange transfusions may be lifesaving.
5. Methylene blue (1% solution in 1.8% sodium sulfate) intravenously SLOWLY; 50 ml. over a period of 10 minutes is the
usual dose.
6. Hospitalization for observation is indicated, especially in infants.

49–55. **ANT PASTES**

These may contain *Arsenic trioxide* (49–63), *Calcium arsenate* (49–108),
Chlordane (49–131), *Sodium arsenite* (49–535), and *Thallium Sulfate*
(49–597). Occasionally *Antimony salts* (49–57) are substituted.

49–56. **ANT POWDERS.** See *Chlordane* (49–131), potassium
cyanide [49–170 (*Cyanides*)] and sodium
fluoride [49–242 (*Fluorides*)].

49–57. **ANTIMONY**

With or without combination with arsenic compounds, antimony is an
active constituent of certain brands of commercial sprays, weed killers, ant
killers and snail baits. It is also a constituent of many medicines. Antimony

oxide is used in glazing cheap "china" and pottery. Poisoning from anti-mony compounds is usually delayed from ½ to 2 hours after ingestion.

A. *Signs and Symptoms*
1. Nausea and vomiting, dehydration and extreme thirst.
2. Weak and rapid pulse.
3. Sensation of choking and tightness in the throat with difficulty in swallowing.
4. Cyanosis.
5. Painful profuse watery (sometimes bloody) diarrhea.
6. Collapse from severe shock.

B. *Treatment*
1. Emetics followed by gastric lavage with warm water.
2. Morphine sulfate subcutaneously for colicky pain and diarrhea.
3. Dextrose, 5% in saline, 500 ml., intravenously. Arterenol bitartrate (Levophed) intravenously, 4 ml. of 0.2% solution in 1000 ml. of 5% dextrose in saline, or metaraminol bitartrate (Aramine) may be necessary in severe cases.
4. Prevention of chilling but avoidance of extreme heat which might cause vasodilation.
5. BAL, 10% solution of dimercaprol in peanut oil and benzyl benzoate, intramuscularly, 0.025 ml. per kilogram of body weight.
6. Hospitalization in severe cases because of a definite tendency toward the development of deferred toxicity.

49–58. ANTIPERSPIRATION REMEDIES. See *Aluminum and Its Salts* (49–36).

49–59. ANTIPYRINE. See *Acetanilid* (49–11) and Topic 59–4.

49–60. ANTU (a-Naphthylthiourea).

This rodenticide is of relatively low toxicity to humans, but ingestion of large doses may cause mild respiratory depression.

A. *Treatment*
1. Emptying of the stomach by emetics or lavage.
2. Oxygen inhalations.

B. *Prognosis.* Complete recovery even after very large doses.

49–61. APOMORPHINE HYDROCHLORIDE

This powerful emetic acts centrally when ingested or injected hypodermically. Doses of not over 5 mg. will cause pronounced vomiting, followed by depression. Larger doses will result in:
1. Extreme pallor.
2. Violent, sometimes projectile, vomiting.
3. Irregular, weak respiration.

    4. Vertigo, sometimes mydriasis.
    5. Muscle weakness; in severe cases, muscle spasm.
    6. Asphyxia.

Treatment
    1. If injected
        a. Limitation of absorption from an extremity by immediate application of a tourniquet.
        b. Oxygen inhalations, preferably by a face mask and rebreathing bag.
        c. Caffeine sodiobenzoate, 0.5 gm., intramuscularly.
        d. Fluid replacement by plasma volume expanders or 5% dextrose in saline intravenously.
    2. If ingested, gastric lavage with 1:2000 potassium permanganate solution followed by the symptomatic measures given above.

Prognosis. Good. Even with very large doses, complete recovery in a few hours usually occurs.

49–62. **ARNICA**

Extracts of this irritant substance are a common constituent of many "patent medicines."

    A. *Locally* it may cause:
        1. Erysipeloid dermatitis.
        2. Cutaneous ulceration and gangrene.
        3. Formation of profuse pus when applied to open wounds. Removal by thorough irrigation is the only treatment required.

    B. *Systemically Following Ingestion* it may result in:
        1. Severe cephalgia.
        2. Nausea and vomiting, sometimes associated with very severe abdominal pain.
        3. Extreme pallor and dryness of the skin.
        4. Rapid, weak pulse.
        5. Irregular, sometimes Cheyne-Stokes, respiration.
        6. Extreme miosis.
        7. Sleepiness, unconsciousness and death through respiratory and cardiac collapse.

    C. *Treatment*
        1. Universal antidote (49–10)
        2. Gastric lavage with 1:2000 potassium permanganate solution followed by magnesium sulfate (Epsom salts) by mouth.
        3. Oxygen inhalations.
        4. Caffeine sodiobenzoate, 0.5 gm., intramuscularly.
        5. Hospitalization if respiratory or circulatory depression has been severe.

49–63. **ARSENIC** (White Arsenic, Arsenic Trioxide)

    A. *Common Uses* of arsenic and its compounds include medicinal preparations, rodenticides, insecticides, metallurgy, and in the textile and chemical industries.

B. *Methods of Absorption*
1. Through the intact skin.
2. By inhalation of dust or fumes.
3. By ingestion.

C. *Signs and Symptoms* of toxicity usually develop in from 15 minutes to 1 hour after ingestion or inhalation of dust or fumes; later, if absorbed through skin.
1. Nausea and vomiting. The vomitus may have a garlicky odor.
2. Acute dysphagia.
3. Acute abdominal pain, sometimes severe enough to simulate an acute surgical abdomen.
4. Diarrhea, often watery.
5. Cyanosis.
6. Weak, rapid pulse and cold, clammy skin.
7. Encephalitis-like symptoms.
8. Severe shock (Topic 15).

D. *Treatment*
1. Immediate emptying of the stomach by
    a. Emetics by mouth, followed if necessary by apomorphine hydrochloride, 3 to 5 mg., subcutaneously.
    b. Gastric lavage with warm water, with or without 30 gm. of sodium thiosulfate.
2. Morphine sulfate, 10 to 15 mg., intramuscularly or intravenously for severe pain and colic.
3. Caffeine sodiobenzoate, 0.5 gm., intramuscularly and/or ephedrine sulfate, 15 mg., intravenously for collapse; repeat as needed every 15 minutes. If these measures do not raise the blood pressure to within 10 mm. of mercury below normal, arterenol bitartrate (Levophed), 4 ml. of 0.2% solution, or metaraminol bitartrate (Aramine), 50 to 200 mg., should be added to 1000 ml. of 5% dextrose in saline and given slowly intravenously with frequent blood pressure checks.
4. Dimercaprol (BAL), 10% solution in peanut oil and benzyl benzoate, intramuscularly, 0.025 ml. per kilogram of body weight. In very severe cases this dosage can be increased to not more than 0.03 ml. per kilogram.
5. Calcium gluconate, 10 ml. of 10% solution, intravenously for abdominal and muscular cramps.
6. Hospitalization, but not until the treatment outlined above has been given.

49–64. ARSENIC COLOR PIGMENTS

Auripigment (arsenic trisulfide), Paris green and Schweinfurt green (copper acetoarsenite) are extensively used in industry and are extremely dangerous.

Treatment. See *Arsenic* (49–63).

49–65. ARSENIC TRICHLORIDE. See *Arsenic* (49–63)

49–66. ARSENIC TRISULFIDE (auripigment) is used in yellow and gold paints and may give symptoms through absorption or ingestion.

Treatment. See *Arsenic* (49–63).

49–67. ARSINE (Arseniuretted Hydrogen)

This colorless, odorless and very dangerous gas may be formed during the burning of lead in industry, from ferrosilicon and from the action of impure sulfuric acid on metals.

    A. Signs and Symptoms. Usually develop 2 to 6 hours after exposure; acute anoxemia if severe. Milder cases are characterized by:
        1. Nausea and vomiting, with severe epigastric pain.
        2. Bronze tinting of the skin due to a combination of jaundice and cyanosis.
        3. Convulsions, delirium and coma.

    B. Treatment
        1. Morphine sulfate or dihydromorphinone hydrochloride (Dilaudid) intramuscularly or intravenously for severe pain.
        2. Dextrose in saline, 500 to 1000 ml. of 5% solution, intravenously, with or without plasma volume expanders. Use of arterenol bitartrate (Levophed) or metaraminol bitartrate (Aramine) intravenously may be necessary if hypotension is extreme.
        3. Oxygen by face mask and rebreathing bag if cyanosis is pronounced.
        4. Hospitalization as soon as the patient's condition permits.

49–68. ASPIDIUM (Male Fern)

Even very small doses of this anthelminthic may give acute toxic symptoms.

    A. Signs and Symptoms
        1. Cephalgia, vertigo; sometimes amblyopia and yellow vision.
        2. Rapid pulse with dyspnea.
        3. Vomiting and diarrhea.
        4. Transient syncope followed by coma.
        5. Acute myalgia and trismus.
        6. Occasional toxic psychoses.

    B. Treatment
        1. Gastric lavage with warm water, leaving 30 gm. of magnesium sulfate (Epsom salts) in the stomach.
        2. Oxygen inhalations by face mask and rebreathing bag.
        3. Caffeine sodiobenzoate, 0.5 gm., intramuscularly and/or ephedrine sulfate, 15 mg., intravenously for circulatory collapse; repeated in 15 minutes if necessary.

4. Hospitalization if gastrointestinal symptoms persist or if shock is severe.

C. *Prognosis.* Good. Fatalities are rare, even with relatively large doses.

49–69. ASPIRIN (Acetylsalicylic Acid)

Two types of toxic reactions to this widely used antipyretic and analgesic are relatively common.

A. *Toxicity from Large Doses.* The minimal lethal dose is usually considered to lie between 0.3 and 0.4 gm. per kilogram of body weight. For signs, symptoms and treatment see *Salicylates* (49–511).

B. *Allergic Sensitivity.* This has been reported to occur in as high as 10% of persons with allergic tendencies. For treatment see Topic 24.

49–70. ASTHMA REMEDIES

A. *Active Agents.* Usually atropine, belladonna, stramonium or hyoscyamine, although aminophylline, antihistaminics, ephedrine, barbiturates, bromides and iodides may be present.

B. *Signs and symptoms* of toxicity and treatment depend upon the active agent.

49–71. ATROPINE SULFATE

Acute atropine poisoning may be caused by skin absorption from belladonna plasters, by ingestion of Jimson weed berries, or by medical use—often from mistaking eye drops containing atropine for nose drops.

A. *Signs and Symptoms*
1. Mouth dry with difficulty in swallowing.
2. Pupils widely dilated.
3. Skin red, hot and dry; body temperature increased.
4. Delirium and collapse.

B. *Treatment*
1. Administration of emetics by mouth if seen early, and if the patient can swallow.
2. Gastric lavage with 1:5000 potassium permanganate solution.
3. Injection of pilocarpine hydrochloride, 10 mg., subcutaneously every ½ hour or until the mouth becomes moist.
4. Sedation by barbiturates orally or intramuscularly.
5. Hospitalization for close observation for at least 24 hours. Relapses may occur after apparent complete recovery.

49–72. AURIPIGMENT (Arsenic Trisulfide). See *Arsenic* (49–63)

.... B ....

49–73. **BABY POWDERS.** See *Zinc Stearate* (49–670) and *Borates* (49–96)

49–74. **BAL** (British Anti-lewisite; Dimercaprol; 2, 3-Dimer-captopropanol; Dithiopropanol)

This was originally developed to neutralize the effects of Lewisite war gas. At the present time its ability to alleviate toxic symptoms caused by antimony, arsenic and certain heavy metals is utilized as a valuable adjunct to emergency therapy.

    A. Uses. BAL has a very definite and effective place in the treatment of:
1. ANTIMONY POISONING
   Dosage, 0.025 ml. of 10% solution per kilogram of body weight every 4 to 6 hours.
2. ARSENIC POISONING
   Dosage, 0.025 to 0.03 ml. of 10% solution per kilogram of body weight every 4 hours.
3. GOLD POISONING
   Dosage, 0.025 to 0.03 ml. of 10% solution per kilogram of body weight every 4 hours.
4. LEWISITE WAR GAS EFFECTS. [See also *War Gases* (49–648) and Topic 64–11.]
   Dosage, a 2 to 5% solution or ointment of BAL is recommended for skin or ophthalmic application. For systemic effects, 0.025 to 0.03 ml. of 10% solution per kilogram of body weight can be given intramuscularly every 4 hours.
5. MERCURY POISONING
   Dosage, intramuscular injection of 0.025 to 0.03 ml. of 10% solution per kilogram of body weight every 4 hours.

    B. Signs and Symptoms of toxicity from BAL are almost always caused by exceeding the recommended maximum dose of 0.05 ml. of 10% solution per kilogram of body weight. They develop within 30 minutes of the time of application, administration or ingestion of the drug. Most of them can be prevented by premedication with ephedrine sulfate, 25 mg., orally.
1. FROM LOCAL APPLICATION
   a. Urticaria and wheals with intense pruritus.
   b. Papular eruptions.
   c. Mottling and increased pigmentation of the skin.
2. FROM INGESTION OR PARENTERAL ADMINISTRATION
   a. Severe headache with conjunctivitis, lacrimation and blepharospasm.
   b. Burning sensation of gums and pharynx.
   c. Nausea and vomiting.
   d. Rapid pulse and elevated blood pressure.
   e. Tetany-like symptoms, with positive Chvostek's and Trousseau's signs (see Topic 44–23).

C. *Treatment*
1. Discontinue local or parenteral use.
2. If ingested, empty the stomach by emetics and/or lavage as soon as possible and administer sedation as needed.

D. *Prognosis.* Complete recovery within a few hours.

49–75. **BANANA OIL.** See *Amyl Acetate* (49–47).

49–76. **BARBITURATES.** [Also see Topic 2–2 (*Addiction*) and Topic 3–10 (*Coma*).]

All of the numerous derivatives of barbituric acid act in approximately the same manner, although there is a marked variation in speed and duration of action and in toxicity. Since they are often prescribed in large amounts, cases of acute poisoning from accidental overdosage and suicide attempts are frequently encountered.

A. *Signs and Symptoms*
1. Disturbances in sensation, especially of the extremities.
2. Slurred speech and other evidences of impairment of coordination.
3. Severe cephalgia.
4. Pupils usually constricted but may be dilated or nonreactive. In early poisoning foggy vision, diplopia and color variations may be present.
5. Respirations at first rapid, then slow and weak from respiratory center depression. Pulmonary edema (Topic 52–2) from increased capillary permeability may develop.
6. Skin cold, clammy and cyanotic.
7. Pulse rapid and weak; extreme hypotension.
8. Anuria.
9. Acute excitement, hallucinations and delirium, followed by increasing sleepiness, coma and death from respiratory failure.

B. *Treatment*
1. Insurance of an adequate airway by postural drainage, suction, insertion of an endotracheal catheter or tracheotomy (Topic 17–11,B).
2. Administration of oxygen under positive pressure by intranasal or endotracheal catheter and rebreathing bag, or tracheotomy tube.
3. Gastric lavage with large quantities of warm water, leaving 60 gm. of magnesium sulfate (Epsom salts) dissolved in a glass (200 ml.) of water in the stomach if the drug has been ingested within 6 hours or if the gag reflex is still present. If suicidal intent (Topic 16) is suspected, the rectum and vagina should be examined and emptied if indicated.
4. Application of external heat by warm blankets or by a bed warmer or cast dryer. DO NOT USE HOT WATER BOTTLES.
5. Slow intravenous injection of 5% dextrose in saline.
6. Protection of the eyeballs from drying by taping the eyelids together.

7. Insertion of a retention catheter with careful measurement of intake and output.
8. Support of the circulation by:
   a. Caffeine sodiobenzoate, 0.5 gm., intramuscularly or intravenously.
   b. Atropine sulfate, 1 mg., intramuscularly or intravenously.
   c. Ephedrine sulfate, 15 mg., injected very slowly intravenously; repeat every 15 minutes if necessary to combat hypotension.
   d. Arterenol bitartrate (Levophed), 4 ml. of 0.2% solution, or metaraminol bitartrate (Aramine), 50 to 100 mg. in 1000 ml. of 5% dextrose in saline, given slowly intravenously, preferably through a plastic intravenous catheter. The average rate of injection should be 0.5 to 1.0 ml. per minute controlled by frequent blood pressure determinations.
9. Reduction of cerebral edema by administration of serum albumin (2 ml. per kilogram of body weight—maximum 80 ml.).
10. Avoidance of the use of all analeptic drugs, including amphetamine sulfate (Benzedrine), pentylenetetrazol (Metrazol) and picrotoxin.
11. Hospitalization of all severe cases, preferably under the care of a competent anesthesiologist or a physician trained in postoperative recovery room care. Peritoneal dialysis (Topic 17–9) may be lifesaving. Painstaking nursing care is an essential part of therapy.

49–77. BARIUM COMPOUNDS

Toxic reactions may follow ingestion of barium carbonate, chloride or sulfide, or inhalation of dust of the carbonate or peroxide. Barium salts are the active ingredient in several brands of commercial rodent poisons. Barium sulfide is used in some depilatories.

Severe toxic effects have been reported following the use of barium sulfate contaminated with barium carbonate in x-ray studies.

A. Signs and Symptoms
1. Dryness and sense of constriction of the mouth and throat; metallic taste.
2. Dilated pupils with loss of accommodation.
3. Irregular, weak pulse—sometimes palpitation.
4. Rapid, shallow breathing with cyanosis.
5. Nausea and vomiting; severe gastritis with acute watery or bloody diarrhea.
6. Gradually increasing sleepiness with mental confusion.

B. Treatment
1. Demulcents such as eggs and milk.
2. Application of external heat.
3. Gastric lavage with 1 to 3% sodium sulfate in warm water.
4. Oxygen by face mask and rebreathing bag if cyanosis is marked.
5. Morphine sulfate, dihydromorphinone hydrochloride (Dilaudid),

or meperidine hydrochloride (Demerol) subcutaneously (or, in severe cases, intravenously) in small doses for severe pain.

6. Atropine sulfate, 0.5 to 1.0 mg., subcutaneously for colic.
7. Magnesium sulfate (Epsom salts), 30 gm., in water by mouth.
8. Oxygen inhalations for dyspnea and cyanosis.
9. Normal salt solution, or 5% dextrose in saline, 500 to 1000 ml., intravenously to combat dehydration.
10. In severe cases cardiac and respiratory stimulants, as well as anticonvulsants, may be needed.
11. Hospitalization as soon as condition permits but not before gastric lavage and administration of magnesium sulfate.

C. *Prognosis.* Good if rapid evacuation of the material from the stomach has been accomplished; guarded if considerable time has elapsed since ingestion. Barium salts rarely cause immediate death but may cause serious, delayed kidney damage.

49–78. **BELLADONNA.** [Also see Topic 59–15 (*Belladonna Alkaloids*).]

The effects and toxicity of belladonna are approximately the same as those of atropine sulfate (49–71). In certain individuals the use of belladonna plasters may result in symptoms through absorption. Children may develop acute toxic symptoms from ingestion of any part of the plant, which is common in many household gardens.

49–79. **BENZEDRINE.** See *Amphetamine Sulfate* (49–45; and Topic 59–6).

49–80. **BENZENE (BENZOL) AND ITS DERIVATIVES**

Acute benzene poisoning is usually caused by inhalation of fumes in industry, where it is used as a solvent, cleanser and fuel.

A. *Signs and Symptoms after Inhalation*
1. Acute conjunctivitis.
2. Severe headache.
3. General malaise and weakness, sometimes preceded by a brief period of exhilaration ("benzene jag").
4. Nausea and vomiting.
5. Facial pallor, with cyanosis of the lips and fingertips.
6. Weak, rapid pulse.
7. Unconsciousness and convulsions.

Treatment
1. Remove from exposure to fumes.
2. Wash eyes with large amounts of water or weak boric acid solution.
3. Give oxygen inhalations for dyspnea and cyanosis.
4. Inject caffeine sodiobenzoate, 0.5 gm., intramuscularly.

Toxic effects appear more rapidly and are much more severe following ingestion than after inhalation.

B. Signs and Symptoms after Ingestion
1. Nausea and vomiting, associated with a burning sensation in the epigastrium.
2. Headache, dizziness and staggering gait.
3. Fixed, nonreactive pupils.
4. Sleepiness, progressing to stupor and loss of consciousness.

Treatment
1. Gastric lavage with 5% sodium bicarbonate solution, followed by olive oil through the lavage tube or by mouth.
2. Oxygen inhalations.
3. Caffeine sodiobenzoate, 0.5 gm., intramuscularly.
4. Treatment of pulmonary edema if present (Topic 52–3).
5. Hospitalization after control of the acute symptoms. Delayed development of tracheobronchitis, lung infection or severe blood changes may occur.

49–81. BENZENE HEXACHLORIDE (BHC, Lindane, 662, Gammexane).

Acute toxic symptoms from this commonly used insecticide usually follow ingestion or absorption through the intact skin although inhalation of dust or fumes may cause toxic symptoms. Commercial preparations contain either a mixture of several isomers in varying proportions, or the gamma isomer alone (Gammexane, Lindane). The latter preparations are more dangerous because they are usually in the form of oily sprays which adhere to the skin.

A. Signs and Symptoms
1. Extreme hyperirritability to outside stimuli, with intermittent muscular spasm and convulsions.
2. Cyanosis followed by extreme, rapidly developing circulatory and respiratory depression.

B. Treatment
1. Remove all contaminated clothing. Wash the body thoroughly with soap and warm water.
2. Empty the stomach (if ingested) by emetics and/or lavage, leaving 30 ml. of magnesium sulfate (Epsom salts) in the stomach.
3. Sedate by rapid-acting barbiturates, chloral hydrate or paraldehyde.
4. Give oxygen under positive pressure, preferably by face mask and rebreathing bag.
5. Support the circulation by caffeine sodiobenzoate, 0.5 gm., intramuscularly or intravenously. Severe cases with marked hypotension may require ephedrine sulfate and/or arterenol bitartrate (Levophed) or metaraminol bitartrate (Aramine) for circulatory support.
6. Hospitalize for close observation. Apparent recovery may be terminated by acute collapse as long as 4 days after initial exposure.

49–82. **BENZIDINE** (Diaminodiphenyl)

Used in the chemical industry and as a laboratory reagent, this drug may cause papillomas of the bladder with secondary carcinomatous degeneration.

49–83. **BENZOL.** See *Benzene and Its Derivatives.* (49–80).

49–84. **BERYLLIUM**

This substance is widely used in industry, especially as the inside coating of fluorescent sign tubes and lamps. The metal itself may be the offending agent, but cases of acute poisoning have also been reported from beryllium carbonate, fluoride, hydroxide, oxide, oxyfluoride, silicate and sulfate. Tremendous variation (from a few hours to several months) in the time lag between exposure and the development of acute symptoms has been noted.

Beryllium disease is of four main types. Each type may be acute or chronic:

- **A. Dermatitis,** contact type, usually from solutions of beryllium salts. This condition is characterized by itching papulovesicular lesions on exposed parts.

  TREATMENT
    a. Removal from exposure.
    b. Alum and lead acetate compresses (10%).
  PROGNOSIS. Good, but re-exposure should be avoided.

- **B. Skin Ulcers** caused by minute lacerations from glass particles carrying beryllium into the skin, with formation of nonhealing ulcers.

  TREATMENT. Surgical excision of the ulcers followed by primary closure.

- **C. Tracheobronchitis,** rarely seen as an emergency. Treatment consists of removal from contact with beryllium. A base line chest film should be obtained for later reference.

- **D. Chemical Pneumonitis.** This condition must be distinguished from acute miliary tuberculosis. If suspected from history or physical findings, immediate hospitalization is indicated, since the reported mortality varies between 18 and 35%.

49–85. **BETHANAPHTHYLAMINE**

Hemorrhagic cystitis, followed by carcinomatous degeneration of polyps of the bladder, may follow inhalation of fumes or absorption through the skin.

49–86. **BHC**. See *Benzene Hexachloride* (49–81).

49–87. **BICHLORIDE OF MERCURY** (Corrosive Sublimate)

A. Signs and Symptoms
  1. Metallic taste, whitish tongue, sensation of choking.
  2. Intense esophageal and gastric pain, with vomiting and bloody diarrhea.
  3. Drowsiness and mental confusion.
  4. Anuria.
  5. Convulsions and coma.

B. Treatment
  1. Induction of vomiting at once.
  2. Application of external heat.
  3. Gastric lavage as soon as possible with large amounts of 5% sodium formaldehyde sulfoxylate solution, leaving about 250 ml. in the stomach.
  4. If seen within 1 hour of ingestion, intravenous administration of 250 ml. of 5% sodium formaldehyde sulfoxylate solution; if over 1 hour has elapsed, 4 ml. of sodium citrate should be given by mouth.
  5. Injection of small doses of morphine sulfate or dihydromorphinone hydrochloride (Dilaudid) subcutaneously or intravenously for pain.
  6. Support of the circulation by intramuscular injection of caffeine sodiobenzoate, 0.5 gm.
  7. Administration of dextrose, 5% in saline, 500 to 1000 ml., intravenously. If signs of collapse are present, 100 to 200 mg. of metaraminol bitartrate (Aramine) or 4 ml. of 0.2% arterenol bitartrate (Levophed) can be added to each liter.
  8. Calcium gluconate (10%), 10 ml., intravenously for severe myalgia and arthralgia.
  9. Dimercaprol (BAL), 10% solution in peanut oil with benzyl benzoate, intramuscularly. In moderate cases the dose should be 0.025 ml. of the 10% solution per kilogram of body weight; in severe cases this should be increased to 0.05 ml. per kilogram.
  10. Hospitalization as soon as condition permits.

49–88. **BISMUTH**

A. Signs and Symptoms
  1. Stomatitis. A purplish line on the gums may be present.
  2. Albuminuria.
  3. Collapse.

B. Treatment
1. Magnesium sulfate, 30 gm., by mouth.
2. Shock therapy (Topic 15–7).
3. In moderate cases intramuscular injections of dimercaprol (BAL), 10% solution in peanut oil and benzyl benzoate, 0.025 ml. per kilogram of body weight. In severe cases this can be increased to not more than 0.035 ml. of the 10% solution per kilogram of body weight.
4. Hospitalization for continuation of BAL therapy.

49–89. BISMUTH SUBNITRATE

The toxicity of this commonly used gastrointestinal remedy is due not to bismuth but to reduction of the nitrate radical to nitrites in the intestinal tract. See *Nitrites* (49–393).

49–90. BISMUTH SUBSALICYLATE

Used as a fungicide, and medicinally as antiluetic treatment, this practically insoluble salt may give signs and symptoms of bismuth (49–88) and/or salicylate (49–511) toxicity in the presence of alkalies.

49–91. BITTER ALMONDS, OIL OF. See *Cyanides* (49–170).

49–92. BLEACHES (Laundry). See *Hypochlorites* (49–284), *Oxalic Acid* (49–425) and sodium perborate [Borates (49–96)].

Contrary to general belief, although nausea and vomiting may be severe, even the most concentrated commercial bleaches do not cause erosions or strictures. In contrast to the effects of alkalies (49–28), complete recovery invariably occurs under symptomatic treatment.

49–93. BLUE VITRIOL. See *Copper* (49–157).

49–94. BLUING (Laundry).

This contains minute amounts only of aniline dyes (49–54) and oxalic acid (49–425).

49–95. BORNYL CHLORIDE (Chlorocamphane, "Turpentine Camphor"). See *Camphor* (49–112)

49–96.   BORATES, BORIC ACID, BORACIC ACID AND BORON.
[Also see 49–503 (*Rocket Fuels*).]

Once considered harmless and found in the form of solutions and powder in many household medicine cabinets, boric acid and salts are now known to be very dangerous, especially to infants and small children. Several series of severe poisonings, with some fatalities, have been reported following accidental oral administration of boric acid solution to hospital nursery infants.

A. Signs and Symptoms. Nausea and vomiting, epigastric pain, diarrhea and collapse may occur. Acute gastroenteritis has been reported through skin or mucous membrane absorption. In severe cases, particularly in children, cyanosis, tachycardia, hypotension, and severe shock may develop. There is generally an erythematous rash extending over the whole body, sometimes involving the pharynx and tympanic membranes. The temperature may be slightly elevated, but usually is subnormal.

Delirium and coma may develop, sometimes delayed for as long as a week, followed by death from central nervous system depression. Chronic and intractable renal damage may occur.

B. Treatment
1. Application of external heat.
2. Gastric lavage with warm water.
3. Sodium bicarbonate by mouth to alkalinize the urine.
4. Hospitalization after treatment of shock (Topic 15–7) because of the danger of severe delayed kidney damage.

49–97.   BOTULISM. (Also see *Food Poisoning,* 49–245.)

Usually a history of eating home canned or preserved foods can be obtained.

A. Signs and Symptoms. Usually delayed for 18 to 36 hours after ingestion. Toxic effects usually develop in the following order:
1. Malaise, constipation, subnormal temperature.
2. Dizziness, headache and disturbances of vision.
3. General muscular weakness.
4. Difficulty in swallowing and speech.
5. Respiratory failure, coma and death.

B. Treatment. Hospitalize at once. Since 18 to 36 hours have usually elapsed, emetics and lavage are of little, if any, value. Stimulants and oxygen therapy usually are necessary before and during transference for hospitalization.

49–98.   BRITISH ANTI-LEWISITE (Dimercaprol). See *BAL* (49–74).

49–99. BROMATES

Deaths from kidney damage have been reported following ingestion of popular brands of cold wave hair preparations containing the potassium salt. The sodium salt, used in the processing of gold ores, is also very toxic.

Treatment
1. Emetics and/or gastric lavage with warm water.
2. Normal salt solution, 1000 ml., intravenously.
3. Caffeine sodiobenzoate, 0.5 gm., intramuscularly.
4. Hospitalization because of the tendency of bromates to cause severe kidney damage.

49–100. BROMIDES

Sodium bromide as well as other basic (alkaline) salts of this halogen cause toxic symptoms by replacement of the chloride radical in the tissues of the body. The toxic picture is a quantitative one and varies markedly depending upon the degree of intoxication which, in turn, varies with the tolerance of the individual.

A. *Mild Intoxication* (from 100 to 200 mg. per 100 ml. of blood)
1. SIGNS AND SYMPTOMS
   a. General listlessness and malaise.
   b. Insomnia.
   c. Inability to concentrate; loss of memory.
2. TREATMENT
   a. Stop administration of bromide-containing medications.
   b. Force fluids by mouth.
   c. Increase the daily intake of sodium chloride to 4 to 8 gm. daily.

B. *Moderate Intoxication* (above 200 mg. per 100 ml. of blood, depending on individual tolerance)
1. SIGNS AND SYMPTOMS
   a. Restlessness and irritability; often insomnia.
   b. Generalized myalgia and arthralgia.
   c. Severe headache, acute depression; sometimes paranoia.
   d. Disorientation, retrograde amnesia and hallucinations—usually visual but sometimes auditory.
   e. Incoordination; tremors.
   f. Vision changes—blurring, diplopia, photophobia, disturbances in color vision. Exophthalmos and ptosis of the lids may be present.
2. TREATMENT
   a. Stop intake of bromides.
   b. Because of an apparent synergistic action, all tranquilizers and barbiturates also should be stopped.

C. *Severe Intoxication* (200 to 500 mg. per 100 ml. of blood)
1. SIGNS AND SYMPTOMS
   a. Dilated fixed pupils.

b. Sallow muddy complexion with or without acne or skin rashes.
c. Fetid breath; tongue dry and coated.
d. Dehydration; often emaciation.
e. Sexual impotence or menstrual irregularities.

2. TREATMENT. As given under Moderate Intoxication (above). Hospitalization may be required for prolonged supportive therapy.

49–101. BRUCINE

This is used as a denaturant. Ingestion may cause a toxic picture similar to strychnine (49–565).

49–102. BULAN

Similar in uses and toxicity to DDT (49–175).

49–103. BUTANE

Inhalation may cause varying degrees of anesthesia. Very explosive. (See *Pentothal Sodium*, 49–444.)

49–104. BUTANOL (n-Butyl Alcohol)

This is more toxic than ethyl alcohol (49–227).

49–105. BUTYN. See *Anesthetics, Local* (49–52) and Topic 59–10.

.... C ....

49–106. CADMIUM AND ITS SALTS

A. Acute Poisoning Occurs in:
1. Manufacturing and use of cadmium alloys.
2. Smelting of ores.
3. Coating of bearings and tools with cadmium.
4. Electroplating, soldering and welding.
5. Process engraving.
6. Manufacturing of storage batteries.
7. Use of cadmium pigment paints.
8. Use of silver polishes containing cadmium carbonate.

B. Methods of Poisoning
1. INHALATION OF VAPOR OR FUMES. These are odorless and do not produce immediate irritation; hence, dangerous amounts may

be inhaled before acute symptoms occur—usually in 2 to 5 hours.
2. INGESTION OF SMALL AMOUNTS. Following ingestion acute symptoms develop within ½ to 1 hour. Use of cadmium-lined food or drink containers and cadmium-plated eating utensils is banned in some localities because of the tendency of cadmium to dissolve in the acids commonly found in food, thereby producing poisonous cadmium chloride.

C. Signs and Symptoms
1. FROM INHALATION (2 to 5 hour lag)
    a. Dry throat, cough.
    b. Headache, nausea, vomiting.
    c. Feeling of constriction in chest, chest pain, dyspnea.
    d. Pneumonia—reported deaths have been due to this condition
2. FROM INGESTION (½ to 1 hour lag)
    a. Salivation and choking.
    b. Vomiting, abdominal cramps and diarrhea.

D. Treatment. Except for the development of pneumonia from the inhalation type, the symptoms from cadmium poisoning disappear spontaneously in from 12 to 15 hours after onset. Symptomatic treatment only is indicated. Dimercaprol (BAL) increases cadmium toxicity—its use is absolutely contraindicated. Hospitalization is rarely necessary.

49–107. CAFFEINE

Acute toxic symptoms may be caused by overdoses of medications containing salts of caffeine or by excessive coffee drinking. Infants and small children are peculiarly susceptible to caffeine, and acute toxic symptoms may be caused by ingestion or therapeutic injection of minute amounts.

A. Signs and Symptoms
1. Vomiting and severe epigastric pain.
2. Dizziness, ringing in the ears.
3. Eye signs (constricted pupils, decreased visual fields, amblyopia, diplopia and photophobia).
4. Headache, occasionally hallucinations and delirium.
5. Palpitation and tight feeling in the chest.
6. In very severe cases trismus, opisthotonus and convulsions.

B. Treatment.
1. Emetics and/or gastric lavage with warm water if due to drinking excessive amounts of coffee.
2. Large amounts of fluids by mouth, or 5% dextrose in saline, 1000 to 2000 ml. intravenously.
3. Barbiturates as necessary for sedation.

C. Prognosis. Complete recovery without residual ill effects.

49–108. CALCIUM ARSENATE AND ARSENITE. See *Arsenic* (49–63).

49–109.   **CALCIUM CYANAMIDE.** See *Cyanides* (49–170).

49–110.   **CALOMEL** (Mercurous Chloride)

This irritant cathartic is sometimes ingested in relatively large doses with resultant extreme abdominal discomfort and greenish black diarrhea. It is almost never fatal. Excessive diarrhea can be controlled by small doses of morphine sulfate (not in infants or small children) or by atropine sulfate.

49–111.   **CAMBOGIA** (Gamboge)

Cambogia is a violent cathartic which in doses of over 3 gm. may cause complete collapse and death. Treatment consists of gastric lavage, with respiratory and circulatory support as needed.

49–112.   **CAMPHOR** (Camphorated Oil, Spirits of Camphor)

Vicks VapoRub, Camphor Ice, and other proprietary medical preparations, and some moth repellents, contain camphor as the active ingredient.
   A. Signs and Symptoms
      1. Headache.
      2. Sensation of warmth.
      3. Characteristic odor of the breath.
      4. Weak, rapid pulse.
      5. Convulsions, often epileptiform in type.
      6. Circulatory collapse.
   B. Treatment
      1. Emetics—apomorphine hydrochloride, 5 mg., hypodermically is best—if seen early.
      2. Gastric lavage with warm water.
      3. External heat.
      4. Oxygen therapy if needed.
      5. Caffeine sodiobenzoate, 0.5 gm., intramuscularly.
      6. Barbiturates as needed for control of convulsions.
      7. Hospitalization if severe convulsions or deep shock occur.

49–113.   **CANDY CATHARTICS.** See *Phenolphthalein* (49–451).

49–114.   **CANTHARIDES** (Spanish Fly, Russian Fly)

This substance is occasionally administered as an aphrodisiac, but its most common use is in hair tonics. Ingestion of even very small amounts may cause nausea, vomiting, abdominal pain and bloody diarrhea, delirium, coma and death from circulatory collapse.

Treatment
1. Administration of demulcents (avoid oils).
2. Immediate emptying of stomach by emetics or gastric lavage.
3. Supportive therapy as required. Shock may be severe.

49–115. CARBARSONE (p-Carbamylaminophenylarsenic Acid)

Used medically in the treatment of amebiasis and trichomonas vaginalis infection, this substance may cause severe toxic symptoms by absorption through the skin.

Treatment. See *Arsenic* (49–63).

49–116. CARBINOL. See *Methyl Alcohol* (49–358).

49–117. CARBOLIC ACID. See *Phenol* (49–450).

49–118. CARBON DISULFIDE

Used as a solvent for fats, oils, waxes, resins and rubber, in the manufacture of rayon and nylon fiber, and as an insecticide. Ingestion or inhalation of concentrated fumes may cause toxic effects.

A. *Signs and Symptoms*
1. Respiratory depression.
2. Nausea and vomiting.
3. Convulsions and death from respiratory failure.

B. *Treatment*
1. Support of the respiration by mouth-to-mouth or manual resuscitation methods after removal from exposure and insurance of a clear airway.
2. If taken by mouth, gastric lavage with warm water followed by mineral oil, 120 ml.
3. Oxygen inhalations.
4. Stimulants and analeptics, especially caffeine sodiobenzoate.

C. *Prognosis.* Rapid recovery without permanent ill effects if signs and symptoms are mild; severe cases often develop severe neuropsychiatric disorders simulating manic depressive and paranoid states.

49–119. CARBON MONOXIDE

This colorless, odorless compound may be inhaled in the presence of fuel gas, illuminating gas and automobile exhaust fumes, and during the use of open circuit diving apparatus (Topic 26–5).

A. *Diagnosis.* History of exposure, cherry or dusky red color to lips, peaceful expression, facial twitchings, temperature elevated, skin pale. Brownish red stippling may be present on the arms or trunk.

B. Treatment
1. Immediate mouth-to-mouth respiration after determining that airway is clear, followed by oxygen inhalations under positive pressure using face mask or endotracheal catheter.
2. Caffeine sodiobenzoate, 0.5 gm., intramuscularly or intravenously.
3. Dextrose solution (50%), 100 ml., slowly intravenously.
4. Prevention of chilling or excitement of any type.
5. Hospitalization as soon as condition will permit.

C. Do not
1. Administer methylene blue solution intravenously.
2. Give morphine, synthetic narcotics, or atropine sulfate.
3. Use heart stimulants (analeptics) unless absolutely necessary.
4. Send the patient home after apparent recovery from the acute phase; close observation for and treatment of deferred toxic effects may be lifesaving.

49–120.   CARBON TETRACHLORIDE

A. Commercial Uses. Fire extinguishers, cleaning fluids, plant forcing preparations, dry shampoos. Toxic effects may arise from inhalation of fumes or skin absorption as well as from ingestion.

B. Signs and Symptoms
1. Headache, mental confusion.
2. Persistent nausea and vomiting.
3. Acute hepatitis.
4. Collapse and coma.

C. Treatment
1. FOLLOWING INHALATION: Fresh air, mouth-to-mouth, manual or mechanical artificial respiration. Administration of air or oxygen under positive pressure may be necessary.
2. FOLLOWING INGESTION:
   a. Gastric lavage with potassium permanganate (1:2000 solution).
   b. Magnesium sulfate (Epsom salts) by mouth as a saline cathartic after lavage.
3. Caffeine sodiobenzoate, 0.5 gm., intramuscularly.
4. Calcium gluconate, 10 ml. of 10% solution, intravenously.
5. Dextrose, 5% in saline, 500 ml., intravenously.
6. Severe cases require hospitalization for blood transfusions and measures to prevent liver and kidney damage.

D. Do not
1. Give fats or oils—they facilitate absorption.
2. Administer epinephrine hydrochloride (Adrenalin); it increases the danger of ventricular fibrillation.
3. Prescribe or administer alcohol in any form; it tends to increase hepatic damage.

49–121. **CARDIAZOL.** See *Metrazol* (49–364).

49–122. **CASHEW NUTS**

The oil from these nuts contains phenols which resemble in structure and action the irritants in poison oak, poison ivy and poison sumac (Topic 54–11).

49–123. **CASTOR BEANS**

Commercial extraction of castor oil leaves a residual pomace containing a very potent toxalbumin (ricin) which is notorious for causing severe allergic reactions, especially severe asthma and bronchospasm.

The attractive varicolored beans, which are found on the ornamental shade trees, may be eaten by children with very serious results (49–694).

49–124. **CASTRIX**

This insecticide if ingested may cause severe convulsions. For treatment see *Strychnine* (49–565).

49–125. **CAUSTIC ALKALIES.** See *Alkalies* (49–28)

49–126. **CHENOPODIUM** (Wormseed)

Medicinal use as an anthelmintic may cause acute toxic symptoms even with very small doses.

   A. *Signs and Symptoms*
      1. Nausea, vomiting, abdominal pain.
      2. Headache, dizziness, impairment of vision and hearing.
      3. Acute depression.
      4. Low back and flank pain from kidney damage.
      5. Delirium; clonic convulsions.
      6. Slow, weak respiration, sometimes Cheyne-Stokes in type. Death may occur from respiratory paralysis.
   B. *Treatment*
      1. Emetics and/or gastric lavage with 1:2000 potassium permanganate solution. Thirty gm. of magnesium sulfate (Epsom salts) in a glass (200 ml.) of water should be left in the stomach.
      2. Oxygen therapy.
      3. Dextrose, 5% in saline, 1000 ml. intravenously.
      4. Caffeine sodiobenzoate, 0.5 gm., intramuscularly.

5. Hospitalization for observation after control of acute symptoms.
C. *Prognosis.* Fair only. Relatively small doses may cause very severe symptoms. Sequelae such as polyneuritis, paresis, and decreased hearing may persist indefinitely.

49–127. **CHINIOFON.** See *Oxyquinoline Derivatives* (49–428).

49–128. **CHLORAL HYDRATE**

"Knockout drops," sometimes administered in alcoholic beverages, usually contain chloral hydrate. See also 49–366.

A. *Diagnosis.* History of intake, all muscles relaxed, pupils constricted, respiration weak and shallow, pulse barely perceptible, skin cold and clammy, temperature and blood pressure below normal.

B. *Treatment*
1. Gastric lavage with warm water or 1:5000 potassium permanganate solution.
2. Stimulants—cardiac and respiratory.
3. Application of external heat.
4. Mouth-to-mouth or manual artificial respiration followed by oxygen under positive pressure by face mask and rebreathing bag.
5. Severe cases with collapse and coma require hospitalization for supportive therapy.

49–129. **CHLORAMINE T**

Several series of cases have been reported in which severe toxic symptoms have followed accidental ingestion of this drinking water disinfectant.

A. *Signs and Symptoms*
1. Rapid onset of respiratory embarrassment and cyanosis.
2. Marked hypotension; subnormal temperature.
3. Abdominal pain.
4. Convulsions.
5. Death from respiratory failure *within a few minutes* if a large amount has been ingested; if the patient survives over 30 minutes the prognosis is usually good.

B. *Treatment*
1. Gastric lavage with large amounts of 1:2000 potassium permanganate solution leaving 30 gm. of magnesium sulfate (Epsom salts) dissolved in 200 ml. (1 glass) of water in the stomach.
2. Oxygen therapy under positive pressure, using a face mask or endotracheal catheter and rebreathing bag.
3. Stimulants and analeptics as indicated.

49–130. CHLORATES

Potassium chlorate is used extensively in industry as an oxidizing agent and medicinally as an antiseptic and astringent.
  A. *Signs and Symptoms*
    1. Dryness of throat.
    2. Severe gastric pain, vomiting and diarrhea.
    3. Yellow sclerae; skin cyanotic due to methemoglobinemia.
    4. Tendency to hemorrhage—epistaxis, metrorrhagia and purpura hemorrhagica.
    5. Respiratory collapse.
  B. *Treatment*
    1. Gastric lavage with large amounts of warm water.
    2. Magnesium sulfate (Epsom salts) by mouth or through the stomach tube.
    3. Dextrose, 5% in saline, 1000 to 2000 ml. intravenously.
    4. Oxygen inhalations under positive pressure.
Methylene blue intravenously should NOT be used.

49–131. CHLORDANE

This has a wide commercial use as an insecticide spray and dust.
  A. *Signs and Symptoms*
    1. Convulsions.
    2. Deep depression, often fatal.
  B. *Treatment*
    1. Oxygen inhalations under positive pressure using a face mask or endotracheal catheter and rebreathing bag.
    2. Insurance of an adequate airway.
    3. Caffeine sodiobenzoate, 0.5 gm., intramuscularly or intravenously.
    4. Barbiturates and/or paraldehyde for sedation.

49–132. CHLORINATED LIME. See *Hypochlorites* (49–284).

49–133. CHLORINE

This very irritant gas, when inhaled, causes acute respiratory irritation which may be followed by pulmonary edema (sometimes delayed), pneumonia and circulatory collapse.
  Treatment
    1. Removal from exposure to gas.
    2. Removal from the skin by copious use of soap and water.
    3. Oxygen under positive pressure.
    4. Maintenance of fluid and electrolyte balance (Topic 7).

5. Control of pain by small dose of morphine sulfate or by inhalation of a mixture of alcohol and ether.
6. Hospitalization because of danger of development of pneumonia or pulmonary edema (Topic 52).

49–134.   CHLOROACETOPHENONE. See *War Gases* (49–648).

49–135.   CHLOROBENZENE (Monochlorobenzene)

This is used in the dry cleaning industry and in the preparation of coal tar pigments and dyes. It may give toxic symptoms through skin absorption, inhalation of fumes, or ingestion. Evidence of poisoning is usually delayed for 2 to 5 hours after exposure.

A. *Signs and Symptoms*
1. Headache; sleepiness deepening into coma.
2. Pallor; later, cyanosis from methemoglobinemia.
3. Fibrillary twitching.
4. Respiratory and circulatory collapse.

B. *Treatment*
1. Removal from exposure to fumes; removal from the skin by washing with soap and water; removal from the stomach by gastric lavage and saline cathartics.
2. Oxygen under positive pressure.
3. Caffeine sodiobenzoate, 0.5 gm., intramuscularly or intravenously.

49–136.   CHLOROETHYLENE. See *Carbon Tetrachloride* (49–120).

49–137.   CHLOROFORM (Trichloromethane)

In addition to its use as a general anesthetic, chloroform is used extensively in industry as a solvent for fats and resins. It is not absorbed through the skin but locally may cause severe erythema and purulent blebs.

Three types of acute chloroform poisoning may require emergency treatment.

A. *Inhalation Type.* Usually due to overdosage during chloroform anesthesia or to ingestion of large amounts of liquid.
1. SIGNS AND SYMPTOMS
   a. Sudden dilation of the pupils; terminally, the corneas become dull and cloudy.
   b. Sudden disappearance of the pulse—good one second, gone the next.
   c. Complete respiratory failure.
   d. Death from circulatory collapse and ventricular fibrillation.
2. TREATMENT
   a. Stop anesthesia if from inhalation; start gastric lavage immediately if from ingestion.

    b. Begin oxygen therapy under positive pressure AT ONCE.

    c. Inject supportive agents such as caffeine sodiobenzoate, 0.5 gm., intramuscularly or intravenously. Epinephrine hydrochloride (Adrenalin) is contraindicated; it may cause acute cardiac dilatation or ventricular fibrillation.

    d. Hospitalize if the patient survives the generally fatal acute stage.

B. Ingestion Type

    1. SIGNS AND SYMPTOMS

      a. Burning sensation in the mouth, throat, esophagus and stomach, with nausea and vomiting.

      b. Cold and clammy skin with cyanosis of extremities and face, and gasping, irregular respiration.

      c. Extreme dilation of the pupils.

      d. Muscular cramping, especially of the masseters.

      e. Progressive hypotension from increasing cardiac weakness and peripheral vasodilation.

      f. Respiratory failure.

    2. TREATMENT. As given for the inhalation type (A,2, above). The prognosis, however, is much better. Hospitalization for observation and treatment of possible liver damage is usually indicated.

C. Delayed Toxicity Type. Delayed toxic reactions to chloroform usually develop 3 to 5 days after administration of an anesthetic to elderly, run-down or cachectic persons and are characterized by severe liver and kidney damage.

    1. SIGNS AND SYMPTOMS

      a. Gradual development of drowsiness and sleepiness.

      b. Nausea and vomiting.

      c. Changes in size of liver—usually enlarged and painful, but may be contracted.

      d. Signs of kidney irritation. The urine may contain acetone and bile pigments.

      e. Delirium and coma.

    2. TREATMENT

      a. Oxygen inhalations.

      b. Caffeine sodiobenzoate, 0.5 gm., intramuscularly or intravenously.

      c. Hospitalization as soon as acute symptoms have been controlled.

49–138. **CHLORONAPHTHALENE** (Halowax)

A. Signs and Symptoms

    1. Acute gastrointestinal irritation.

    2. Jaundice.

    3. Convulsions.

    4. Coma.

    5. Possible severe liver damage.

B. Treatment

    1. Control of convulsions by ether inhalations or rapidly acting barbiturates.

2. Gastric lavage.
3. Oxygen therapy as required.
4. Hospitalization for measures against possible liver damage.

49–139. CHLORONITROBENZENE. See *Nitrobenzene* (49–394).

49–140. CHLOROPICRIN

Developed originally as a war gas, chloropicrin (trichloronitromethane) is now used occasionally as a fumigant. Vomiting is the chief symptom of toxicity. For treatment see under *War Gases* (49–648).

49–141. CHLOROQUINE PHOSPHATE (Aralen Diphosphate)

Long-term use of this antimalarial drug has been reported to cause retinopathy and blindness.

Accidental ingestion by children of even small amounts has a very high mortality rate. Fatalities have been caused by as little as 1 gm.

A. Signs and Symptoms (Develop rapidly—usually within 30 minutes)
   1. Headache, very severe.
   2. Visual disturbances.
   3. Convulsions.
   4. Respiratory and cardiac arrest; develops suddenly and without warning.

B. Treatment
   1. Emptying of stomach by emetics (49–4,D) *at home,* followed by lavage at a hospital after control of convulsions by rapidly acting barbiturates.
   2. Oxygenation and, if necessary, closed cardiac massage (Topic 17–2,A).
   3. Vasopressors as needed.
   4. Ammonium chloride by mouth if the patient survives the acute phase; should be continued for at least 48 hours in hospital.

49–142. CHLOROTHIAZIDE (Diuril). See under *Diuretics* (Topic 59–69).

49–143. CHLORTHION. See *Organic Phosphates* (49–421).

49–144. CHOKECHERRY

Sometimes eaten in large quantities by children, campers and tourists, this wild fruit may cause serious and even fatal toxic symptoms. The toxicity is due to the presence of amygdalin. The treatment is the same as outlined under cyanides (49–170).

49–145. CHROMATES, CHROMIC ACID, CHROMIUM TRIOXIDE

This acid and its salts are used medicinally, in paints, and in the chemical and leather industries.

A. Modes of Toxicity

1. EXPOSURE TO DUST may cause chronic sloughs of the nasal cartilages with epistaxis and an acute macular dermatitis. Acute allergic reactions, sometimes very severe, may also occur (Topic 24).
2. INGESTION may cause:
   a. Yellow discoloration of the mouth and pharynx.
   b. Cold, clammy, cyanotic skin.
   c. Dysphagia from corrosion and edema of the posterior pharynx, glottis and esophagus.
   d. Severe gastric burning, with vomiting of yellowish and greenish material, often followed by watery, bloody diarrhea.
   e. Acute myalgia.
   f. Acute kidney damage, with residual permanent changes.
   g. Coma.

B. Treatment

1. If ingested, immediate gastric lavage with large amounts of warm water.
2. Oxygen under positive pressure by face mask and rebreathing bag for cyanosis.
3. Normal salt solution intravenously.
4. Caffeine sodiobenzoate, 0.5 gm., intramuscularly.
5. Calcium gluconate, 10 ml. of 10% solution, intravenously for acute muscular cramps.
6. Morphine sulfate or dihydromorphinone hydrochloride (Dilaudid) in small doses subcutaneously or intravenously for relief of acute pain.
7. Tracheotomy (Topic 17–11,B) if swelling of the glottis is progressive and possible interference with breathing is anticipated.

49–146. CHRYSAROBIN

Accidental ingestion of this substance, sometimes used in the treatment of fungous infections, has caused severe nausea, vomiting, gastric pain and diarrhea. It apparently acts only as a simple irritant. Treatment consists of demulcents and emetics by mouth followed by magnesium sulfate (Epsom salts). Complete recovery without residual ill effects is the rule.

49–147. CIGARETTES AND CIGARS

These may be ingested by children or may cause acute toxic symptoms in nonaccustomed persons through inhalation. The toxic effects are due to nicotine (49–389).

49–148. CINCHOPHEN

Cinchophen is used in rheumatism remedies and as an antipyretic.

  A. Signs and Symptoms
   1. Tinnitus, vertigo and deafness.
   2. Nausea and vomiting.
   3. Hepatic tenderness and pain.
   4. Coma. If terminal, acute fatty degeneration of the liver is usually found.

  B. Treatment
   1. Gastric lavage with 1:5000 potassium solution.
   2. Caffeine sodiobenzoate, 0.5 gm., intramuscularly.
   3. Magnesium sulfate (Epsom salts) by mouth in large doses.
   4. Hospitalization if large amounts have been ingested because of possible serious liver damage.

49–149. CINEOL

Cineol is the chief toxic substance in oil of cajeput and oil of eucalyptus. [See *Oil, Essential* (49–407).]

49–150. CLEANING FLUIDS AND COMPOUNDS

These liquids are readily available in most households and account for many cases of severe poisoning in children. Common offenders are:
   1. Benzene (benzol) and its derivates [naphtha, toluene, toluol, xylene and xylol (49–80)].
   2. Carbon tetrachloride (49–120).
   3. Gasoline (49–254).
   4. Kerosene (49–303).
   5. Oxalic acid (49–425).
   6. Stoddard solvent (49–561).

49–151. COBALT. See *Metal Fumes* (49–348).

49–152. COCAINE (Methyl-benzoyl-ecgonine hydrochloride)

Cocaine ("snow") and its salts may cause severe toxic symptoms in a number of ways.

  A. By Absorption from Skin or Mucous Membrane Following Local Medicinal Use. See 49–52 (*Anesthetics, Local*) and Topic 59–10.

  B. By Use in the Eyes
   1. SIGNS AND SYMPTOMS
      a. Acute conjunctivitis, sometimes with hemorrhage.

    b. Chemosis, lacrimation and photophobia.
    c. Edema of the lids.
    d. Corneal ulceration and keratitis.
    e. Glaucoma.
    f. Acute systemic symptoms as given under C below.

2. TREATMENT
    a. Discontinue use of the medication at once.
    b. Treat the systemic symptoms (C, below).
    c. Hospitalize if local or general symptoms are severe or if the patient does not respond satisfactorily to treatment.

C. By Self-administration. Cocaine and its salts in certain individuals cause euphoria, elation and increased mental and physical activity. Sniffing of the powder, ingestion and hypodermic injection may result in symptoms which will cause the user to be brought for examination and treatment. Tolerance to tremendous doses is rapidly attained, but the remarkable absence of acute withdrawal symptoms results in few, if any, cases of true addiction (Topic 2). Continued use, however, may result in mental and moral deterioration, cachexia, insomnia, diplopia, transient anesthesias, hallucinations, and mania—sometimes homicidal. Self-administration is reportable AT ONCE to the proper authorities.

1. SIGNS AND SYMPTOMS (following overdosage by any method)
    a. Widely dilated pupils.
    b. Weak, rapid pulse.
    c. Severe chills; skin pale and clammy.
    d. Burning and feeling of constriction in the pharynx, with or without dysphagia.
    e. Nausea, vomiting and severe gastric pain, with tenesmus and/or diarrhea, sometimes severe enough to be mistaken for an acute surgical abdomen.
    f. Acute dyspnea; occasionally Cheyne-Stokes respiration.
    g. Acute central nervous system symptoms—headache, dizziness, excitement, confusion, hallucinations, illusions, etc. Loss of the senses of taste and smell is fairly common.
    h. Slowly developing coma with death from respiratory failure.

2. TREATMENT
    a. If the drug has been recently injected subcutaneously or intramuscularly, absorption sometimes can be controlled to some extent by application of a tourniquet or packing the extremity in ice. If the drug has been injected intravenously, the absorption is so rapid and the onset of toxic effects so speedy that a tourniquet is of no value. If ingested, the universal antidote (49–10), tannic acid solution (strong tea), or weak potassium iodide solution should be given by mouth, followed by thorough gastric lavage with 1:5000 potassium permanganate solution. If the patient will not cooperate sufficiently to allow safe passage of a stomach tube, apomorphine hydrochloride, 3 to 5 mg., should be given subcutaneously followed by as much warm water as the patient will drink.

b. Acute cocaine intoxication, no matter what its cause, should be treated as follows:

  (1) Phenobarbital sodium, 0.3 gm., intramuscularly or intravenously. Paraldehyde, 4 ml., in normal saline intramuscularly may be substituted. Sedatives should be administered *only if necessary* and with great caution.

  (2) Atropine sulfate, 1 mg., subcutaneously or intravenously.

  (3) Caffeine sodiobenzoate, 0.5 gm., intramuscularly or intravenously.

  (4) Hospitalization as soon as condition permits because of the danger of delayed collapse.

49–153. CODEINE (Methylmorphine)

This widely used narcotic is relatively safe. It practically never causes addiction. Large oral or parenteral doses may have toxic effects.

A. Signs and Symptoms

1. Slowing of the pulse, which usually remains regular and of good quality.
2. Flushing of the face, associated with a feeling of tightness in the head, especially in the occipital region; extreme generalized vasodilation.
3. Nausea and vomiting; gastric pain.
4. Temporary anuria; constipation and impaction.
5. Extreme miosis in early stages, followed by terminal mydriasis. Exophthalmos may be present. Smaller doses sometimes have a temporary mydriatic effect.
6. Muscle fibrillation, tremors, occasionally generalized convulsions.
7. Respiratory paralysis.

B. Treatment

1. Emetics followed by gastric lavage with 1:5000 potassium permanganate solution if ingested.
2. Magnesium sulfate (Epsom salts) by mouth; relief of impaction may be required.
3. Oxygen therapy under positive pressure.
4. Caffeine sodiobenzoate, 0.5 gm., intramuscularly.
5. Hospitalization in severe cases as soon as the patient's general condition permits.

49–154. COLCHICINE

Colchicine is an active and toxic alkaloid occurring in a common plant, meadow saffron. Ingestion of any part of the plant may cause acute poisoning. Used medicinally as an antirheumatic remedy it may cause severe toxic signs and symptoms coming on about 2 hours after ingestion.

A. Signs and Symptoms

1. A sensation of suffocation and tightness in the chest with difficulty in swallowing.
2. Nausea and violent vomiting followed by watery or bloody diarrhea.

    3. Severe generalized myalgia and arthralgia with twitching of iso-
        lated muscle groups. The muscles of the calves are especially
        affected.
    4. Cyanosis.
    5. Dilated pupils.
    6. Persistent consciousness until death occurs from generalized ex-
        haustion in from 10 to 36 hours.

B. Treatment
    1. Emetics followed by gastric lavage with 1:5000 potassium per-
        manganate solution.
    2. Rapidly acting barbiturates intravenously for sedation.
    3. Calcium gluconate, 10 ml. of 10% solution, intravenously for
        myalgia.

49–155. COLOCYNTH (Bitter Apples)

A. Signs and Symptoms
    1. Visual and auditory disturbances.
    2. Vertigo.
    3. Confusion and disorientation.
    4. Severe abdominal pain.
    5. Watery and bloody diarrhea.
    6. Kidney irritation with polyuria and oliguria.
    7. Liver and pancreas damage.
    8. Circulatory disturbances (weakness, faintness, clammy skin,
        etc.) followed by collapse.

B. Treatment
    1. Evacuation of stomach contents by emetics if possible; if un-
        successful, by gastric lavage with 1:5000 potassium per-
        manganate solution.
    2. Caffeine sodiobenzoate, 0.5 gm., intramuscularly.
    3. Hospitalization if signs of kidney, liver or pancreas damage are
        present.

49–156. CONIINE (Hemlock, Horseradish)

The leaves containing this alkaloid may be confused with parsley, celery and parsnip.

A. Signs and Symptoms
    1. Nausea and vomiting, salivation.
    2. Acute dysphagia.
    3. Dilated pupils, diplopia and amblyopia.
    4. Impaired hearing.
    5. Convulsions.
    6. Progressive weakening of skeletal musculature, respiratory mus-
        cles last of all.
    7. Complete consciousness until death from respiratory failure.

B. Treatment
    1. Evacuation of stomach contents as soon as possible by emetics
        and/or gastric lavage.

    2. Administration of saline cathartics.

    3. Oxygen therapy as needed, preferably under positive pressure.

  C. Prognosis. Good if the patient survives for 2 hours. No permanent ill effects are to be anticipated.

49–157. COPPER

Chronic copper poisoning gives a toxic picture similar to lead poisoning (49–313).

  A. The following salts of copper may cause acute poisoning characterized by vomiting and acute gastroenteritis:

    1. Copper acetoarsenite (verdigris, Paris green). Arsenic poisoning symptoms [see *Arsenic* (49–63)] are also caused by this pigment.

    2. Copper oxides [also see *Metal Fumes* (49–348)].

    3. Copper sulfate (bluestone, blue vitriol).

  B. Treatment

    1. Demulcents—milk, white of eggs.

    2. Potassium ferrocyanide, 0.5 gm., in water by mouth.

    3. Lavage with 1000 ml. of water containing milk of magnesia.

49–158. CORROSIVE ACIDS. See *Acids* (49–19).

49–159. CORROSIVE SUBLIMATE. See *Bichloride of Mercury* (49–87).

49–160. CORTISONE. [Also see Topic 59–2 (*ACTH*).]

This crystalline hormonal substance may cause many types of toxic symptoms, especially through sodium retention and the production of alkalosis through metabolic imbalance. Among the symptoms which may bring the patient for emergency care are hypertension, sleepiness, nervousness, extreme weakness, psychosis, and pain and hemorrhage from the upper gastrointestinal tract. Except for stopping the cortisone and administering sedation, the only treatment required is arrangement for thorough evaluation, preferably under hospital control.

49–161. COSMETICS

Although an almost endless variety of substances are used in cosmetics, antimony and arsenic-containing compounds are the main offenders in the production of toxic symptoms. See *Antimony* (49–57) and *Arsenic* (49–63). The use of "indelible" lipsticks may cause soreness of the tongue and throat, coryza, sinusitis, as well as dermatitis and urticaria. Patch tests may be necessary to identify the offending substance.

49–162. CRAYONS

Most varieties of children's chalk and wax crayons are required by law to be harmless. In spite of this, ingestion of some types of wax crayons may cause toxic symptoms from paranitraniline and/or benzidine. In addition, toxic symptoms from arsenic salts, chromium, copper and lead have been reported. Some marking crayons, such as those used by carpenters, may be dangerous. Aniline dyes are usually the toxic substance.

Treatment. See *Aniline Dyes* (49–54).

49–163. CREOLIN

This is a compound containing about 15% cresols. For signs and symptoms of toxicity and treatment see *Phenol* (49–450).

49–164. CREOSOTE

The toxic properties of this substance are the result of its cresol content. For toxic picture and treatment see *Phenol* (49–450).

49–165. CRESOL. See *Phenol* (49–450).

49–166. CROTON OIL

Acute and sometimes dangerous toxic signs and symptoms caused by this irritant cathartic and purgative are sometimes encountered following ingestion in an alcoholic drink (the so-called "Mickey Finn") used occasionally by bartenders to get rid of obstreperous customers.

A. Signs and Symptoms
1. A burning sensation in the mouth.
2. Severe stomach pain with nausea and vomiting.
3. Severe purging; diarrhea may be bloody.
4. Collapse and coma.

B. Treatment
1. Egg white or flour mixed with water by mouth.
2. Emetics such as mustard in warm water or syrup of ipecac; if unsuccessful, apomorphine hydrochloride, 5 mg., subcutaneously.
3. Stimulants—strong coffee, aromatic spirits of ammonia (4 ml. in water) by mouth or caffeine sodiobenzoate, 0.5 gm., intramuscularly.
4. Shock therapy if indicated (Topic 15–7).
5. Hospitalization in severe cases.

49–167. CUBEB

At one time cubeb was commonly used as a urinary antiseptic and in the form of cigarettes for asthma and bronchitis. Inhalation or ingestion of this oleoresin may cause severe toxic symptoms.

   A. *Signs and Symptoms*
   1. Nausea and vomiting; abdominal pain and diarrhea.
   2. Severe muscle and joint pain; muscular fibrillation and twitching.
   3. Miosis.
   4. Delirium, followed by coma and death from respiratory failure.
   B. *Treatment*
   1. Emetics followed by gastric lavage with 1:5000 potassium permanganate solution.
   2. Oxygen therapy.
   3. Calcium gluconate, 10 ml. of 10% solution, given slowly intravenously.
   4. Large amounts of fluids by mouth or intravenously.

49–168. CURARE (Intocostrin, Metubine Iodide, d-Tubocurarine Chloride)

Acute toxic signs and symptoms may follow parenteral injection of any derivatives of curare as adjuncts to anesthesia or as muscle relaxants, and are characterized by prolonged apnea, bradycardia, and vascular collapse.

   Treatment
   1. Oxygen therapy.
   2. Neostigmine methylsulfate, 1 to 2 mg., subcutaneously.
   3. Atropine sulfate, 0.5 mg., subcutaneously or intravenously.
   4. Avoidance of massage or local heat to the site of injection.

49–169. CUTICLE REMOVERS

These commonly used cosmetic preparations may contain potassium hydroxide and/or trisodium phosphate. See *Alkalies* (49–28).

49–170. CYANIDES

   A. *Signs and Symptoms.* Victims of acute cyanide poisoning are practically always either dead or in deep coma when first seen by the physician. Occasionally, recognition of the known exposure, with odor of bitter almonds on the breath, may give time for administration of pure oxygen under pressure, followed by animal charcoal and hydrogen peroxide (1:5) and sodium thiosulfate, 5% solution, by mouth. If the patient receives the oxygen therapy while vital signs are present, he has some chance of recovery. Following this, the routine treatment below should be given AT ONCE.

B. Routine Treatment
1. Amyl nitrite inhalations alternating with oxygen therapy. A syringe containing epinephrine hydrochloride (Adrenalin), 1:1000 solution, should be ready at all times to combat a sudden drop in blood pressure.
2. Immediate intravenous injection—VERY SLOWLY—of 20 ml. of a 5% solution of sodium thiosulfate, alternating every 10 minutes with intravenous injection of 50 ml. of a 1% solution of methylene blue containing 1.8% sodium sulfate (Geiger's formula). This may be repeated until 500 ml. of sodium thiosulfate and 200 ml. of methylene blue solution have been given.
3. Caffeine sodiobenzoate, 0.5 gm., intravenously. Atropine sulfate, pentylenetetrazol (Metrazol), and strophanthin may be tried but are of questionable value.
4. Hospitalization for whole blood transfusions and follow-up care because of the danger of sudden relapse.

C. Prognosis. If the patient is alive 1 hour after exposure to fumes or ingestion of the cyanide compound there is some chance he may recover. Sudden, unexplained and fatal relapses may occur 4 to 5 hours after apparent improvement.

49–171.   **CYCLOPROPANE.** See Topic 59–8 (*Anesthetics, Inhalation*).

. . . . D . . . .

49–172.   **DAPHNE** (Wild Pepper, Dwarf Bay). See 49–703.

49–173.   **DD COMPOUNDS** (Chlorinated Propylene-propanes)

All of these compounds are used full strength as fumigants. They are very toxic by ingestion, absorption through the intact skin and inhalation but, fortunately, have a garlic-like odor which is very offensive and repellent even to small children.

A. Signs and Symptoms
1. Blistering of the skin on contact.
2. Acute irritation of the eyes and upper respiratory tract from fumes.
3. Substernal pain, dyspnea and cyanosis.
4. Acute gastroenteritis.
5. Pulmonary edema (Topic 52).

B. Treatment
1. IF ON THE SKIN
   a. Remove contaminated clothing and wash the skin thoroughly with mild soap and water.

    b. Treat blisters as second degree chemical burns (Topic 28–10).
  2. IF INHALED
    a. Remove from exposure.
    b. Start artificial respiration at once, followed as soon as possible by oxygen inhalations under positive pressure using a face mask and rebreathing bag.
    c. Inject theophylline ethylenediamine (aminophylline) SLOWLY intravenously if bronchospasm is present.
    d. Give sedative cough mixtures.
    e. Treat pulmonary edema (Topic 52–3) if present.
    f. Hospitalize for at least 24 hours for observation.
  3. IF INGESTED
    a. Administer nonoily demulcents.
    b. Empty the stomach immediately by gastric lavage with large amounts of water.
    c. Control gastrointestinal pain with narcotics as needed.
    d. Support the respiration with oxygen therapy.
    e. Hospitalize for supportive and symptomatic care.

49–174.   **DDD** (Tetrachlorodiphenylethane). For toxicity and treatment see *DDT* (49–175).

49–175.   **DDT** (Dichlorodiphenyltrichlorethane, Chlorophenothane)

    Used extensively as an insecticide, DDT has undoubtedly often been credited with the production of serious conditions—especially pulmonary edema (Topic 52)—caused in fact by the solvents used in the insect sprays, usually petroleum derivatives. However, in strong concentrations, or if ingested, DDT has a definite toxic action which usually comes on 2 to 4 hours after exposure.

  A. Signs and Symptoms
    1. Vomiting from gastric irritation.
    2. Acute depression and apprehension.
    3. Incoordination and giddiness; paresthesias of the face and lips.
    4. Muscular tremors and convulsions, both tonic and clonic.
    5. Dyspnea and cyanosis, followed by respiratory failure. Death may occur from sudden ventricular fibrillation.

  B. Treatment
    1. Demulcents by mouth followed by gastric lavage with large amounts of water.
    2. Magnesium sulfate (Epsom salts), 30 gm., by mouth.
    3. Oxygen therapy under positive pressure by face mask and rebreathing bag or intranasal catheter if signs of respiratory distress are present.
    4. Caffeine sodiobenzoate, 0.5 gm., intramuscularly or intravenously.
    5. Calcium gluconate, 10 ml. of a 10% solution, intravenously.
    6. Phenobarbital sodium, 0.06 to 0.2 gm., intravenously if convulsions are present.

7. Hospitalization for at least 24 hours under close observation because of the tendency toward relapse.

C. **Chronic Exposure** to DDT has been reported as causing blurred speech, loss of coordination and other neurologic signs and symptoms.

49–176. DELPHINIUM (Larkspur). See 49–705.

49–177. DEMEROL (Meperidine, Isonipecaine, Dolantin, Dolosal, Pethidine, Endolat)

This commonly used synthetic narcotic is similar in action and addictive tendencies to the narcotic opium derivatives, although it is a much weaker anodyne. See Topic 2–3 (*Addiction*); Topic 9 (*Narcotics*) and *Morphine* (49–370).

49–178. DEMETON (Systox). See *Organic Phosphates* (49–421).

49–179. DEODORANTS AND DEODORIZERS

Preparations used to neutralize body odor may contain *alcohol* (49–22 and 23), *aluminum salts* (49–36), or *boric acid* or *borates* (49–96). Deodorizers used in the home may contain *formaldehyde* (49–246), *essential oils* (49–407), *p-dichlorobenzene* (49–183), *naphthalene* (49–381) or *isopropyl alcohol* (49–300). Although most deodorant preparations contain only small amounts of toxic materials, ingestion of more than a minute quantity calls for emptying the stomach by emetics or gastric lavage.

49–180. DEPILATORIES (Hair Removers)

These cosmetics usually contain a mixture of inert ingredients with barium, calcium and sodium sulfide or thallium. See *Sodium Sulfide* (49–550) and *Thallium* (49–597).

49–181. DETERGENTS. See *Alkyl Sodium Sulfates* (49–31).

49–182. DIALKYLPHOSPHATE

Although this substance is sometimes used medicinally in glaucoma and myasthenia gravis because of its anticholinesterase activity, its use as an insecticide causes most of the cases of acute poisoning. The signs and symptoms of toxicity and treatment are the same as outlined under *Organic Phosphates* (49–421).

49–183. DICHLOROBENZENE

Both the ortho isomer (used as a wood preservative) and the para isomer (used in mothproofing sprays) are toxic when inhaled or ingested. Signs and symptoms of toxicity and treatment are approximately the same as for naphthalene (49–381).

49–184. DICHLOROETHANE

A. *Use.* As a solvent for fats, gums, rubber and resins.
B. *Signs and Symptoms* may be caused by inhalation or ingestion.
  1. Nausea and vomiting; diarrhea.
  2. Somnolence; weakness.
  3. Respiratory and circulatory collapse.
C. *Treatment*
  1. If inhaled, immediate removal from the area contaminated with fumes to the fresh air. If ingested, emptying of the stomach by emetics and/or gastric lavage followed by saline cathartics.
  2. Oxygen therapy.
  3. Caffeine sodiobenzoate, 0.5 gm., intramuscularly. Shock therapy (Topic 15–7) may be necessary.
  4. Hospitalization in severe cases because of the tendency toward serious liver and kidney damage.

49–185. 2, 4-DICHLOROPHENOXYACETIC ACID (2–4–D).

This acid is used in the preparation of herbicides utilized principally in the control of broad-leafed weeds. Although no proved cases of acute toxicity in man following ingestion have been reported, experimental studies indicate that it is a potentially dangerous substance. Peripheral neuropathy following exposure to the diethylamine salt during manufacture has been reported, with spontaneous recovery.
  Treatment
  1. Immediate gastric lavage.
  2. Support of the circulatory system.
  3. Oral administration of quinidine sulfate to combat extreme muscle weakness and to prevent development of ventricular fibrillation.

49–186. DICODID (Eucodal)

This is used medicinally as a sedative and analgesic, and gives toxic reactions similar to morphine. Addiction (Topic 2–3) has been reported. For treatment see *Morphine* (49–370).

49–187. **DICUMAROL**

Because this anticoagulant causes bleeding for some time after discontinuance of therapeutic use, emergency care may be required for some or all of the toxic effects listed below. 4-Hydroxycoumarin [*Warfarin* (49–647)], used as a rodenticide only, is even more toxic, especially to children.

A. Signs and Symptoms
1. Generalized ecchymoses; hemorrhagic purpura, hematuria, hemorrhage from the nose, gums or gastrointestinal tract.
2. Menorrhagia.
3. Extreme weakness from secondary anemia.

B. Treatment
1. Stop the anticoagulant if still being given. If ingested, empty the stomach immediately.
2. Transfer for hospitalization for vitamin K therapy, fluid replacement (Topic 7) and possibly transfusions.

49–188. **DIELDRIN** (Hexachloro-epoxy-octahydroendo, Exo-dimethane naphthalene)

A. Uses. As an insecticide where long-continued action is desirable, usually in combination with kerosene (49–303) and xylene (49–660), both of which may complicate the toxic picture.

B. Absorption may be through the intact skin, by inhalation, or through the gastrointestinal tract, with the primary site of toxic action the central nervous system.

C. Signs and Symptoms (usually delayed ½ to 10 hours after ingestion)
1. Severe headache and vertigo.
2. Nausea and vomiting.
3. Muscular twitching and tremors.
4. Severe epileptiform convulsions; these may be the first manifestations of poisoning and may occur without premonitory symptoms.
5. Acute respiratory depression, sometimes terminal.

D. Treatment
1. Removal of all contaminated clothing; thorough washing of skin with soap and water. THE ATTENDANT MUST WEAR GLOVES.
2. Prevention or control of convulsions by large doses of rapid-acting barbiturates, intravenously if necessary.
3. If ingested, emptying of the stomach by lavage with large amounts of warm water.
4. Administration of oxygen under positive pressure, preferably by face mask or endotracheal catheter and rebreathing bag.
5. Hospitalization as soon as possible with continued treatment and observation for at least a week after the last convulsion. Recovery is usually slow but complete.

49–189. **DIETHYLENE GLYCOL** (Diethylene Ether)

Rather commonly used in industry as a solvent, lubricant and hygroscopic agent, this liquid, if ingested, may have very serious immediate and delayed effects.

A. Signs and Symptoms
1. Ataxia and vertigo.
2. Nausea, vomiting and abdominal cramping, often associated with diarrhea.
3. Heartburn.
4. Extreme generalized weakness and myalgia, especially of the lumbar muscles.
5. Coma, sometimes preceded by convulsions. Death occurs from respiratory failure.
6. Severe kidney damage with albuminuria and oliguria; sometimes uremia in severe cases which recover from coma.

B. Treatment
1. Immediate emptying of the stomach by emetics and/or gastric lavage.
2. Administration of oxygen under positive pressure by face mask or intranasal catheter and rebreathing bag if respiratory depression is acute.
3. Normal salt solution, 1000 ml., intravenously.
4. Hospitalization because of the tendency of diethylene glycol to cause delayed and severe kidney damage.

49–190. **DIETHYLSTILBESTROL**

Therapeutic doses, or overdosage, of this estrogenic agent may cause toxic reactions.

A. Signs and Symptoms
1. Extreme lassitude.
2. Nausea and vomiting.
3. Abdominal pain followed by bloody diarrhea.
4. Temporary psychoses.

B. Treatment
1. Discontinue administration of the estrogen.
2. Administer sedation as needed.
3. Refer for gynecologic consultations as soon as possible.

49–191. **DIGITALIS**

A. Signs and Symptoms
1. Headache, nausea and vomiting.
2. Loss of appetite, tiredness, general malaise and drowsiness.
3. Slow pulse; bigeminal rhythm.

4. Visual disturbances (amblyopia, blurring, diplopia, bizarre color vision changes).
5. Characteristic ECG changes.

B. Treatment
1. If seen early before toxic symptoms are marked, emptying of the stomach by emetics and/or gastric lavage with 500 ml. of 1:1000 potassium permanganate solution or strong tea (tannic acid solution, 1%).
2. Oral or intravenous administration of potassium.
3. Application of external heat.
4. Atropine sulfate, 0.5 to 1.0 mg., subcutaneously or intravenously.
5. Inhalations of oxygen.
6. Sedation by cautious use of barbiturates.

49–192. DILAN

This insecticide is similar in action and toxicity to DDT. (49–175).

49–193. DILANTIN (Sodium Diphenylhydantoinate).

Usual doses, as well as overdosage, of this drug used for prevention of epileptic attacks may cause a severe toxic picture.

A. Signs and Symptoms
1. Feelings of apprehension, tension and tremulousness.
2. Dizziness and ataxia.
3. Nausea and vomiting.
4. Blurring of vision and diplopia.
5. Generalized lymphadenopathy and hepatosplenomegaly.

B. Treatment
1. Discontinue therapeutic use, or decrease the size of the dose, of the drug.
2. Impress on the patient or his family the need for further medical treatment. The patient should be made to understand that stopping the drug may cause an increase in the number and severity of the attacks of epilepsy.

49–194. DILAUDID (Dihydromorphinone Hydrochloride)

The signs and symptoms of acute toxicity, addictive tendencies (Topic 2–3) and treatment are approximately the same as outlined under morphine (49–370).

49–195. DIMERCAPROL (2, 3-Dimercaptopropanol). See *BAL* (49–74).

49–196.   **DIMETHYL KETONE.** See *Acetone* (49–14).

49–197.   **DIMETAN**

This is used as an aphicide. Skin absorption does not occur, but ingestion may cause a toxic picture similar to that caused by DDT (49–175).

49–198.   **DIMETHYLPHTHALATE** is used as an insect repellent. Ingestion may cause toxic effects.

   A. *Signs and Symptoms*
     1. Burning sensation of mucous membranes of the mouth, throat and pharynx.
     2. Coma, usually delayed 1 to 2 hours after ingestion.
   B. *Treatment*
     1. Universal antidote (49–10) or demulcents by mouth.
     2. Emptying of the stomach as soon as possible by emetics and/or gastric lavage.
     3. Dextrose, 5% in saline, 500 to 1000 ml., intravenously.
     4. Caffeine sodiobenzoate, 0.5 gm., intramuscularly or intravenously.

49–199.   **DINITROBENZENE**

Evidence of acute toxicity may come on suddenly or may develop following several weeks' exposure in industry. Symptoms may be brought on by prolonged exposure to sunlight or by overindulgence in alcoholic beverages.

   A. *Signs and Symptoms*
     1. Complaint of a taste like bitter almonds in the mouth.
     2. Headache, vertigo, fatigue.
     3. Dyspnea.
     4. Nausea and vomiting with severe gastric pain.
     5. A peculiar cyanosis, ranging from pale yellow to a grayish black. Jaundice may be present.
     6. Marked blood picture changes.
   B. *Treatment*
     1. Gastric lavage with normal salt solution.
     2. Saline cathartics.
     3. Dextrose, 5% in saline, 500 to 1000 ml., intravenously.
     4. Oxygen therapy.
     5. Methylene blue (1% solution in 1.8% sodium sulfate solution), 50 ml., intravenously for cyanosis.
     6. Hospitalization because of the tendency toward late development of serious heart, liver and blood damage.

49–200. **DINITROCRESOL**

Uses. Fungicide and insecticide. For symptoms and signs of toxicity and treatment see *Dinitrophenol* (49–201).

49–201. **DINITROPHENOL**

Prescription or sale of this substance for use as a weight reducing medication is prohibited by law. It is used extensively in the explosives industry and as a fungicide, insecticide and weed-killer.

A. *Signs and Symptoms*
1. EXTREME TEMPERATURE ELEVATION to 110° F. (43.3° C.).
2. Profuse perspiration, extreme thirst and fatigue.
3. Flushing of the skin followed by development of a yellow color.
4. Rapid, deep breathing; restlessness; acute anxiety, sometimes convulsions.
5. Coma followed by death from respiratory failure.

B. *Treatment*
1. Gastric lavage with large amounts of 1:2000 potassium permanganate or 5% sodium bicarbonate solution.
2. Reduction of temperature by cold packs, cold water enemas or alcohol rubs.
3. Dextrose, 5% in saline, 1000 ml., intravenously.
4. Oxygen by face mask and rebreathing bag.
5. Caffeine sodiobenzoate, 0.5 gm., intramuscularly or intravenously.

49–202. **DINITROTOLUENE**

This may cause arthralgia, dyspnea and cyanosis, severe headache, dizziness, nystagmus and severe chest pain, usually in persons handling the material. Ingestion of alcohol in any form accentuates the toxic picture.

Treatment. See *Nitrobenzene* (49–394).

49–203. **DIODRAST**

Diodrast is used in intravenous pyelography. Mild allergic reactions (Topic 24) are relatively common; rarely, death may occur from acute hypersensitivity.

All patients should be tested for sensitivity before injection of the contrast medium.

49–204. **DISULFIRAM** (Antabuse). See Topic 59–11.

49–205. **DITHIOCARBAMATES** (Maneb, Nabam, Ferbam, Zeneb, Zerlate, Ziram). See under *Zerlate* (49–664).

49–206. **DJENKOL BEANS**

These beans are used as a food by natives of Java and Sumatra and, as a rule, are well tolerated. However, occasionally they may cause acute and very uncomfortable effects, even in persons accustomed to them for years.

   A. Signs and Symptoms
      1. Musty odor to the breath.
      2. Severe bladder and inguinal pain; milky urine with a very offensive odor; hematuria, anuria.
      3. Intense colic with flatulence, vomiting and diarrhea.

   B. Treatment
      1. Large amounts of fluids by mouth.
      2. Sodium bicarbonate, 2 to 4 gm., orally three to four times a day.
      3. Morphine sulfate or dihydromorphinone hydrochloride (Dilaudid) in small doses subcutaneously for severe pain.

  Prognosis. Fatalities are rare. Complete recovery in 3 to 4 days is the usual course.

49–207. **DOG PARSLEY.** See 49–706.

49–208. **DORIDEN** (Glutethimide)

This drug, although not a barbiturate, has similar actions and toxicity. See *Barbiturates* (49–76).

49–209. **DYES**

   A. Aniline Dyes. See 49–54.
   B. Azo Dyes. The most commonly used azo dyes are alizarine blue S, brilliant vital red, Chicago blue, chlorazol fast pink, indigo carmine, Pyridium (a commonly used urinary antiseptic which may cause methemoglobinemia if given in large doses), scarlet red and toluidine blue. All the members of this group have approximately the same toxicity as *Scarlet Red* (49–517) and require the same treatment.
   C. Benzidine Dyes have been used extensively as trypanocides. The most commonly used members of this group are diamidinostilbene, pentamidine, tryptan blue and tryptan red. All are toxic if large

amounts are ingested and all have a cumulative toxic action if therapeutic doses are continued over a long period.

1. SIGNS AND SYMPTOMS
   a. Fever.
   b. Acute dermatitis, often generalized, may be exfoliative.
   c. Acute or chronic kidney irritation.
   d. Occasional agranulocytosis.
2. TREATMENT consists of withdrawal of the drug, although symptoms may persist for as long as 6 weeks afterward. Ingestion of large amounts requires immediate emptying of the stomach by emetics and/or gastric lavage followed by vigorous catharsis.

D. Coal Tar Dyes

This general heading includes all dyes derived from benzene (49–80), and includes all the headings listed in this section, and.

E. Flavins (acridine dyes) are derived from a coal tar base and, before the development of the sulfa drugs and antibiotics, were frequently used in 1:1000 to 1:10,000 solutions to check surface infection. The two most common preparations are acriflavine and proflavine. Neither is toxic if applied to raw surfaces or ingested. Industrial exposure has been reported as causing acute conjunctivitis, lacrimation and acute dermatitis.

F. Gentian Violet (methylrosaniline chloride) is a triphenylamine dye. Large amounts of gentian violet, as well as the other common triphenyl dyes (brilliant green, acid fuchsin and basic fuchsin) can be ingested without danger to life, although in some persons nausea, vomiting and diarrhea may occur.

1. TREATMENT
   a. Removal of large amounts from the stomach by emetics and/or gastric lavage.
   b. Administration of magnesium sulfate (Epsom salts) by mouth to clear the lower gastrointestinal tract.
   c. Assurance of the patient or family that the color of the skin, sclerae and mucous membranes will slowly return to normal.

G. Hair Dyes. See 49–260.

H. Methylene Blue (tetramethylthionine chloride) is a coal tar dye which is often used medicinally (and usually ineffectively) for its supposed parasiticidal, antiseptic and analgesic action. It has a very low toxicity. A 1% solution in 1.8% sodium sulfate solution (Geiger's formula) is used intravenously in the treatment of acute methemoglobinemia from nitrite, acetanilid and sulfanilamide poisoning because of its ability to decrease the methemoglobin and to increase the oxygen-carrying capacity of the red blood corpuscles. Conversely, in acute cyanide poisoning its tendency toward forming methemoglobin to bind the cyanide is utilized.

Ingestion of large amounts of methylene blue may cause gastrointestinal and bladder irritation, depression of the parasympathetic receptive system similar to that caused by atropine (49–71) and temperature elevation by central action.

Treatment
1. Emptying of the stomach as soon as possible by emetics and/or gastric lavage with 1:5000 potassium permanganate solution.
2. Administration of oxygen by mask and rebreathing bag if respiratory depression is present.
3. Injection of pilocarpine hydrochloride, 10 mg., subcutaneously every ½ hour or until the mouth becomes moist.
4. Sedation by barbiturates.
5. Hospitalization for observation if a large amount has been ingested. Transfusion may be indicated for hemolysis and/or methemoglobinemia.

I. Phthalein Dyes
1. EOSIN (tetrabromofluorescein) is harmless if ingested, even in large amounts. Use of lipsticks containing eosin may cause acute dermatitis or gastrointestinal symptoms in certain sensitive individuals.
2. FLUORESCEIN SODIUM (Uranine) is used locally in a 1 or 2% solution to demonstrate defects in the conjunctiva and cornea. The eye should be anesthetized with a few drops of ½% tetracaine (Pontocaine) before testing, and all fluorescein removed after examination by thorough irrigation with saline.

   Fluorescein in a 20% solution can be given orally and intravenously for diagnosis of intraocular disease and for determination of renal function. If large amounts have been ingested, emptying of the stomach by emetics and/or gastric lavage may be indicated to prevent the characteristic yellowish discoloration of the sclerae and skin, which may be very disturbing to the patient. No other treatment is necessary.
3. PHENOLPHTHALEIN. See 49–451.
4. PHENOLTETRACHLORPHTHALEIN AND PHENOLSULFONPHTHALEIN, used in tests for liver function, are harmless.
5. TETRABROMPHENOLPHTHALEIN, used in gallbladder visualization, is usually nontoxic although a few serious allergic reactions have been reported.

J. Shoe Dyes. Ingestion may cause very severe toxic reactions, as may absorption through the skin from recently dyed shoes. See *Aniline Dyes* (49–54) and *Nitrobenzene* (49–394).

K. Triphenyl Dyes (acid fuchsin, basic fuchsin, brilliant green, gentian violet) are relatively nontoxic.

. . . . E . . . .

49–210. EMETINE

This alkaloid occurs in ipecac and is used medicinally in the treatment of amebic dysentery and, in small doses, as an emetic and expectorant.

A. Signs and Symptoms
1. Nausea and vomiting.
2. Difficulty in swallowing, with a sensation of tightness in the chest.

    3. Acute stomach pain, intestinal cramping and diarrhea.

    4. Cardiac depression and collapse.

B. Treatment

    1. Absolute rest.

    2. Stimulation with analeptic drugs, especially caffeine sodiobenzoate and amphetamine sulfate (Benzedrine) parenterally.

49–211. **ENORIN**

This is an insecticide similar in action to, but more toxic than, Dieldrin (49–188).

49–212. **EPHEDRINE** (Racephedrine, I-sedrine)

Excessive use of nose drops or nasal sprays containing ephedrine may cause transient symptoms (Topic 59–26) which clear rapidly when the medication is discontinued. Ingestion may cause toxic effects.

A. Signs and Symptoms

    1. Extreme nervousness with tonic and clonic convulsions.

    2. Cold and clammy skin.

    3. Mydriasis.

    4. Dysphagia.

B. Treatment

    1. Emptying of the stomach, preferably by emetics, but if necessary by gastric lavage.

    2. Control of extreme nervousness and convulsions by sedation with barbiturates or paraldehyde.

C. Prognosis. Complete recovery usually occurs even after ingestion of very large amounts, although a few fatalities have been reported.

49–213. **EPILEPSY "CURES"**

These proprietary compounds usually contain barbiturates (49–76), bromides (49–100) or sodium diphenylhydantoinate [*Dilantin* (49–193)].

49–214. **EPINEPHRINE** (Adrenalin)

In certain hypersensitive persons even minimal therapeutic doses (Topic 59–27) may produce great discomfort.

A. Signs and Symptoms

    1. Tenseness, restlessness and acute anxiety.

    2. Tremors and dizziness.

    3. Respiratory distress, palpitation.

These symptoms are usually more uncomfortable than serious and in most instances can be cleared up rapidly by sedation with barbiturates. Severe, sometimes fatal, reactions from inadvertent, ill-advised or excessive intravenous injections of epinephrine hydrochloride have been reported. Persons with hyperthyroidism, cardiovascular disease and angina pectoris are notoriously susceptible. Aggravation of pre-existent psychomotor symptoms and activation of psychoses may take place. When epinephrine is given intravenously its action is so rapid that no emergency measures are of any benefit. Severe reactions, almost always caused by the accidental injection of a very large dose or by ingestion, are characterized by:

1. Cerebrovascular accidents (Topic 60–2).
2. Acute pulmonary edema (Topic 52–2).
3. Cardiac dilatation.
4. Ventricular fibrillation (Topic 29–3,A).

B. Treatment
1. Limitation of absorption by application of a tourniquet to an extremity proximal to the site of injection if the error in the amount injected is realized in time.
2. If ingested, emptying of the stomach AT ONCE by gastric lavage.
3. Sedation with paraldehyde or barbiturates, preferably given parenterally.
4. Oxygen inhalations by face mask and rebreathing bag.
5. Treatment of pulmonary edema (Topic 52–3).
6. Hospitalization for observation after acute symptoms have been controlled.

C. Prognosis. Good if the patient survives the first half hour. No permanent ill effects are to be anticipated.

49–215. EPN. See *Organic Phosphates* (49–421).

49–216. EPOXY RESINS

Used as concrete adhesives, these substances may cause severe contact dermatitis. The catalysts or hardeners used with these epoxy compounds may cause erythema, pruritus, periorbital and facial edema and, apparently, permanent hypersensitivity. Inhalation of the fumes may result in severe and persistent bronchospasm.

49–217. EQUANIL. See *Meprobamate* (49–336).

49–218. ERGOT

A. Signs and Symptoms
1. Extreme pallor of the face with cyanosis of the extremities.
2. Small, weak, rapid pulse.
3. Visual, auditory and sensory disturbances.
4. Hallucinations.
5. Myocardial infarction.

B. Treatment
1. Induction of vomiting followed by gastric lavage with 500 ml. of 1:2000 potassium permanganate solution if ingested.
2. Papaverine hydrochloride, 0.03 gm., subcutaneously.
3. Application of external heat.
4. Forced respiration of oxygen by face mask and rebreathing bag.
5. Hospitalization for observation. Gangrene of the extremities may occur.

49–219.   **ERGOTAMINE** (Gynergen). See *Ergot* (49–218).

49–220.   **ERYTHRITYL TETRANITRATE**

This is used commercially in the explosives industry and medicinally in the treatment of hypertension. Its toxic symptoms and signs and treatment are similar to those outlined under *Nitrites* (49–393).

49–221.   **ESERINE.** See *Physostigmine* (49–463).

49–222.   **ESSENTIAL OILS.** See *Oil, Essential* (49–407).

49–223.   **ETHANOL.** See *Ethyl Alcohol* (49–227).

49–224.   **ETHER.** See *Anesthetics, Inhalation* (Topic 59–8).

49–225.   **ETHIDE** (Dichloronitroethane)

Used as a grain fumigant. Inhalation of fumes or ingestion may cause severe toxic symptoms. The treatment is the same as for oxides of nitrogen (49–426).

49–226.   **ETHINE.** See *Acetylene* (49–17).

49–227.   **ETHYL ALCOHOL.** (Also see Topic 2–1, Topic 3–13, Topic 18–1, and Topic 36–1.)

Ethyl alcohol and isopropyl alcohol vary in some side effects but give practically the same toxic picture following ingestion. The amounts necessary to produce toxic symptoms vary markedly in different individuals. Both are commonly used in rubbing alcohol compounds, and ethyl alcohol is the active agent in intoxicating beverages. The denaturing substances commonly used to make rubbing compounds nonpotable give unpleasant symptoms but, as a rule, are harmless in themselves.

Treatment
1. Gastric lavage with a large volume of water.
2. Application of external heat.
3. Caffeine sodiobenzoate, 0.5 gm., and/or amphetamine sulfate (Benzedrine), 15 mg., intramuscularly or intravenously.
4. Prevention of aspiration of vomitus by postural drainage and suction.

49–228.   **ETHYL CHLORIDE.** See *Anesthetics, Inhalation* (Topic 59–8).

49–229.   **ETHYL GASOLINE**

The symptoms and treatment following ingestion are the same as for gasoline (49–254). Tetraethyl lead apparently is relatively nontoxic in the concentrations commonly found in ethyl gasoline, although persons concerned with its manufacture or who experience prolonged cutaneous contact may develop the clinical picture of acute or chronic lead poisoning [see *Lead Salts* (49–313)] from absorption through the intact skin.

49–230.   **ETHYLENE.** See *Anesthetics, Inhalation* (Topic 59–8).

49–231.   **ETHYLENE GLYCOL** (Diethylene Glycol, Antifreeze, Prestone)

These very toxic liquids are commonly used in automobile "permanent" antifreeze mixtures, hence are often available for ingestion by children. Toxic effects are due to breaking down of these liquids to oxalic acid (49–425). The appropriate measures outlined below should be carried out if ingestion is even suspected; DO NOT WAIT FOR SYMPTOMS TO DEVELOP.

A. Signs and Symptoms (usually delayed 1 to 2 hours after ingestion)
1. Temporary exhilaration followed by development of progressively deepening coma.
2. Rapid, weak pulse.
3. Acute respiratory distress.
4. Muscular paralysis, loss of reflexes; a positive Babinski may be present.
5. Anuria and uremia; if either develops, the condition is generally fatal.

B. Treatment
1. Induction of vomiting.
2. Gastric lavage with large amounts of a 1:5000 potassium permanganate solution.

    3. Administration of oxygen under positive pressure, preferably by a face mask and rebreathing bag.
    4. Injection of caffeine sodiobenzoate, 0.5 gm., intramuscularly. Shock therapy (Topic 15–7) may be necessary.
    5. Hospitalization as soon as possible.

49–232.   **EUCAINE.** See *Anesthetics, Local* (49–52) and Topic 59–10.

49–233.   **EUCALYPTOL.** [Also see *Oil, Essential* (49–407).]

  Oil of eucalyptus (50% eucalyptol) is an ingredient of many widely used household remedies. Ingestion of even small amounts may have serious effects.

A. Signs and Symptoms
    1. Nausea, vomiting, abdominal pain and diarrhea.
    2. Miosis.
    3. Dizziness and mental confusion.
    4. Dysuria and hematuria.
    5. Convulsions in children.
    6. Dyspnea and cyanosis.
    7. Circulatory collapse, followed by coma.
    8. Late development of pulmonary edema (Topic 52) and bronchopneumonia.

B. Treatment
    1. Force the patient, if conscious, to swallow 60 to 120 ml. of liquid petrolatum.
    2. Empty the stomach by emetics and/or gastric lavage.
    3. Start oxygen inhalations at once.
    4. Administer saline cathartics.
    5. Hospitalize if a large amount has been ingested or if marked circulatory or respiratory depression has been present.

49–234.   **EUCODAL.** See *Dicodid* (49–186) and *Morphine* (49–370). Addiction (Topic 2–3) has been described.

49–235.   **EUDERMOL** (Nicotine Salicylate). See *Nicotine* (49–389).

49–236.   **EUONYMIN**

  This is a digitalis-like substance found in the fruit of many varieties of bushes and trees (arrowwood, bitter ash, burning bush, strawberry tree, etc.).

A. Signs and Symptoms
  1. Vomiting with watery diarrhea.
  2. Hallucinations.
  3. Somnolence deepening to coma.
B. Treatment
  1. Emetics followed by gastric lavage.
  2. Saline cathartics.
  3. Supportive measures as required.

. . . . F . . . .

49–237. FAVA BEANS

  Chills, fever, nausea, vomiting, jaundice, red-brown or black urine, gastrointestinal bleeding, and hemoglobinemia may be caused by ingestion of green or incompletely cooked, broad (Windsor) beans or horse beans, or by inhalation of the pollen or dust from grinding. Different individuals show wide variations in susceptibility; in addition, the same individuals may vary in susceptibility at different times.

Treatment
      Immediate hospitalization for supportive therapy and blood transfusions.

49–238. FERRIC AND FERROUS SALTS. See *Iron Salts* (49–296).

49–239. FINGER NAIL POLISH. See *Acetone* (49–14) and *Aniline Dyes* (49–54).

49–240. FIRE EXTINGUISHERS

  Toxic ingredients depend on the type.
    1. Dry type—magnesium stearate, tricalcium phosphate.
    2. Foam type—aluminum sulfate, methyl bromide.
    3. Gas type—compressed carbon dioxide gas.
    4. Liquid type—carbon tetrachloride, dichloromethane, chlorobromethane, and trichlorethylene.
  For treatment see under the specific toxic constituents.

49–241. FIREWORKS

  Many acutely toxic substances may be present in the fuel, binders, oxidizers and coloring agents of fireworks. In some instances, mild transient toxic signs and symptoms may be caused by inhalation of fumes.
  Among commonly used toxic constituents are:

Antimony salts (49–57)	Mercury (49–343)
Arsenates (49–63)	Nitrates (49–391)
Barium salts (49–77)	Perchlorates (See *Chlorates,* 49–130)
Chlorates (49–130)	Phosphorus (49–462)
Copper salts (49–157)	Strontium salts
Lead salts (49–313)	Thiocyanates (49–600)

Ingestion by children may be fatal if the stomach is not emptied at once and careful symptomatic follow-up care administered.

49–242. **FLUORIDES**

Sodium, barium and zinc fluorides are often the active toxic ingredients in roach, ant, insect and rodent poisons. Ingestion (especially by children) and inhalation of the dust during manufacture and use have caused many cases of acute and serious poisoning.

A. Signs and Symptoms
1. Nausea and vomiting associated with abdominal pain, burning, and cramps—often very severe.
2. Bluish gray cyanosis.
3. Muscular tremors and myalgia, especially of the calf muscles.
4. Convulsions.

B. Treatment
1. If inhaled, removal from exposure.
2. If ingested, immediate induction of vomiting, followed by gastric lavage with large amounts of calcium chloride or lime water.
3. Application of external heat.
4. Calcium gluconate (10% solution), 10 ml., intravenously for severe myalgia; repeat in 30 minutes if necessary.
5. Oxygen inhalations under positive pressure.
6. Hospitalization because of the danger of serious liver and kidney damage.

49–243. **FLUOROACETATES**

These compounds, sometimes used as rodenticides, are very toxic in a different manner from other fluoride derivatives, apparently because of blocking of cellular energy production resulting in the slow development of convulsions.

A. Signs and Symptoms
1. Acute apprehension and anxiety.
2. Nausea and vomiting.
3. Aberrations of special senses, especially auditory, visual (nystagmus) and mental (hallucinations).
4. Paresthesias (usually facial).
5. Muscle twitching.
6. Epileptiform convulsions, often followed by development of cardiac abnormalities (pulsus alternans, ectopic beats, ventricular tachycardia and fibrillation).

B. Treatment
1. Immediate emptying of the stomach by emetics and gastric lavage if fluoroacetic poisoning is even suspected.
2. Control of convulsions by rapidly acting barbiturates intravenously.
3. Administration of oxygen under positive pressure by face mask and rebreathing bag.
4. Glyceryl monoacetate (monacetin), 0.5 ml. per kilogram of body weight, intramuscularly; repeat in ½ hour if necessary.
5. Hospitalization for close observation and symptomatic care.

49–244. **FLUOROSILICATES** (Silicofluorides)

These salts have approximately the same toxicity and require the same treatment as fluorides (49–242).

49–245. **FOOD POISONING**

A. Botulism (49–97). Evidence of toxicity usually does not develop until 18 to 36 hours after eating improperly processed canned foods; in some instances, much longer. The toxic picture is caused by an exotoxin produced under anaerobic conditions by *C. botulinus*. The prognosis depends upon the amount of toxin ingested in relation to body weight. For treatment see 49–97, above.

B. Bacterial. From enterotoxins in food produced by the growth of staphylococci or by organisms themselves (salmonella, streptococcus). Signs and symptoms of toxicity from staphylococcic enterotoxins develop 2 to 6 hours after ingestion; from streptococci, 2 to 12 hours.

1. SIGNS AND SYMPTOMS
   a. Vertigo, weakness, general malaise, increased salivation.
   b. Nausea and vomiting with acute gastric pain, tenesmus and diarrhea.
   c. Muscular cramps.
   d. Shock—usually transient, but may be severe and resistant to treatment (Topic 15–7).

2. TREATMENT
   a. Empty the stomach AT ONCE by emetics or gastric lavage.
   b. Control severe pain by morphine sulfate or dihydromorphinone hydrochloride (Dilaudid) subcutaneously, intramuscularly or intravenously, depending on the severity.
   c. Give castor oil, 30 ml., or calomel (mercurous chloride), 0.2 gm., by mouth.
   d. Decrease tenesmus and diarrhea by bismuth subcarbonate, 1 gm., or kaolin, 7.5 gm., by mouth. Camphorated tincture of opium (paregoric), 4 to 8 ml., may be given orally after each bowel movement.
   e. Hospitalize if severe shock or dehydration is present; usually it is not necessary.

C. **Chemical.** Ingestion of acid foods stored in containers lined with antimony, cadmium or zinc may result in nausea, vomiting and diarrhea lasting 2 or 3 days if not treated. Food preservatives and salt substitutes may give toxic signs and symptoms. See *Nitrites* (49–393).

Treatment
1. Emetics if profuse vomiting has not occurred, followed by gastric lavage.
2. Saline cathartics.
3. Atropine sulfate, 0.5 mg., subcutaneously.
4. Bismuth subcarbonate by mouth.
5. Specific treatment as outlined under the offending metal.

D. **Radioactive Contamination.** See Topic 64–4 and 5 (*Wartime Emergencies*).

49–246. FORMALDEHYDE

A solution of this pungent gas is the active ingredient in many commonly used household antiseptics, deodorizers and fumigants. It is also used to wrinkle-proof clothing. Inhalation of fumes or ingestion of solutions of the gas such as formalin (49–247) may cause an acute toxic picture.

A. **Signs and Symptoms**
1. Characteristic odor on the breath.
2. If inhaled, acute irritation of the eyes, nose and upper respiratory tract. Bronchospasm and/or laryngeal edema may occur.
3. If ingested, soreness of the mouth and throat with difficulty in swallowing.
4. Nausea and vomiting; sometimes hematemesis.
5. Severe abdominal pain with diarrhea, often bloody.
6. Severe shock.
7. Convulsions and coma.
8. Respiratory collapse and death.

B. **Treatment**
1. Have the patient swallow aromatic spirits of ammonia, 8 ml. in water. Follow with demulcents such as raw eggs and milk.
2. Induce vomiting by emetics followed by gastric lavage with 0.2% ammonia in water.
3. Inject morphine sulfate subcutaneously for severe pain if respiratory depression is not acute.
4. Combat dyspnea by oxygen under positive pressure.
5. Begin treatment of shock (Topic 15–7) as soon as possible.
6. Hospitalize if convulsions have occurred or respiratory depression has developed.

49–247. FORMALIN

This is an aqueous solution containing 40% formaldehyde and small amounts of ethyl and/or methyl alcohol. For treatment of poisoning see *Formaldehyde* (49–246).

49–248. **FOWLER'S SOLUTION.** See *Arsenic* (49–63).

49–249. **FREONS**

These chlorinated-fluorinated hydrocarbons are used in refrigerators and as the propelling agents in insecticide "bombs." Inhalation of fumes may cause transient upper respiratory irritation and mental confusion. The chief danger, however, lies in contact of the containers with fire in the home. At high temperatures freons may break down into chlorine, fluorine, hydrogen fluoride, and phosgene—all dangerous in even low concentrations.

49–250. **FUMIGATING GASES.** See *Benzene* (49–80), *Carbon Tetrachloride* (49–120), *Cyanides* (49–170), *Formaldehyde* (49–246), *Nicotine* (149–389) and *Sulfides* (49–280).

49–251. **FURNITURE POLISH**

Ingestion of these preparations by children may cause severe illness and even death due to toxic effects of mineral seal oil. These effects are similar to, but more severe than, gasoline (49–254) and kerosene (49–303).

. . . . G . . . .

49–252. **GADOLINIUM CHLORIDE**

This by-product of the uranium industry has caused cardiovascular collapse in laboratory animals, but no cases of human toxicity have been reported.

49–253. **GAMMEXANE** (Gamma Benzene Hexachloride). See *Benzene Hexachloride* (49–81).

49–254. **GASOLINE**

Its wide use as a motor fuel and as a cleansing agent makes gasoline one of the main present-day causes of poisoning. Toxic signs and symptoms may follow contact with the skin over large areas of the body, inhalation of fumes, or ingestion. Addiction to gasoline fumes has been reported.

A. Skin Contact

1. Repeated or prolonged washing of the skin with gasoline results in removal of the protective fat layer, with subsequent lowering of resistance to infection.
2. Exposure of large areas of skin to gasoline may cause severe toxic symptoms from absorption similar to those given below for inhalation of high concentrations. Acute symptoms from skin absorption are sometimes encountered following automobile accidents in which the clothing has been saturated with gasoline.

TREATMENT

   a. Remove all contaminated clothing at once.
   b. Wash the skin thoroughly with soap and water.
   c. Give symptomatic therapy as outlined below.

B. Inhalation

1. LOW OR MEDIUM CONCENTRATIONS of gasoline fumes will cause:
   a. Flushing of the skin.
   b. Staggering gait, confusion, incoherence and disorientation— may be mistaken for alcoholic intoxication.
   c. Acute dysphagia.

TREATMENT

   a. Removal from exposure.
   b. Fresh air or inhalations of oxygen.

PROGNOSIS. Complete recovery in a short time.

2. HIGH CONCENTRATIONS may cause:
   a. Muscular twitching; tonic and clonic convulsions.
   b. Dilated and nonreactive pupils.
   c. Delirium followed by sudden loss of consciousness.
   d. Death from ventricular fibrillation or complete respiratory arrest.

TREATMENT

   a. Removal from exposure.
   b. Oxygen inhalations under positive pressure by face mask and rebreathing bag.
   c. Caffeine sodiobenzoate, 0.5 gm., intramuscularly for circulatory failure. DO NOT give epinephrine hydrochloride (Adrenalin) because of the danger of inducing ventricular fibrillation.
   d. Hospitalization as soon as possible. The acute stage may be followed in 2 to 3 hours by peripheral and retrobulbar neuritis, epileptiform seizures, paresthesias and pneumonitis.

PROGNOSIS. Fair if the patient survives the initial exposure. Permanent mental changes as well as serious kidney damage may develop.

C. Ingestion may cause:

1. Burning sensation in mouth and throat.
2. Nausea, vomiting and diarrhea.
3. Extreme restlessness, with muscular twitching and incoordination.
4. Chemical pneumonitis which may develop into pneumonia from aspiration of fumes.

TREATMENT
    a. Gastric lavage as soon as possible with 120 ml. of olive oil, followed by warm water.
    b. Caffeine sodiobenzoate, 0.5 gm., intramuscularly.
    c. Oxygen inhalations, preferably by means of a face mask and rebreathing bag.
    d. Antibiotics to lessen the chance of development of an aspiration pneumonia.
    e. Hospitalization to minimize the chance of development of respiratory tract, kidney or brain damage.

PROGNOSIS. Good if the stomach is emptied within a short time after ingestion; poor if several hours have elapsed.

49–255. **GELSEMIUM** (Yellow Jasmine)

Used medicinally in some localities as an antineuralgic and antispasmodic, the alkaloid (gelsemine) may cause acute poisoning.

A. Signs and Symptoms
1. Great weakness, unsteady gait.
2. Vertigo and headache.
3. Aphasia.
4. Paralysis of the tongue with inability to swallow.
5. Lowered body temperature.
6. Pale and clammy skin, later becoming olive green, finally flushed and cyanotic.
7. Dilated, nonreactive pupils. Ptosis of the eyelids is often present.

B. Treatment
1. Induction of vomiting by emetics; followed, if necessary, by gastric lavage with 1:2000 potassium permanganate solution.
2. Local heat.
3. Caffeine sodiobenzoate, 0.5 gm., intramuscularly.
4. Oxygen therapy.
5. Insurance of an open airway by suction, traction on the tongue, or insertion of a nasopharyngeal catheter or airway. Tracheotomy (Topic 17–11,B) may be necessary.
6. In severe cases, hospitalization is indicated.

49–256. **GLUTETHIMIDE** (Doriden)

This nonbarbiturate hypnotic is a central nervous system depressant which may cause coma and death from respiratory failure.
    Treatment consists of lavage, insurance of an adequate airway, hydration and respiratory support.

49–257. **GOLD SALTS**

All of the gold salts commonly used medicinally in the treatment of arthritis and lupus erythematosus are very toxic. These salts are:
1. Gold sodium thiosulfate (Sanochrysine).

2. Sodium aurothiomalate (Myochrysine).
3. Aurothioglucose (Solganal).
4. Aurothioglycolanilide (Lauron).

Apparently there is very great variation in personal tolerance of these drugs, not only in different individuals but also in the same person at different times, and the patient may suffer acute toxicity.

A. Signs and Symptoms
1. Fever, also associated with characteristic facial puffiness.
2. Various skin disorders, some with intense pruritus.
3. Nausea, vomiting, acute abdominal pain and diarrhea.
4. Polyneuritis affecting almost exclusively the motor nerves.
5. Signs of liver and kidney damage in addition to blood changes.

B. Treatment
1. Stop administration of the offending drug.
2. Give sedatives, anodynes or narcotics as needed for pain.
3. Hospitalize at once for the usual heavy metal poisoning therapy.
   [See *Arsenic* (49–63).]

C. Prognosis. Good unless agranulocytosis has developed—then a mortality of about 30 per cent.

49–258. GUAIACOL

Toxic signs and symptoms and treatment are similar to those listed under phenol (49–450).

49–259. **GYNERGEN.** See *Ergot* (49–218).

. . . . H . . . .

49–260. **HAIR DYES AND SPRAYS**

Many of the hair dyes in common use contain alcohol (49–22 and 23) borates (49–96), cadmium salts (49–106), caustic hydroxides [*Alkalies* (49–28)], copper salts (49–157), dichromates [Chromates (49–145)], and ether (49–224). All may cause systemic poisoning of varying severity through absorption from the scalp and surrounding skin or by ingestion, in addition to the localized damage to the hair and scalp. Among the more complex constituents which may give toxic reactions are:

Aminoanisole	Henna
Aminodiphenylamines	Nitrodiamino compounds
Chloroaminophenols	Phenetols
Chlorodiamines	Polyvinylpyrrolidones
Diaminophenols	Pyrogallol

Treatment

In mild cases the only treatment required is to stop use of the dye. Severer cases may require symptomatic treatment as outlined under pyrogallol (49–486).

49–261. **HALLUCINOGENS**

Plants containing small amounts of these psychotomimetic (sometimes called "consciousness-expanding") drugs have been used for many years as a means of escape from reality in Asia and the Orient [e.g., hashish or marihuana (49–332)] and in religious rites in southwestern United States and Mexico where sliced peyote nuts [*Mescal* (49–347)] and certain varieties of mushrooms containing psilocybin (49–373) are chewed by participants. A synthetic derivative of lysergic acid, the diethylamide (LSD), has a similar, but more powerful, effect. Illegal sale and use of sugar cubes saturated with LSD have been reported during the last few years with several incidents of severe toxic signs and symptoms following ingestion.

The toxic effects (hallucinations, increased perception, personality dissociation, etc.) are temporary and last from 6 to 8 hours to 2 to 3 weeks. They leave no known permanent ill-effects provided the person ingesting the substance is familiar with, or has been informed of, the effects of hallucinogens. However, if ingestion is accidental, it may lead to severe psychotic decompensation, even attempts at self-destruction.

Hallucinations also occur in chronic mercury fume poisoning ("Mad-Hatter's syndrome") and from use of solutions of epinephrine hydrochloride (Adrenalin) which have degenerated after prolonged exposure to air and light.

True addiction to these drugs does not occur.

49–262. **HEADACHE REMEDIES**

These proprietary compounds generally contain acetanilid (49–11) combined with caffeine (49–107), bromides (49–100) and salicylates (49–511).

49–263. **HELLEBOREIN**

This is one of several glucosides found in the roots and seeds of plants of the Helleborus family.

Ingestion of even small amounts may result in rapid development of toxicity.

A. Signs and Symptoms
   1. Nausea, vomiting, abdominal pain and diarrhea.
   2. Headache and vertigo; occasionally tinnitus.
   3. Dilation of the pupils, photophobia and visual disturbances.
   4. Myalgia, especially of the calves.
   5. Delirium, convulsions and coma.
   6. Death from respiratory collapse.

B. Treatment
   1. Emetics followed by gastric lavage with large amounts of water.
   2. Artificial respiration by mouth-to-mouth or manual methods (Topic 17–1) followed by administration of air or oxygen

under positive pressure by face mask if respiratory depression is acute.

3. Administration of 10% calcium gluconate intravenously for acute myalgia.

4. Hospitalization as soon as possible for close observation for at least 24 hours after apparent complete recovery.

49–264. **HELVELLA**

This is a variety of mushroom which is generally considered to be edible, but which occasionally causes very severe delayed toxic symptoms coming on from 6 to 8 hours after ingestion. For signs and symptoms of toxicity and treatment see *Mushroom Poisoning* (49–373).

49–265. **HEMLOCK.** See *Coniine* (49–156).

49–266. **HEPARIN**

Purpura, ecchymosis and hematuria from the use of this anticoagulant may be severe enough to require immediate shock therapy (Topic 15–7). Plasma volume expanders should be given for temporary support and the patient should be hospitalized at once for thorough investigation and possible blood transfusions. [Also see *Dicumarol* (49–187).]

49–267. **HEPTACHLOR**

This is a complex insecticide which by inhalation, skin absorption or ingestion can give a toxic picture similar to that produced by chlordane. In addition, severe and permanent liver damage may occur. For signs and symptoms of toxicity and treatment see *Chlordane* (49–131).

49–268. **HEROIN** (Diacetylmorphine)

This powerful narcotic is more toxic and addictive than any of the other opiates. The signs and symptoms of toxicity, as well as the treatment, are the same as outlined for morphine (49–370). Prescription or administration of heroin is forbidden in the United States, but because of its potency it is common in the illegitimate narcotic market. [See Topic 2–3 (*Addiction*).]

49–269. **HETP.** See *Organic Phosphates* (49–421).

49–270. **HEXAETHYL TETRAPHOSPHATE** (HETP). See *Organic Phosphates* (49–421).

49–271. **HEXAMETHYLENETETRAMINE** (Methenamine, Urotropin)

In acid urine, this drug slowly releases formaldehyde. Excessively large
doses may give mild toxic symptoms. See *Formaldehyde* (49–246).

49–272. **HEXYLRESORCINOL**

Use of high concentrations or large doses by mouth may give a picture
suggestive of mild phenol poisoning. The treatment is the same as outlined
under *Phenol* (49–450).

49–273. **HISTAMINE**

Medical use of excessive amounts may cause severe, sometimes fatal,
shock. For treatment see Topic 15–7.

49–274. **HOMATROPINE**

Therapeutic use in ophthalmology may cause a slow pulse, dysphagia,
vertigo, weakness, excitement and collapse, as well as the expected mydriasis. Complete recovery in a short period is the rule. No special treatment
is required.

Overdosage has been reported as causing excitement, confusion and
coma, with very slow respiration, rapid pulse and hypotension.

   A. Treatment
     1. Stop the medication.
     2. If ingested, empty the stomach by immediate gastric lavage.
   B. Prognosis. Complete recovery in 12 to 24 hours.

49–275. **HORSERADISH.** See *Coniine* (49–156).

49–276. **HYDROCHLORIC ACID.** See *Acids* (49–19).

49–277. **HYDROCYANIC ACID.** See *Cyanides* (49–170).

49–278. **HYDROFLUORIC ACID**

This extremely corrosive solution (hydrogen fluoride, 47%, in water) is
used in etching and engraving. It may cause severe toxic symptoms by:
     1. Contact with the skin or nails.

2. Contact with the eyes.
3. Inhalation of the fumes.
4. Ingestion.

A. Skin Contact. Even small amounts of hydrofluoric acid on the skin or nails will cause severe damage. The onset is insidious; after the acid is removed the skin or nails will appear to be normal for about an hour. Erythema, followed by vesication and tissue destruction, then develops rapidly, resulting in a nonhealing ulcer that sometimes extends to the bone. Fingernails and nail beds may be completely destroyed.

Treatment
1. Immediate washing with water for 1 to 2 HOURS.
2. After lengthy washing, application of a paste made from equal parts of magnesium oxide and magnesium sulfate (Epsom salts).
3. Injection of calcium gluconate (10% solution) into, under and around the affected area. Nails should be partially cut away and the nail bed injected as above. Small ulcers should be excised en bloc and the base injected with 10% calcium gluconate.

Following injection, the areas should be painted with Berwick's or other triple dye solution and treated as an open wound or third degree chemical burn.

B. Contact with the Eyes may cause serious and permanent damage.

Treatment
1. IMMEDIATE washing with large amounts of water.
2. Instillation of 1% tetracaine hydrochloride (Pontocaine) to control pain, followed by 1% atropine sulfate to dilate the pupil.
3. Application of an eye patch.
4. IMMEDIATE reference for ophthalmologic care.

C. Inhalation of Fumes

Treatment
1. Removal from exposure.
2. Inhalation of 1% calcium chloride solution sprayed into the respiratory tract with an atomizer.
3. Hospitalization if marked irritation of the respiratory tract is present.

D. Ingestion

Treatment
1. Milk or white of egg by mouth.
2. Morphine sulfate or dihydromorphinone hydrochloride (Dilaudid) subcutaneously for pain.
3. Immediate gastric lavage with large quantities of lime water even if evidence of corrosion is present.
4. Hospitalization.

49–279. HYDROGEN SELENIDE

This is a colorless gas used in industry. Even very low concentrations may cause toxic reactions.

A. Signs and Symptoms
1. Severe throat irritation—cough, hoarseness, dysphagia.

   2. Rhinitis and anosmia.
   3. Urticaria.
   4. Extreme hypotension.
   5. Dyspnea and cyanosis, followed by pulmonary edema.
   B. Treatment
   1. Removal from exposure.
   2. Oxygen by face mask and rebreathing bag.
   3. Antihistaminics if urticaria is marked.
   4. Support of the circulation by plasma volume expanders intra-
      venously.
   5. Treatment of pulmonary edema (Topic 52–3).

49–280. HYDROGEN SULFIDE

   Poisoning from this foul-smelling gas, formed by putrefaction of sulfur-
containing material, is fairly common among petroleum and sewer workers.
   A. Low Concentrations are irritant only and may cause:
   1. Acute conjunctivitis, photophobia and colored rings around bright
      lights.
   2. Rhinitis with decrease or loss of the sense of smell.
   3. Tracheitis, bronchitis, pneumonia (Topic 53–14), and pulmonary
      edema (Topic 52).
   B. Treatment
   1. Removal from exposure.
   2. Instillation of olive oil into the eyes for conjunctivitis.
   3. Oxygen therapy under positive pressure.
   C. High Concentrations are very depressant and may cause:
   1. Nausea and vomiting.
   2. Progressively increasing somnolence, amnesia and transient un-
      consciousness coming on especially after exertion.
   3. Dysphagia.
   4. Rapid pulse, low blood pressure.
   5. Eye signs (strabismus, diplopia, exophthalmos, fixed nonreactive
      pupils).
   6. Delirium and hallucinations, followed by convulsions.
   7. Death from respiratory failure.
   Treatment
   1. Removal from exposure.
   2. Prolonged artificial respiration—preferably oxygen inhalations
      by mask or endotracheal catheter.
   3. Caffeine sodiobenzoate, 0.5 gm., intramuscularly. In severe cases
      intravenous administration of 4 ml. of 0.2% arterenol bitar-
      trate (Levophed) in 1000 ml. of 5% dextrose in saline may
      be necessary for circulatory support. Metaraminol bitartrate
      (Aramine), 50 to 100 mg., may be added to the dextrose
      solution in place of Levophed.
   4. Atropine sulfate, 0.6 mg., subcutaneously.
   5. Hospitalization for prevention or treatment of delayed sequelae
      (pneumonia, pulmonary edema, cardiac dilatation, severe
      gastrointestinal symptoms and peripheral polyneuritis)

Prognosis. Good if the patient survives the initial acute respiratory de-
depression.

49–281. **HYDROQUINONE**

Most of the cases of acute poisoning from hydroquinone arise from its
use as a photographic developer.

A. *Signs and Symptoms*
1. Dizziness; ringing in the ears.
2. Rapid respiration; profuse sweating.
3. Nausea and vomiting.
4. Restlessness; muscular twitching.
5. Cyanosis, probably due to methemoglobinemia.
6. Collapse.

B. *Treatment*
1. Emetics; if unsuccessful, gastric lavage with 1:2000 potassium
permanganate solution.
2. Oxygen by face mask and rebreathing bag if cyanosis is extreme.
3. Saline cathartics.
4. Hospitalization for thorough study because of the relatively frequent late development of a severe hemolytic anemia.

49–282. **HYOSCINE.** See *Atropine Sulfate* (49–71).

49–283. **HYOSCYAMUS** (Henbane)

This flowering garden plant may cause severe toxic symptoms similar
to those from atropine in children if the foliage or stalks are chewed. For
toxic picture and treatment see *Atropine Sulfate* (49–71).

49–284. **HYPOCHLORITES** (Chlorinated Lime, Clorox, Bleach-
ing Powder, Labarraque's Solution, Dakin's
Solution, Emergency Water Sterilizers)

Concentrated solutions have severe caustic alkali actions; more diluted
solutions cause only mild gastrointestinal symptoms. Although the antiseptic and bleaching actions depend on the chlorine content, this is too low
to give toxic symptoms and can be disregarded in treatment.

Treatment
1. Administration of demulcents (olive oil, crushed bananas, starch,
egg albumen).
2. Emptying of the stomach by emetics or gastric lavage (unless
there is definite evidence of corrosion or perforation).
3. Hospitalization if evidence of extensive or severe mucous membrane erosion is present. Opiates for control of pain as well
as extensive therapy for shock (Topic 15–7) may be necessary before transfer.

. . . . I . . . .

49–285.   **IMPERIAL GREEN** (Copper Acetoarsenite). See *Arsenic*
             (49–63).

49–286.   **INDELIBLE INKS, PENCILS AND STAINS.** See *Aniline
             Dyes* (49–54) and Topic 42–7 (*Puncture
             Wounds of the Hand*).

49–287.   **INDIGO**

Ingestion of small amounts of natural or synthetic indigo may cause
toxic effects.
  A. Signs and Symptoms
     1. Retching, vomiting, abdominal pain and diarrhea.
     2. Fever.
     3. Muscle twitching and pain.
     4. Renal colic.
  B. Treatment
     1. Emetics followed by gastric lavage with 1:5000 potassium per-
        manganate solution.
     2. Intravenous injection of 5% dextrose in saline.
     3. Calcium gluconate (10% solution) intravenously.
  C. Prognosis. Complete recovery in 1 to 2 days.

49–288.   **INK.** See *Aniline Dyes* (49–54). Marking inks may
             contain silver salts (49–530).

49–289.   **INK ERADICATORS.** See *Hypochlorites* (49–284) and
             Oxalic Acid (49–425).

49–290.   **INSULIN.** See Topic 3–3 (*Diabetes Mellitus*).

49–291.   **IODIDES**

These are relatively nontoxic, but excessive doses or prolonged use of
therapeutic doses can cause iodism [see *Iodine* (49–292)] as well as enlargement of the salivary glands which may be mistaken for mumps
(Topic 32–17).

49–292. **IODINE**

A. Local Application
1. Skin, mahogany-brown; marked erythema, desquamation and vesication.
2. Mucous membranes corroded.

B. Exposure to Fumes
1. Conjunctivitis, lacrimation, sparkling before the eyes.
2. Headache, somnolence.
3. Swelling of parotid glands [see *Iodides* (49–291)].
4. Severe cough.

C. Ingestion
1. Metallic iodine taste with severe pain and burning in the esophagus and stomach often associated with brownish discoloration of the mucous membranes of the mouth and throat (from tincture).
2. Faintness.
3. Nausea and vomiting (blue color of vomitus if the patient has been given starch).
4. Extreme thirst.
5. Convulsions.

Treatment
1. Give large amounts of starch solution by mouth.
2. Empty the stomach by gastric lavage with 1% sodium thiosulfate solution; repeat until the returned fluid no longer shows any blue color.
3. Control convulsions by rapidly acting barbiturates.
4. Apply external heat.
5. Inject caffeine sodiobenzoate, 0.5 gm., intramuscularly.

49–293. **IODOFORM**

Acute toxic symptoms may develop from wounds packed with iodoform gauze or from ingestion.

A. Symptoms
1. Nausea and vomiting.
2. Rapid pulse.
3. Acute excitement; sometimes convulsions.

B. Treatment
1. Removal of packing (or emptying of the stomach if ingested).
2. Control of excitement by rapidly acting barbiturates.

49–294. **IPECAC**

This excellent and rapidly acting emetic has caused death when the fluidextract (14 times as powerful as the syrup) has been administered by error. In addition to its emetic action, ipecac is a very efficient sedative.

49–295.   **IRON OXIDE.** See *Iron Salts* (49–296) and *Metal Fumes* (49–348).

49–296.   **IRON SALTS**

Since most of the common salts of iron oxidize rapidly on exposure to air to form basic ferric sulfate, acute poisoning from this source may be encountered. Most of the cases of acute toxicity, however, are caused by children's ingestion of candy-coated ferrous sulfate tablets, with a mortality rate of about 30 per cent.

    A. Signs and Symptoms
        1. Metallic taste in mouth, vomiting of bluish green material.
        2. Rapid, weak pulse; hypotension.
        3. Diarrhea with black stools, often persistent enough to cause acute dehydration.
        4. Very severe shock, especially in children.
    B. Treatment
        1. Administration of demulcents (raw eggs, starch solution, milk) by mouth followed by emetics and gastric lavage with sodium bicarbonate solution.
        2. Oxygen therapy under positive pressure.
        3. Treatment of shock (Topic 15–7).
        4. Immediate hospitalization for fluid replacement (Topic 7) and in severe cases for therapy with a chelating agent such as desferrioxamine B.

49–297.   **ISODRIN**

A powerful rodenticide. See *Dieldrin* (49–188).

49–298.   **ISOLAN**

An insecticide. See *Organic Phosphates* (49–421).

49–299.   **ISONIAZID**

Large doses of this drug used in the treatment of tuberculosis may be very toxic, especially in children.

    A. Signs and Symptoms
        1. Nausea and vomiting.
        2. Cyanosis of extremities.
        3. Generalized convulsions and coma.
    B. Treatment
        1. Emetics or gastric lavage.

2. Oxygen therapy under positive pressure.
3. Plasma volume expanders and 5% dextrose in saline intravenously.
4. Barbiturates intramuscularly.
5. Pyridoxine hydrochloride (vitamin B_6) therapy.

49–300. ISOPROPYL ALCOHOL (Avantine, Dimethylcarbinol)

A. Common Uses
1. As a rubbing compound—usually with a denaturant to make it unpotable. [See 49–65 (*"Waterfront Cocktails"*).]
2. As a solvent for waxes and resins.
3. In the production of safety glass, paints and varnishes.
4. In the manufacture of perfumes and cosmetics.

B. Signs and Symptoms (usually following ingestion but may be caused by inhalation of concentrated fumes)
1. Dizziness, muscular weakness and incoordination but no exhilaration as with ethyl alcohol.
2. Severe headache.
3. Slow pulse with low blood pressure.
4. Acute gastrointestinal irritation with bloody vomitus and diarrhea.
5. Anuria and uremia.

C. Treatment
1. Immediate gastric lavage with large quantities of water.
2. Caffeine sodiobenzoate, 0.5 gm., intramuscularly.
3. Barbiturates for sedation, preferably intravenously.
4. Hospitalization for possible transfusion is indicated in severe cases, since very severe liver and kidney damage may occur.

. . . . J . . . .

49–301. JEQUIRITY BEANS

These beans contain a very poisonous alkaloid, aldrin.
   Signs and Symptoms following ingestion are similar to those listed under castor beans (49–123).

49–302. JUTE

Processing of jute fibers in the manufacture of bags, mats, ropes, etc., may cause severe allergic reactions: asthma, bronchitis, bronchospasm, laryngitis and tracheitis.
   Treatment
1. Removal from exposure.
2. Management as outlined under Topic 24 (*Allergic Reactions*).

. . . . K . . . .

49–303. **KEROSENE** (Coal Oil)

This common petroleum distillate has a wide use as a household fuel, solvent and cleanser and also as the "inert ingredient" in many types of household and garden sprays. Although often considered as being of low toxicity, the exact opposite is true; the mortality is close to 10% following ingestion, probably owing in great part to aspiration during ingestion, vomiting and gastric lavage. Inhalation of the fumes may cause transient excitement, headache, hallucinations and delirium, but these signs and symptoms clear rapidly when the concentration of the fumes is lowered by adequate ventilation. It is after these transient and uncomfortable symptoms clear up that the serious pathologic condition (pneumonitis, pneumonia) becomes apparent.

A. Signs and Symptoms from Ingestion
1. Gastrointestinal irritation.
2. Circulatory disturbances.
3. Severe depression, coma, sometimes convulsions.
4. Pulmonary symptoms, especially aspiration pneumonia.

B. Treatment
1. Gastric lavage immediately unless profuse vomiting has taken place. The lavage tube should be pinched off before withdrawal in order to minimize aspiration of stomach contents.
2. Saline cathartics.
3. Oxygen under positive pressure by face mask and rebreathing bag.
4. Caffeine sodiobenzoate intramuscularly. (Dosage according to age, Topic 5.) Do NOT administer to children under 6 years of age.
5. Hospitalization as soon as possible.

49–304. **KNOCKOUT DROPS.** See *Chloral Hydrate* (49–128).

. . . . L . . . .

49–305. **LACTIC ACID**

A. Ingestion may cause:
1. Severe burning of the mouth, pharynx, esophagus and stomach.
2. Nausea and vomiting; sometimes bloody emesis.
3. Rapid, weak pulse; cold perspiration.
4. Dyspnea and cyanosis.
5. Death from dehydration and exhaustion secondary to acute gastroenteritis.

B. Treatment
1. Universal antidote (49–10).
2. Gastric lavage with large quantities of lime water.
3. Large amounts of fluid by mouth or intravenously.
4. Hospitalization after lavage and administration of fluids.

49–306. **LARKSPUR.** See *Delphinium* (49–705).

49–307. **LAUDANUM** (Tincture of Opium). See *Morphine* (49–370).

49–308. **LAURON.** See *Gold Salts* (49–257).

49–309. **LEAD ACETATE.** See *Lead Salts* (49–313).

49–310. **LEAD ARSENATE AND ARSENITE**

Both of these substances, commonly used as insecticides, may cause toxic symptoms through inhalation. See *Lead Salts* (49–313).

49–311. **LEAD CHROMATE** (Chrome Yellow). Very toxic. See *Lead Salts* (49–313).

49–312. **LEAD OXIDE.** See *Lead Salts* (49–313) and *Metal Fumes* (49–348).

49–313. **LEAD SALTS**

In addition to exposure in industry, signs and symptoms of toxicity may occur in children from ingestion of old-fashioned paints and from use of improperly glazed china and other ceramics.
- **A. Signs and Symptoms**
  1. Sweetish metallic taste, with dryness of the throat and extreme thirst.
  2. Dizziness.
  3. Severe abdominal pain and cramping; constipation.
  4. Convulsions.
  5. Coma.
- **B. Treatment**
  1. Gastric lavage with 1% sodium sulfate solution.
  2. Magnesium sulfate (Epsom salts), 30 gm., by mouth.
  3. Application of external heat.
  4. Control of abdominal pain and cramping by morphine sulfate subcutaneously in adults or camphorated tincture of opium by mouth in children [dosage according to age (Topic 5)].
  5. Control of convulsions by intramuscular or intravenous injection

of rapidly acting barbiturates, chloral hydrate by mouth or rectally, or paraldehyde intramuscularly.
6. Hospitalization.

49–314. LEMON GRASS OIL

This is a volatile (essential) oil which is not only very toxic if ingested [see *Oil, Essential* (49–407)], but which causes a dermatitis similar to poison oak (Topic 54–11) on contact with the skin.

49–315. LETHANE

Lethane is used as a contact insecticide and may give acute toxic signs and symptoms if ingested. See *Thiocyanates* (49–600,D).

49–316. LEVOPROPOXYPHENE

This recently introduced antitussive drug may, in large doses, cause nausea, urticaria, dizziness, drowsiness, coma and cardiac arrest. Recovery usually follows lavage and supportive therapy.

49–317. LIME

A. Quicklime (burnt lime, unslaked lime, calcium oxide) is a very powerful caustic which liberates heat when exposed to moisture. It may cause serious damage if ingested or allowed to come in contact with any portion of the eyes.
   1. BY MOUTH the signs, symptoms and treatment are approximately the same as for any strongly caustic alkali. [See *Alkalies* (49–28).]
   2. IN THE EYES it may cause:
      a. Hyperemia, edema and corneal ulceration.
      b. Extensive erosion, sometimes with resultant permanent opacities and complete loss of vision.
   3. TREATMENT consists of IMMEDIATE washing with large amounts of water, followed by reference to an ophthalmologist.
B. Slaked Lime is harmless.

49–318. LINDANE. See *Benzene Hexachloride* (49–81).

49–319. LIPSTICKS

See *Cosmetics* (49–161). In general, the more "kiss-proof," the more chance of toxic reactions.

49–320. **LITHIUM CHLORIDE**

This is one of the substances which in very minute amounts may cause acute toxic signs and symptoms in certain individuals. Apparently, the tolerance of different persons varies tremendously. Since in addition to its commercial use in fireworks and in soldering aluminum, it is a constituent of some mineral waters and sodium chloride substitutes, familiarity with its toxic effects is important.

A. Signs and Symptoms
1. Tinnitus and vertigo; blurred vision.
2. Sleeplessness; generalized weakness.
3. Tremors of the extremities often associated with muscular twitching.
4. Bizarre shifting disturbances in sensation.
5. Acute dysphagia.
6. Mental confusion, coma, and occasionally death.

B. Treatment. Hospitalization for thorough investigation and possible extensive intravenous therapy, especially M/6 lactic acid solution, is indicated in all cases when the history and findings suggest lithium poisoning. Marked hypersensibility to stimuli, if present, should be controlled by intravenous barbiturates or intramuscular paraldehyde before transfer.

C. Prognosis. Guarded on account of the marked variation in reaction and response to therapy.

49–321. **LOCAL ANESTHETICS.** See *Anesthetics, Local* (49–52), and Topic 59–10.

49–322. **LSD.** See *Hallucinogens* (49–261).

49–323. **LYE**

Lye originally was made by bleaching wood ashes, but the term is now used for several of the strong alkalies, especially sodium and potassium hydroxide and carbonate. All act as severe caustics on direct contact with exposed parts of the body, and all may cause severe, often fatal, damage if ingested. Because lye is available in most households (washing powders, drain pipe cleaners, paint removers, etc.), contact with the skin or ingestion by accident or with suicidal intent is relatively common.

A. In the Eyes lye may cause severe conjunctivitis, chemosis, ulceration and loss of vision. It is more dangerous than most acids.

Treatment
1. Wash with large amounts of cold water.
2. Apply on eye patch.
3. Refer to an ophthalmologist immediately.

B. On the Skin lye may cause deep chemical burns with sloughing and loss of tissues.

Treatment
1. Wash with large amounts of cold water followed by a 10% solution of acetic acid (diluted vinegar will do).
2. Apply a petrolatum gauze burn dressing under sterile precautions (see Topic 28–2).
3. Control severe pain by codeine sulfate or morphine sulfate subcutaneously.

C. If Ingested
Signs and Symptoms
1. Whitish discoloration of mucous membranes of the mouth and throat, later becoming brownish.
2. Severe burning pain in the mouth, esophagus and stomach; bloody vomitus.
3. Rapid respiration with feeble pulse.
4. Collapse and coma.
5. Death. If within a few hours to one day, death is usually due to hemorrhage and shock or to edema of the glottis; later deaths are caused by lung lesions, pericarditis or peritonitis.

Treatment
1. Give demulcents by mouth—white of egg or olive oil.
2. Neutralize with diluted vinegar or 5% acetic acid.
3. Apply external heat.
4. Lavage with large amounts of water unless marked erosion or corrosion is present. In that case, DO NOT WASH STOMACH OR GIVE EMETICS.
5. Inject morphine sulfate subcutaneously or intravenously as necessary for pain.
6. Give caffeine sodiobenzoate, 0.5 mg., intramuscularly.
7. Hospitalize as soon as the patient's condition will allow.

49–324. LYSERGIC ACID DIETHYLAMIDE (LSD). See *Hallucinogens* (49–261).

. . . . M . . . .

49–325. MAGNESIUM

Metallic magnesium is used in the manufacture of light metal alloys; grinding may cause fine, sharp fragments which perforate the skin and cause marked swelling and crepitus from formation of hydrogen bubbles.
Treatment. Surgical excision.

49–326. MAGNESIUM OXIDE. See *Metal Fumes* (49–348).

49–327. **MAGNESIUM SULFATE** (Epsom Salts)

Ingestion of excessive amounts, absorption through the rectum, or intravenous injection may result in severe toxic symptoms.

  A. *Signs and Symptoms*
    1. Vomiting with acute gastric pain.
    2. Dilation of the pupils.
    3. Cyanosis.
    4. Generalized weakness.
    5. Collapse from respiratory and cardiac failure.

  B. *Treatment*
    1. Artificial respiration and/or oxygen under positive pressure by face mask or endotracheal catheter and rebreathing bag.
    2. Calcium gluconate, 10 ml. of 10% solution, intravenously.
    3. Physostigmine salicylate, 0.5 mg., subcutaneously.
    4. Administration of large amounts of fluids by mouth and/or intravenously.

49–328. **MALATHION**

This is one of the few organic phosphate insecticides approved for household use. In spite of its relatively low toxicity, treatment may be necessary if exposure has been excessive. See *Organic Phosphates* (49–421).

49–329. **MALE FERN.** See *Aspidium* (49–68).

49–330. **MANGANESE**

Toxic symptoms following inhalation of manganese dust may occur in workers in the steel and battery industries and among ore handlers. Signs and symptoms are usually low grade and chronic, but severe acute muscular cramps (especially in the calves), uncontrollable laughter, slurred speech, and staggering gait may require emergency therapy. Both the chronic and acute pictures can easily be mistaken for drug addiction (Topic 2).

  Treatment. Hospitalization for thorough investigation is indicated if the history or symptoms suggest manganese poisoning, as the incidence of a subsequent peculiarly virulent type of pneumonia is relatively high.

49–331. **MANGANESE OXIDE.** See *Metal Fumes* (49–348).

49–332.   **MARIHUANA** (Indian hemp, *Cannabis sativa,* Hashish, Bhang)

  A. Signs and Symptoms (same for ingestion or smoking)
1. Inebriation characterized by motor excitement, restlessness, euphoria and gaiety, sometimes anxiety, usually coming on about 1 hour after smoking or ingestion.
2. Extreme thirst.
3. Wide dilation of the pupils with sluggish reaction to light.
4. Aphrodisiac effects, probably much less marked than usually believed.
5. Vertigo and transient collapse with a soft, irregular pulse.
  B. Treatment
1. Symptomatic only—spontaneous recovery in a short time always occurs.
2. Psychiatric reference to determine the underlying causative factors. Contrary to wide publicity, no relationship to criminal offenses, sexual or otherwise, has ever been established. Addiction does not occur.

49–333.   **MATCHES**

Most present-day matches contain phosphorus trisulfide or sesquisulfide which are almost inert chemically and therefore relatively nontoxic. "Safety matches" have no toxic ingredients in harmful amounts in the heads (the phosphorus compound is on the friction surface on the box or book); therefore, children who suck or eat the heads need no treatment except disciplining. Ingestion of large numbers of the heads of "strike anywhere" matches requires treatment because many brands contain potassium chlorate and antimony sulfide in addition to a phosphorus compound. Old-fashioned "sulfur matches" contain yellow phosphorus and are very dangerous; ingestion of 16 has been reported as fatal to an adult.

For toxic signs and symptoms and treatment see *Phosphorus* (49–462).

49–334.   **MECHOLYL** (Methacholine)

This is sometimes used in the treatment of urinary retention and cardiac arrhythmias. Therapeutic doses, as well as overdosage, may give a toxic picture.

  A. Signs and Symptoms
1. Nausea and vomiting.
2. Generalized weakness.
3. Precipitation of asthmatic attacks in susceptible persons.
4. Momentary heart block.
  B. Treatment. Atropine sulfate intravenously in large doses (up to 2 mg.).

49–335. **MENTHOL**

A. *Ingestion* may cause
   1. Nausea and vomiting with severe abdominal pain.
   2. Dizziness; staggering gait.
   3. Slow respiration, flushed face.
   4. Sluggishness, sleepiness and, in large amounts in children, coma.
B. *Treatment*
   1. Emetics and/or gastric lavage.
   2. Magnesium sulfate (Epsom salts) as a saline cathartic.
C. *Prognosis.* Complete recovery within a few hours.

49–336. **MEPROBAMATE** (Equanil, Miltown)

A. *Usual Doses.* See Topic 59–41.
B. *Excessive Doses.* (above 5 gm.) may cause:
   1. Shallow respiration with cyanosis.
   2. Muscular weakness, loss of reflexes, hypotension.
   3. Acute mental depression.
Treatment
   1. Artificial respiration (mouth-to-mouth, manual or mechanical after clearing the airway).
   2. Emptying of the stomach by emetics, or gastric lavage if ingested in large amounts.
   3. Support of the circulation by caffeine sodiobenzoate or ephedrine sulfate intravenously. Severe cases may require slow intravenous injection of 4 ml. of a 0.2% solution of arterenol bitartrate (Levophed) or 50 to 100 mg. of metaraminol bitartrate (Aramine) in 1000 ml. of 5% dextrose in saline.
   4. Hospitalization for observation and supportive therapy.
C. *Sudden Discontinuance* can cause acute, serious withdrawal symptoms and signs, often magnified by the fact that many habitual users of tranquilizing drugs have prepsychotic tendencies.
Withdrawal Signs and Symptoms
   1. Severe headache; persistent insomnia.
   2. Excessive salivation.
   3. Epileptiform convulsions.
   4. Activation of psychotic tendencies, especially acute depression states; may be suicidal.
Treatment
   1. Mild cases need only symptomatic care with close supervision and observation at home.
   2. Severe cases require hospitalization for careful psychiatric evaluation and control.

49–337. **MERBROMIN** (Mercurochrome). See *Mercury Antiseptics* (49–344).

49–338. MERCAPTANS

These are released during the process of petroleum refining. Inhalation of high concentrations may cause fever, dyspnea, cyanosis, convulsions and coma.

Treatment
1. Removal from exposure.
2. Air or oxygen by face mask and rebreathing bag.
3. Hospitalization for observation for at least 24 hours; delayed pulmonary edema (Topic 52) may occur.

49–339. MERCOCREOSOL (Mercresin). See *Mercury Antiseptics* (49–344).

49–340. MERCURIC CHLORIDE. See *Bichloride of Mercury* (49–87).

49–341. MERCUROCHROME (Merbromin). See *Mercury Antiseptics* (49–344).

49–342. MERCUROUS CHLORIDE. See *Calomel* (49–110).

49–343. MERCURY

About 100 occupations offer definite industrial hazards, usually through inhalation of fumes or dust containing mercury. Fatalities in the home have occurred from fumes from gas heaters and radiators painted with "aluminum" paint. Mercury may cause toxic effects by absorption through the intact skin, open wounds, the lungs and the gastrointestinal tract.

Toxic Signs and Symptoms in industry are generally chronic and may be unrecognized until an acute picture develops or is superimposed. For signs and symptoms and treatment of acute toxicity see *Bichloride of Mercury* (49–87).

49–344. MERCURY ANTISEPTICS

A wide variety of commercial compounds intended to utilize the antiseptic action of mercury are available. The most common are mercocreosol (Mercresin), merbromin (Mercurochrome), and thimerosal (Merthiolate). All are practically nontoxic.

Treatment (if a large amount has been ingested)
1. Empty the stomach by emetics and/or gastric lavage.
2. Give saline cathartics by mouth.

49–345. MERCURY DIURETICS

The effective irritant diuretic action of certain mercury compounds has led to the medical use of mersalyl (Salyrgan), mercurophylline (Mercuzanthin) and many others. All may cause acute toxic signs and symptoms if given too frequently or in excessive doses.

A. Allergic Reactions are characterized by chills, fever, urticaria and, occasionally, bronchospasm and laryngeal edema. For treatment see Topic 24.

B. Immediate Toxicity. Acute symptoms may come on during intravenous injection of the same dose to which the patient is accustomed.

Signs and Symptoms
1. Apprehension, substernal pain.
2. Dyspnea and cyanosis.
3. Bradycardia and hypotension.
4. Mental confusion, sometimes delirium.
5. Collapse, probably due to ventricular fibrillation.

Treatment
1. Stop the medication at once.
2. Limit absorption and extension if possible by application of a tourniquet.
3. Administer oxygen therapy by mask and rebreathing bag.
4. Give caffeine sodiobenzoate, 0.5 gm., intramuscularly.
5. Hospitalize for observation.

Prognosis. Good unless the initial onset has been overwhelming.

C. Deferred Toxicity. Coming on from 1 to 3 hours after injection, this type is characterized by:
1. Chills and fever.
2. Dyspnea and cyanosis.
3. Asthmatic symptoms.
4. Pulmonary edema (Topic 52).
5. Evidence of sodium deficiency.

Treatment
1. Oxygen under positive pressure by face mask or endotracheal catheter and rebreathing bag.
2. Epinephrine hydrochloride (Adrenalin) (1:1000) subcutaneously in SMALL DOSES for asthmatic symptoms.
3. Administration of sodium.
4. Hospitalization.

49–346. MERTHIOLATE (Thimerosal). See *Mercury Antiseptics* (49–344).

49–347. **MESCAL** (Peyote)

Intoxication from ingestion of this substance, derived from a certain type of cactus, is sometimes encountered, especially in Mexicans, Indians and Negroes. Also see *Hallucinogens* (49–261).
- A. *Signs and Symptoms*
  1. Rapid fall in blood pressure.
  2. Hallucinations similar to schizophrenia.
- B. *Treatment.* Symptomatic only. Complete recovery without permanent ill effects occurs in 6 to 8 hours.

49–348. **METAL FUMES**

Inhalation of high concentrations of freshly formed metallic oxide fumes from smelting, brazing, galvanizing and welding may give rise to a type of poisoning known variously as metal fume fever, brass chills, metal ague, foundry workers' ague, zinc chills, spelter shakes, or Monday morning fever. The clinical picture, treatment and prognosis are completely different from the toxic symptoms from ingestion of the different metals. The following metallic oxides may cause the condition

Antimony	Lead
Beryllium	Magnesium
Cadmium	Manganese
Cobalt	Zinc (most common)
Copper	

- A. *Signs and Symptoms* (usually coming on from 1 to 3 hours after exposure)
  1. A peculiar metallic taste in the mouth; dryness of the throat; cough; tightness in the chest.
  2. Nausea and vomiting; severe general malaise and exhaustion.
  3. Temperature elevated but rarely above 39° C. (102.2° F.).
  4. Profuse perspiration.
- B. *Treatment*
  1. Absolute bed rest.
  2. Codeine sulfate and acetylsalicylic acid (aspirin) by mouth every 4 hours.
  3. Dextrose, 5% in saline, 500 to 1000 ml., intravenously.
- C. *Prognosis.* Complete recovery in 1 to 2 days. Never fatal.

49–349. **METALDEHYDE**

This very toxic substance is a constituent of many snail baits. In the form of compressed tablets it is used as fuel for small heaters.
- A. *Signs and Symptoms* (usually a 1 to 3 hour time lag after ingestion before onset)
  1. Salivation, nausea and vomiting, with severe abdominal pain.

2. Flushed face, high temperature.
3. Muscle twitching and incoordination.
4. Coma, sometimes fatal in 5 to 8 hours.

B. Treatment
1. Warm salt water or other emetics, followed if necessary by gastric lavage.
2. Magnesium sulfate (Epsom salts), 30 ml., by mouth.
3. Application of external heat.
4. Caffeine sodiobenzoate, 0.5 gm., intramuscularly.
5. Hospitalization for prevention and/or treatment of liver and kidney damage.

49–350. METALLIC OXIDES. See *Metal Fumes* (49–348).

49–351. METAPHEN. See *Mercury Antiseptics* (49–344).

49–352. METHANOL. See *Methyl Alcohol* (49–358).

49–353. METHEDRINE (Methamphetamine). See *Amphetamine Sulfate* (49–45) and *"Speed-balls"* (49–555).

49–354. METHENAMINE (Hexamethylenetetramine, Urotropin)

A. Toxic Signs and Symptoms are due to slow decomposition of methenomine into formaldehyde.

B. Ingestion of Large Doses may cause:
1. Severe diarrhea.
2. Pain in the kidney and bladder with painful urination and albumin and blood in the urine.

C. Treatment
1. Emetics and/or gastric lavage.
2. Codeine sulfate or morphine sulfate subcutaneously for control of severe pain.
3. Large amounts of fluid by mouth and/or intravenously.

D. Prognosis. Complete recovery without residual ill effects.

49–355. METHOPHENOBARBITAL (Mephobarbital). See *Barbiturates* (49–76).

49–356. **METHOXYCHLOR**

This insecticide is slightly less toxic than DDT, although signs and symptoms of toxicity are more prolonged. Muscular twitching, tremors and acute depression may require symptomatic treatment. No fatal cases of poisoning from methoxychlor have been reported. For treatment see *DDT* (49–175).

49–357. **METHYL ACETATE**

Through inhalation of fumes, or by ingestion, this solvent for nitrocellulose, resins and oils may give severe toxic signs and symptoms similar to methyl alcohol (49–358).

49–358. **METHYL ALCOHOL** (Methanol, Methyl Hydrate, Carbinol, Wood Alcohol, Wood Spirit, Wood Naphtha, Columbia Spirit, Colonial Spirit)

Widespread use of this very dangerous liquid as a solvent in industry, in antifreeze mixtures, in the chemical industry and as a fuel makes accidental ingestion fairly common. In addition, many serious cases have been caused by ingestion, by accident or intent, of methyl in place of ethyl alcohol. There is a wide variation in susceptibility of different individuals, but as little as 60 ml. has been fatal. Inhalation of the fumes also may give an acute toxic picture.

A. Signs and Symptoms
Mild Cases
1. Severe headaches; aching pain in the extremities.
2. Nausea and vomiting; gastric pain.
3. Dilated, sluggish pupils.
4. Visual disturbances with temporary, sometimes permanent, blindness.
5. Slow and labored respiration, often with dyspnea and cyanosis. If marked dyspnea is present, the prognosis is unfavorable.

Severe Cases
1. All the signs and symptoms given above in greater degree.
2. Severe abdominal pain.
3. Increased reflex hyperexcitability, with trismus, opisthotonos and convulsions.
4. Hypotension with a weak, rapid pulse.
5. Hallucinations; sometimes mania.
6. Acute visual disturbances and eye signs. These usually do not become acute until 18 to 24 hours after ingestion.
   a. Dilated, fixed pupils—sometimes responsive to convergence tests but rarely to light.
   b. Eyeballs sensitive to pressure; motion of eyes painful; ptosis of lids.

       c. Retrobulbar neuritis with partial or complete permanent loss of vision.
    7. Acute peripheral neuritis.

B. Treatment
    1. Administration of emetics. In adults, apomorphine hydrochloride, 5 mg., subcutaneously, followed if necessary by gastric lavage with 4% sodium bicarbonate solution, is the most effective method. Apomorphine should not be used in small children because of its secondary respiratory depressant effect.
    2. Magnesium sulfate (Epsom salts) by mouth or by lavage.
    3. Control of severe pain by opiates as needed. Hyoscine hydrobromide, 0.3 mg. subcutaneously, may be useful in controlling acute restlessness.
    4. Oxygen for dyspnea and cyanosis, preferably by face mask and rebreathing bag.
    5. Caffeine sodiobenzoate, 0.5 gm., intramuscularly to support the circulation.
    6. Intravenous sodium bicarbonate solution.
    7. HOSPITALIZATION OF ALL CASES—even those which appear to be relatively mild. Proper and prompt treatment may prevent permanent blindness. Peritoneal dialysis may be life-saving or sight-saving.

C. Prognosis. Poor; the mortality is high even if relatively small amounts of methyl alcohol have been ingested. Death may be due to respiratory or cardiac failure or to very severe kidney damage.
    If recovery occurs, it is a prolonged process. Residual eye, kidney and heart damage is common.

49–359. METHYL BROMIDE

Acute toxic signs and symptoms from this very dangerous volatile liquid used in fire extinguishers, as a refrigerant, and as an insecticide do not develop for from 4 to 12 hours after inhalation of the fumes. On the skin, methyl bromide causes itching, prickling and blistering, followed by a sensation of cold and the development of the systemic toxic picture after 4 to 6 hours.

A. Signs and Symptoms
    1. Transient blurred and double vision, sometimes followed by temporary blindness.
    2. Nausea, vomiting and abdominal pain.
    3. Sleepiness, loss of memory, profound weakness.
    4. Slurred speech.
    5. Muscular twitching, incoordination and temporary paralysis.
    6. Mental confusion, sometimes psychoses or mania.
    7. Epileptiform convulsions.
    8. Pulmonary edema (Topic 52).
    9. Circulatory and/or respiratory collapse.

B. Treatment
    1. Remove from exposure. Undress the victim and wash contaminated areas of the body with soap and water.
    2. Clear the airway and begin artificial respiration by mouth-to-

mouth or manual methods immediately. Substitute administration of oxygen under positive pressure by face mask and
rebreathing bag as soon as possible.
3. Protect against injury (tongue-biting, etc.) during convulsions.
4. Administer rapid-acting barbiturates for control of acute excitement or convulsions, preferably intravenously. Oversedation
should be avoided.
5. Give caffeine sodiobenzoate, 0.5 gm., intramuscularly or intravenously. Arterenol bitartrate (Levophed) or metaraminol
bitartrate (Aramine) in 1000 ml. of 5% dextrose in saline
intravenously may be necessary if circulatory collapse is
profound.
6. Hospitalize for observation for at least 48 hours, even if the
toxic picture is relatively mild, because of the tendency
toward late development of pulmonary edema (Topic 52).

49–360. **METHYL CHLORIDE**

This very toxic gas is used in refrigeration systems and in the chemical
industry.
For signs and symptoms of toxicity and treatment see *Methyl Bromide*
(49–359).

49–361. **METHYLETHYLKETONE**

This is an industrial solvent that on brief contact can cause extreme
thickening of the fingernails, with permanent destruction of the nail beds.
Treatment is symptomatic only.

49–362. **METHYL FORMATE**

Widely used as a solvent in industry, methyl formate may cause severe
toxic effects through absorption from the respiratory tract or by ingestion.
A. Signs and Symptoms
1. Feeling of suffocation and constriction of the chest; acute dyspnea.
2. Visual disturbances—amblyopia and nystagmus.
B. Treatment. As outlined under *Methyl Alcohol* (49–358).

49–363. **METHYL SALICYLATE** (Oil of Wintergreen)

This pleasant-smelling liquid is used as an aromatic flavoring extract,
as a rubefacient in rubbing liniments and ointments, and medicinally as
an antirheumatic and antiseptic agent. Because of its attractive smell and
taste, it is frequently ingested by infants and children, with a very high
mortality (about 55%). Absorption through the intact skin also can cause
an acute toxic picture. Methyl salicylate is from ten to twenty times as toxic

as acetylsalicylic acid but is much more slowly absorbed from the gastrointestinal tract.

A. Signs and Symptoms
1. Odor of wintergreen or acetone on the breath.
2. Sleepiness.
3. Profuse perspiration.
4. Nausea and persistent vomiting; dehydration and thirst.
5. Disturbances in sight and hearing.
6. Labored, rapid, "panting dog" respiration; cyanosis.
7. Convulsions and coma.
8. Circulatory and respiratory depression. Death is usually caused by respiratory collapse.

B. Treatment. See *Salicylates* (49–511).

C. Prognosis. Fair in adults; poor in infants and children, especially if hyperpnea is present. Nephritis, toxic hepatitis and acidosis are frequent sequelae.

49–364.   **METRAZOL** (Cardiazol, Pentylenetetrazol)

In hypersensitive individuals use of pentylenetetrazol (Metrazol) in therapeutic doses as an analeptic may result in brief but extremely violent convulsions and in auricular fibrillation. No treatment is indicated except protection against injury (fractures, dislocations, tongue biting, etc.) until the convulsion ceases. The auricular fibrillation is transient and not dangerous. Pentylenetetrazol is probably the safest of the potent analeptics.

49–365. **MEXICAN JUMPING BEANS**

Diarrhea of varying degrees of intensity, probably caused by surface contaminants, may make a child who eats several of these peculiarly acting beans very uncomfortable and the parents very apprehensive. However, larvae in the beans which cause the "jumping" are harmless. Administration of a laxative and reassurance of the parents are generally all that is required.

49–366. **"MICKEY FINN"**

Two formulas are occasionally (and illegally) added to alcoholic beverages in some disreputable cocktail lounges and bars to get rid of obstreperous or offensive customers:
1. Drops: 1 to 2 ml. of croton oil.
2. Powders: A mixture of powdered jalap and milk sugar.

Both are very effective, although in different ways, and, in certain instances, very dangerous. Neither should be confused with "knockout drops," which contain chloral hydrate (49–128) and which usually are administered with a more sinister purpose.

A. Signs and Symptoms
1. Acute burning sensation in the mouth.

2. Nausea and violent vomiting associated with tenesmus, severe abdominal pain and violent diarrhea.
3. Cold and clammy skin; weak pulse; hypotension.
4. Collapse and sometimes death from respiratory and/or circulatory failure if an excessive dose has been given.

B. Treatment

1. Give demulcents (white of eggs, flour, etc.) by mouth as soon as possible.
2. Empty the stomach (if vomiting has not been profuse) by emetics or lavage.
3. Institute artificial respiration by mouth-to-mouth, manual or mechanical means if respiratory depression is severe.
4. Give large amounts of black coffee or strong tea by mouth, or inject caffeine sodiobenzoate, 0.5 gm., intramuscularly. In extreme cases support the circulation by intravenous ephedrine sulfate, arterenol bitartrate (Levophed) or metaraminol bitartrate (Aramine).
5. Hospitalize if respiratory or circulatory depression is profound. Sudden collapse may occur several hours after apparent control of acute signs and symptoms of toxicity.

49–367.　**MILTOWN.** See *Meprobamate* (49–336) and Topic 59–41.

49–368.　**MISSILE PROPELLANTS.** See *Rocket Fuels* (49–503).

49–369.　**MONOCHLOROBENZENE.** See *Chlorobenzene* (49–135).

49–370.　**MORPHINE.** [Also see Topic 2–3 (*Addiction*), Topic 3–13 (*Coma*) and Topic 9 (*Narcotics in Emergency Cases*).]

A. Acute Morphinism may follow ingestion, subcutaneous, intramuscular or intravenous injection, or ((occasionally) absorption through mucous membranes. If subcutaneous or intramuscular injections are given to a patient whose circulatory system is much depressed, overwhelmingly cumulative, even lethal-toxic, effects may occur when the circulation improves.

Signs and Symptoms

1. Pinpoint nonreactive pupils.
2. Subnormal temperature.
3. Gradually slowing respiration with slowly increasing cyanosis and increasing somnolence deepening into coma.
4. Convulsions—common in children, rare in adults.
5. Collapse from respiratory failure.

Treatment

1. Keep the patient awake and moving if possible. Muscular activity such as walking is beneficial in mild cases but can be detrimental if respiratory depression is acute.
2. Give strong black coffee by mouth, or caffeine sodiobenzoate, 0.5 gm., intramuscularly or intravenously.
3. If ingested, induce vomiting as soon as possible; then lavage with 1:2000 potassium permanganate solution, provided the patient is not in deep coma.
4. If only a few moments have elapsed after injection into an extremity, apply a tourniquet proximal to the injection site— tight enough to shut off the venous return, but not tight enough to interfere with the arterial pulse.
5. Inject atropine sulfate, 0.5 mg., subcutaneously or intravenously.
6. Combat anoxia and cyanosis by administration of oxygen under positive pressure by face mask or endotracheal catheter and rebreathing bag.
7. Apply external heat by warm blankets, a bed warmer or cast dryer. HOT WATER BAGS SHOULD NOT BE USED UNLESS OTHER MEANS OF APPLYING HEAT ARE NOT AVAILABLE.
8. If the measures outlined above have been tried and found ineffective, inject 1 ml. (5 mg.) of nalorphine hydrochloride (Nalline) intravenously PROVIDED THE PATIENT IS NOT AN ADDICT and that the toxic substance has been positively identified. Nalorphine hydrochloride is also spectacularly effective as a physiologic antagonist to synthetic narcotics.
9. Hospitalize for supportive therapy after control of acute symptoms.

Prognosis. If the patient can be kept alive for 6 to 8 hours, he will generally make a complete recovery, although remissions sometimes occur from reabsorption from the gastrointestinal tract.

B. Chronic Morphinism with Withdrawal Symptoms. (Also see Topic 2–3.) This serious condition is a true emergency. Since many states and countries consider prescribing opiates of any type for an addict as a crime except in extreme emergency or as a life-saving measure, symptomatic supportive therapy and sedation through barbiturates, paraldehyde and/or phenothiazines is indicated until the patient can be transferred for treatment to a properly accredited institution. A generally recognized exception to this rule is that if the patient has been booked and is in police custody, narcotics may be administered for control of acute withdrawal symptoms. Also, it is becoming increasingly recognized in several parts of the world that persons who seek relief from addiction or from withdrawal symptoms should be treated as patients and not as criminals.

49–371. **MOTH REPELLENTS**

These may be of several strengths. For very slightly toxic repellents, see *Paradichlorobenzene* (49–436); moderately toxic, *Camphor* (49–112); and extremely toxic, *Naphthalene* (49–381).

49–372. **MUSCARINE**

This very toxic substance occurs in certain varieties of poisonous mushrooms ("fly mushrooms") and toadstools, but not in most fungi.

A. Signs and Symptoms
1. Rapid onset and course with acute symptoms lasting only 1 to 3 hours. Death from cardiac arrest or complete collapse may occur in a few hours. In nonfatal cases, complete recovery usually occurs in 1 to 2 days.
2. Toxic symptoms and signs are due to parasympathetic stimulation characterized by lacrimation, salivation, miosis, sweating, dyspnea, abdominal pain, vomiting, diarrhea and intense excitement, followed by circulatory and respiratory depression.

B. Treatment
1. Induction of vomiting.
2. Gastric lavage with 1:2000 potassium permanganate solution.
3. Subcutaneous or intravenous injection of atropine sulfate, the physiologic antagonist of muscarine. Doses up to 1 mg. may be necessary; repeat until the muscarine effect has been neutralized.
4. Administration of magnesium sulfate (Epsom salts), 30 gm., by mouth.

49–373. **MUSHROOM POISONING**

A. Rapid Poisoning. Acute toxic signs and symptoms developing from a few minutes to 3 hours after ingestion and occasionally causing death are usually due to the muscarine contained in *Amanita muscaria* and *pantherina*. Considerable variation in the degree of toxicity in different localities has been noted; for example, in Switzerland *A. muscaria* ("fly agaric") is considered to be very dangerous, while in Alaska it is eaten by Eskimos as a source of pleasurable intoxication. For treatment see 49–372 (Muscarine).

B. Delayed Poisoning. Toxic signs and symptoms coming on 6 to 24 hours after ingestion are almost invariably due to *Amanita phalloides* and allied forms in the United States and to *A. verna* in Europe. These varieties of bulb agarics account for about 90% of all fatalities from mushroom poisoning; ingestion of the "amanita toxins" has a mortality rate of 50%. A less frequent offender is the Helvella (false morel) which may cause acute toxic signs and symptoms coming on from 6 to 8 hours after ingestion.

C. Identification. Members of the amanita family are responsible for practically all cases of serious mushroom poisoning; hence, one simple rule may be lifesaving: NEVER EAT A MUSHROOM

THAT HAS TWO SWELLINGS ON THE STALK! These two enlargements—the annulus just below the gills, and the volva at or slightly beneath ground level—are characteristic of the deadly amanita family only; other mushrooms may have one, but no other important variety has both.

D. Signs and Symptoms (after a latent period of 6 hours or more)

1. Sudden, very severe abdominal pain associated with nausea and vomiting. The vomitus may be bloody.
2. Diarrhea with blood and mucus followed by extreme thirst, dehydration and rapidly developing weakness.
3. Apparent marked improvement, usually lasting a few hours, then sudden development of acute cyanosis with coldness of the skin of the extremities and collapse of the circulatory system with progressive central nervous system involvement. Death usually occurs 48 to 72 hours after ingestion.

E. Treatment

1. Induction of vomiting by whatever means are necessary, including apomorphine subcutaneously. This is essential so that fragments of the ingested mushroom can be recovered for identification. Vomiting, even if profuse, should be followed by lavage with 1:2000 potassium permanganate solution.
2. Administration of morphine sulfate or dihydromorphinone hydrochloride (Dilaudid) subcutaneously or intravenously for severe pain and apprehension. Codeine sulfate or meperidine hydrochloride (Demerol) may be of value in less severe cases.
3. Intravenous injection of 500 to 1000 ml. of 10% dextrose in saline to combat dehydration.
4. Emptying of the bowel by magnesium sulfate (Epsom salts).
5. Hospitalization as soon as possible even if apparent improvement has been noted.

F. Hallucinogenic Effects

Psilocybin, an unsaturated indole, is the active toxic agent in certain varieties of mushrooms used in religious rites in Mexico because of their peculiar ability to produce hallucinations (49–261). Recovery in 8 to 10 hours after ingestion is to be expected. No specific treatment is required.

49–374. MUSHROOM "MIASMA"

In certain localities crews engaged in dumping compote and cleaning the bins used in growing mushrooms have developed:

1. Dryness of the nose and throat lasting about 8 hours.
2. Nausea and restlessness with a burning sensation in the nose and throat.
3. After 24 hours, fever, rapid pulse, dry cough and dermatitis usually involving the nose, below the eyes and the scrotum.
4. Fever, sweating, chills and chest pain lasting until about the 8th day after exposure.
5. Gradual abatement of signs and symptoms in about 2 weeks.

The cause is not known. Symptomatic treatment only is required. No fatalities have been reported.

49–375. **MUSSEL POISONING**

Poisonous heat-stable alkaloids are present in certain seafoods during certain months. Mussels, clams, oysters or abalone may be affected.

   A. Signs and Symptoms. Acute progressive respiratory paralysis coming on without warning generally causes the patient to be brought for emergency care. The diagnosis depends wholly upon the history—usually several members of the same family or party are affected.

   B. Treatment

     1. Animal charcoal or the universal antidote (49–10).

     2. Apomorphine hydrochloride, 4 to 5 mg., subcutaneously, as an emetic. As much as 8 mg. may be given to an adult if necessary, but the original dose should never be repeated; if apomorphine does not cause vomiting it may produce extreme respiratory depression.

     3. Magnesium sulfate (Epsom salts) as a purgative.

     4. Long-continued administration of oxygen under positive pressure by face mask or endotracheal catheter and rebreathing bag. Recovery from respiratory paralysis with establishment of normal breathing may occur after several hours.

     5. Hospitalization as soon as normal respiration has been re-established. Relapses are common.

49–376. **MUSTARD GAS.** See *War Gases* [*Vesicants* (49–648,D)].

49–377. **MYOCHRYSINE.** See *Gold Salts* (49–257).

. . . . N . . . .

49–378. **NAIL POLISH.** See *Acetone* (49–14) and *Aniline Dyes* (49–54).

49–379. **NAIL POLISH REMOVERS.** See *Acetone* (49–14).

49–380. **NAPHTHA.** See *Benzene* (49–80).

Do not confuse with *Naphthol* (49–382).

49–381. NAPHTHALENE

This is the most toxic of the insect repellents commonly found in moth balls. It is also a constituent of some brands of deodorant cakes. Toxic signs and symptoms may be caused in children by clothes that have been stored in mothballs.

A. *Signs and Symptoms*
 1. Characteristic odor on the breath.
 2. Nausea and vomiting, gastroenteritis.
 3. Profound depression.
 4. Development after 3 to 7 days of symptoms due to hemolysis.

B. *Treatment*
 1. Give demulcents such as white of egg.
 2. Induce vomiting by strong salt water, mustard, ipecac or other emetics. Apomorphine hydrochloride subcutaneously is very effective but should not be used in small children.
 3. Place the patient at absolute rest with application of external heat.
 4. Force fluids by mouth or give 500 to 1000 ml. normal salt solution intravenously.
 5. Give caffeine sodiobenzoate, 0.5 gm., intramuscularly (except in small children).
 6. Avoid fatty substances, including milk.
 7. Hospitalize severe cases; deferred hemolysis may require repeated transfusions.

49–382. NAPHTHOL

Both the alpha and beta isomers of naphthol may give severe toxic signs and symptoms by ingestion as well as by absorption through the intact skin.

A. *Signs and Symptoms*
 1. Nausea and vomiting.
 2. Convulsions and coma.
 3. Severe liver, kidney and spleen damage, with jaundice, albuminuria and anemia.

B. *Treatment*
 1. If ingested, gastric lavage with 1:2000 potassium permanganate solution.
 2. Hospitalization of all cases for observation because of the possibility of serious liver, kidney and spleen damage.

49–383. NAPHTHYLAMINE

The beta isomer of naphthylamine may cause severe bladder irritation after ingestion or inhalation of fumes.

A. *Signs and Symptoms*
 1. Elevated temperature.

2. Dysuria and hematuria from small punctate hemorrhages in the bladder wall which may form multiple premalignant papillomas.

B. Treatment
1. If inhaled, oxygen therapy by face mask and rebreathing bag using positive pressure.
2. If ingested, emetics or gastric lavage with 1:2000 potassium permanganate solution.
3. Referral to a urologist if hematuria or acute dysuria is present.

49–384. **NARCYLENE.** See *Acetylene* (49–17).

49–385. **NEOCINCHOPHEN.** See *Cinchophen* (49–148).

49–386. **NIACIN.** See *Nicotinic Acid* (49–390).

49–387. **NICKEL**

Acute dermatitis, gingivitis and stomatitis may be caused by nickel and its salts. Removal from contact and symptomatic treatment usually result in rapid recovery. [For exceptions see *Nickel Carbonyl* (49–388).]

49–388. **NICKEL CARBONYL**

This liquid is used extensively in industry. Inhalation of fumes may result in acute poisoning. More than one part of fumes to a million of air may cause very severe, even fatal, toxic effects.

A. Signs and Symptoms of Toxicity during Exposure
1. Nausea and vomiting.
2. Dizziness and severe cephalgia.

Treatment
    Removal of the patient to fresh air usually results in apparent recovery, but observation for 2 to 3 days is absolutely necessary.

B. Delayed Toxic Signs and Symptoms (latent period of 12 to 30 hours)
1. Pain and feeling of constriction in the chest.
2. Severe cough.
3. Slow pulse; rapid respirations.
4. Dyspnea and cyanosis.
5. Convulsions.
6. Enlargement of the liver.

Treatment
1. Oxygen inhalations under positive pressure.
2. Caffeine sodiobenzoate, 0.5 gm., intramuscularly.
3. Calcium gluconate, 10 ml. of 10% solution, intravenously very slowly.

      4. Dimercaprol (BAL) intramuscularly, 0.025 ml. of 10% solution
         per kilogram of body weight, every 4 hours.
      5. Hospitalization for observation because of the possibility of de-
         layed development of severe brain, lung and liver damage.
  C. Prognosis. Good in most cases. If convulsions or cyanosis are pres-
      ent, the chances of terminal bronchopneumonia are much in-
      creased.

49–389. **NICOTINE.** Also see *Cigarettes* and *Cigars* (49–147), and *Tobacco* (49–611).

A. Signs and Symptoms
    1. Depression, muscular weakness and prostration.
    2. Pupils first contracted, then dilated.
    3. Nausea and vomiting followed by profuse diarrhea.
    4. Dyspnea and tachycardia.
    5. Muscular tremors followed by convulsions.

B. Treatment
    1. Universal antidote (49–10) followed AT ONCE by gastric lavage
       with 1:2000 potassium permanganate solution. Speed is essen-
       tial because nicotine is absorbed very rapidly.
    2. Caffeine sodiobenzoate, 0.5 gm., intramuscularly or intrave-
       nously.
    3. Application of heat.
    4. Artificial respiration and oxygen therapy started as soon as pos-
       sible and continued until dyspnea has cleared.

49–390. **NICOTINIC ACID** (Niacin)

Used as a preservative in foods and as a medication, nicotinic acid may give toxic signs and symptoms in both therapeutic and excessive doses.

A. Signs and Symptoms
    1. A sensation of heat starting in the face and spreading to arms
       and hands, then to the body, especially the perianal region.
    2. Flushing of the face.
    3. Gradual subsidence of the stinging and tingling of the involved
       parts.
    4. Generalized itching.
    5. Vague, nonlocalized, abdominal discomfort.

Although the effects are uncomfortable, complete recovery in 1 to 1½ hours always takes place.

49–391. **NITRATES**

Nitrates are used for many purposes in industry, especially in the proces-sing and pickling of meat products. Contamination of well water with or-ganic matter may cause sufficient concentration of nitrates to give toxic signs and symptoms. Fatalities have been reported from inhalation of silage gases. .

A. Signs and Symptoms

  1. SMALL DOSES may cause methemoglobinemia and resultant cyanosis. Breaking down of nitrates to nitrites by bacterial action in the intestine is the causative factor. For signs and symptoms of the nitrite toxicity see *Nitrites* (49–393).
  2. LARGE DOSES may cause:
     a. Nausea and vomiting with tenesmus, bloody diarrhea and generalized weakness.
     b. Cardiac irregularities.
     c. Dysuria and hematuria.
     d. Convulsions and collapse; sometimes death.

B. Treatment. See *Nitrites* (49–393).

49–392. **NITRIC OXIDE** (NO). See *Oxides of Nitrogen* (49–426).

49–393. **NITRITES.** [Also see *Nitrates* (49–391).]

Poisoning from nitrites may occur through inhalation or through ingestion.

A. Signs and Symptoms

  1. Flushing of the face, dyspnea and cyanosis.
  2. Slow, weak and irregular pulse.
  3. Sudden collapse with extreme hypotension.

B. Treatment

  1. Gastric lavage with 1:2000 potassium permanganate solution if ingested.
  2. Oxygen inhalations for dyspnea and cyanosis.
  3. Shock therapy (Topic 15–7).
  4. Methylene blue, 1% solution in 1.8% sodium sulfate solution, 50 ml., intravenously.
  5. Hospitalization in severe cases or if methylene blue solution has been given.

49–394. **NITROBENZENE**

Nitrobenzene is a common ingredient in shoe polishes and dyes, often in combination with aniline and aniline dyes.

A. Signs and Symptoms

  1. Tinnitus, vertigo and incoordination.
  2. Nausea and vomiting.
  3. Dyspnea and cyanosis.
  4. Convulsions and coma.

B. Treatment

  1. Gastric lavage with normal salt solution.
  2. Oxygen inhalations.

3. Dextrose, 5% in saline, 500 to 1000 ml., intravenously.
4. Methylene blue, 1% solution in 1.8% sodium sulfate solution, 50 ml., intravenously for cyanosis.
5. Saline cathartics.
6. Hospitalization because of the tendency toward delayed development of cardiac, hepatic and renal damage.

49–395. NITROCHLOROBENZENE

A. *Ingestion* may cause rapid onset of:
1. Staggering gait.
2. Pallor or cyanosis from the formation of methemoglobinemia.
3. Dyspnea.
4. Excitement and hallucinations.
B. *Inhalation* may cause the same picture except that symptoms usually are less severe and do not become apparent for 1 to 2 hours.
C. *Treatment.* As given for *Nitrobenzene* (49–394).

49–396. NITROGEN DIOXIDE (NO$_2$). See *Oxides of Nitrogen* (49–426).

49–397. NITROGEN TETROXIDE (N$_2$O$_4$). See *Oxides of Nitrogen* (49–426).

49–398. NITROGLYCERIN. See *Nitrites* (49–393).

49–399. NITROUS OXIDE (N$_2$O). See *Anesthetics, Inhalation* (Topic 59–8).

49–400. NOVOCAIN (Procaine). See *Anesthetics, Local* (49–52), and Topic 59–10.

49–401. NUX VOMICA. See *Strychnine* (49–565).

. . . . O . . . .

49–402. OBESITY CURES. See *Amphetamine Sulfate* (49–45) and Topic 59–6; and *Dinitrophenol* (49–201).

49–403.   **OIL OF ALMONDS** (Artificial). See *Nitrobenzene* (49–394).

49–404.   **OIL OF BETULA.** See *Methyl Salicylate* (49–363).

49–405.   **OIL OF BITTER ALMONDS.** See *Amygdalin* (49–46) and *Cyanides* (49–170).

49–406.   **OIL, COAL.** See *Kerosene* (49–303).

49–407.   **OIL, ESSENTIAL.** Oils of absinthe, apiol, cajeput, cedar, eucalyptus, menthol, nutmeg, pennyroyal, rue, savin and tansy are complex mixtures of alcohols, esters, ethers, ketones and hydrocarbons. Ingestion of very small amounts (less than 30 ml.) may be fatal. The signs and symptoms of toxicity are similar to those outlined under *Eucalyptol* (49–233) and *Turpentine* (49–633). The treatment is the same.

49–408.   **OIL OF GAUTHERIA.** See *Methyl Salicylate* (49–363).

49–409.   **OIL OF LEMON GRASS.** See *Lemon Grass Oil* (49–314).

49–410.   **OIL OF MIRBANE.** See *Nitrobenzene* (49–394).

49–411.   **OIL OF PEPPERMINT.** See *Menthol* (49–335).

49–412.   **OIL OF PINE.** See *Pine Oil* (49–467).

49–413.   **OIL OF ROSEMARY.** See *Rosemary* (49–504).

49–414. **OIL OF SWEET BIRCH.** See *Methyl Salicylate* (49–363).

49–415. **OIL OF TUNG.** See *Tung Oil* (49–632).

49–416. **OIL OF VITRIOL.** See *Acids* (49–19).

49–417. **OIL, VOLATILE.** See *Oil, Essential* (49–407).

49–418. **OIL OF WINTERGREEN.** See *Methyl Salicylate* (49–363).

49–419. **OLEANDER.** See 49–736.

49–420. **OPIUM** [Laudanum (Tincture of Opium); Paregoric (Camphorated Tincture of Opium)]

See Topic 2–3 (*Addiction*); Topic 9 (*Narcotics*); and *Morphine* (49–370).

49–421. **ORGANIC PHOSPHATES**

These compounds, originally designed for war-time use, are now utilized as insecticides by spraying and dusting, often by airplane.

A. Most Common Compounds

CHLORTHION (o,o-Dimethyl-o-3-chloro-4-nitrophenyl thiophosphate). Moderately toxic—minimal skin penetration.

DEMETON (Systox) (Ethyl-mercaptoethyl-diethyl thiophosphate). Very toxic.

DIALKYLPHOSPHATE

DIPTERIX. Moderately toxic.

EPN (Ethyl p-nitrophenyl thionobenzenephosphonate). Moderately toxic.

MALATHION. The least toxic of the organic phosphates and the only one approved for household use.

METACIDE (Dimethyl p-nitrophenyl thionophosphate), Very toxic.

OMPA (Octamethyl pyrophosphoramide). Very toxic.

PARAOXON (Diethyl-p-nitrophenyl phosphate). Extremely toxic.

PARATHION (Diethyl-p-nitrophenyl thionophosphate). Extremely toxic.

PHOSDRIN. Very toxic.

SULFOTEPP (Tetraethyl dithiopyrophosphate). Extremely toxic.

TEPP (Tetrin) (Tetraethyl pyrophosphate). Extremely toxic.

THIMET. Very toxic.

TRITHION. Moderately toxic.

B. **Mode of Action.** In all of these compounds the organic phosphorus-containing portion of the molecule is strongly cholinesterase inhibiting. Since the function of the cholinesterase in the body is to hasten the hydrolysis of acetylcholine, the accumulation of acetylcholine may result in stimulation of the entire parasympathetic nervous system [muscarine effect and nicotine effect, see *Muscarine* (49–372) and *Nicotine* (49–389)].

Acquired sensitivity to, or tolerance for, these compounds is unknown, and skin lesions do not occur. There is a marked variation in the amounts required to cause toxic effects in different individuals.

C. **Entrance into the Body** may be through the *intact* skin, by inhalation or by ingestion.

D. **Incidence of Poisoning.** Anyone who comes in contact with dust-spraying or dusting apparatus or plants or vegetables to which the organic phosphates have been applied *within 30 days*, may develop toxic signs and symptoms. Included in this category are the following:

1. Agricultural, greenhouse and nursery workers, formulators, packagers and distributors.
2. Crop dusters—pilots, flagmen and mechanics; persons servicing equipment used in application.
3. Occupants of houses in or near treated areas, especially to the leeward, and children playing in treated areas.
4. Travelers passing the fields during application; casual trespassers.
5. Beekeepers.

E. **Time of Onset of Toxic Effects** varies from 15 minutes to 24 hours. Exposure may not take place until a workman changes his contaminated clothing at the end of the day's work. Onset of symptoms most commonly occur within ½ hour of exposure or while in bed at night.

If an individual gives a history of exposure to any of the organic phosphates within 24 hours and presents, even mildly, any of the signs and symptoms listed below (especially severe headache and fixed contracted pupils), treatment should be begun AT ONCE.

Laboratory tests are of no value as an emergency measure.

F. **Signs and Symptoms**

1. PREMONITORY indications of organic phosphate poisoning are severe headache and profuse salivation, lacrimation and perspiration.
2. ACUTE TOXIC SYMPTOMS AND SIGNS (following the premonitory stage by ½ to 1 hour)
   a. Dim vision, with fixed miosis.
   b. Dizziness and fainting; severe headache.
   c. Nausea and vomiting with or without persistent diarrhea.
   d. Dyspnea and increasing cyanosis.

    e. Incontinence of urine and feces.

    f. Muscular twitching and tonic convulsions.

    g. Respiratory failure followed by pulmonary edema (Topic 52).

    h. Total collapse and death.

G. Treatment

  1. Atropine sulfate in large doses, 1 to 2 mg., intravenously or sub-cutaneously, repeated hourly if necessary. Combatting of the effects of organic phosphates on skeletal muscle by administration of 2-pyridine aldoxime methiodide has been reported, but only as an adjunct to, not a substitute for, large doses of atropine.

  2. Removal of excess secretions by postural drainage, suction or intratracheal tube followed by oxygen therapy by face mask or endotracheal tube and rebreathing bag, using positive pressure. Continuation for several hours may be necessary.

  3. If the material has been ingested, gastric lavage WITH WARM WATER ONLY.

  4. Hospitalization as soon as possible if during the prodromal or premonitory stage. The patient should be accompanied by a physician or registered nurse, since onset of acute toxic symptoms may be terminal if proper symptomatic treatment is not given AT ONCE. Close observation for at least 24 hours after the disappearance of acute symptoms, or after the last injection of atropine sulfate, is essential.

H. Do Not Give

  1. Morphine sulfate, codeine sulfate, meperidine hydrochloride (Demerol), methadone hydrochloride (Dolophine) or other natural or synthetic narcotics.

  2. Large doses of barbiturates. If sedation is necessary, chloral hydrate orally or rectally or paraldehyde orally or intramuscularly in the smallest effective doses should be used. Need for extreme sedation indicates that atropinization is not adequate.

  3. BAL.

  4. Sodium thiosulfate or potassium permanganate solution.

  5. Calcium gluconate.

  6. Apomorphine hydrochloride or ipecac as an emetic.

  7. Aminophylline, theophylline or chlorotheophylline.

I. Prognosis. Poor, unless the condition is recognized and given proper emergency treatment at once. Good, if proper immediate treatment is given. Complete recovery without residual ill effects may occur after even very severe exposure. After recovery the patient can usually be allowed to return to his regular work with the warning that any exposure to organic phosphates should be avoided for several months.

49–422. **ORTHO-DICHLOROBENZENE**

Used as a wood preservative. For signs and symptoms and treatment see *Naphthalene* (49–381).

49–423. **OUABAIN**

The toxic effect of this rarely used digitalis-like alkaloid is much greater than the more frequently used preparations. See *Digitalis* (49–191).

49–424. **OXALATES.** See *Oxalic Acid* (49–425) and *Potassium Oxalate* (49–475).

49–425. **OXALIC ACID**

This acid is the active agent in many household bleaching and cleansing preparations and in some ink eradicators. It also occurs in the leaves and blades (*not* the stalks) of rhubarb plants (49–501). TREATMENT OF OXALIC ACID INGESTION DOES NOT FOLLOW THE OUTLINE GIVEN UNDER ACIDS (49–19).

A. Signs and Symptoms
1. Burning of the mouth, throat and esophagus; dysphagia.
2. Rapid, weak pulse; cold, clammy skin.
3. Bloody vomitus caused by erosion of the gastric mucosa.
4. Violent diarrhea with subsequent acute dehydration.

B. Treatment
1. Have the patient swallow large amounts of calcium lactate, chalk (or plaster off the wall if necessary), egg white, liquid petrolatum or olive oil. DO NOT PASS A STOMACH TUBE if concentrated oxalic acid has been swallowed. DO NOT GIVE the usual alkalies used to neutralize strong acids; they form salts with oxalic acid which may be more corrosive than the acid itself.
2. Inject apomorphine hydrochloride, 5 mg., subcutaneously at once.
3. Apply external heat.
4. Support the circulation with caffeine sodiobenzoate, 0.5 gm., intramuscularly. Ephedrine sulfate, metaraminol bitartrate (Aramine) or arterenol bitartrate (Levophed) intravenously may be necessary if circulatory collapse is extreme.
5. Control severe pain by morphine sulfate subcutaneously.
6. Hospitalize as soon as the patient's condition will allow. Acute edema of the glottis may require tracheotomy (Topic 17–11,B) before transfer.

49–426. **OXIDES OF NITROGEN**

All of these substances are volatile and all can cause acute toxic symptoms following inhalation of relatively small amounts.

A. Exposure to Toxic Concentrations may occur in:
1. Commercial production of explosives, nitrocellulose and photographic and x-ray films.

2. Photoengraving.
3. Metal etching and pickling.
4. Welding and oxyacetylene operations.
5. Use of the carbon arc.
6. Silo cleaning. Decomposition of nitrates in silage may result in a fatal concentration of nitrogen oxides.

B. Modes of Toxic Action
1. ANESTHETIC ACTION [see *Anesthetics, Inhalation* (Topic 59–8)]. This is unimportant in industry since nitrous oxide is never present in high enough concentrations to cause anesthetic symptoms.
2. NITRITE ACTION [see *Nitrites* (49–393)], resulting from breaking down of NO, NO_2 and N_2O_4 in the lungs.
3. LOCAL IRRITATIVE AND CORROSIVE ACTION in the lungs due to NO_2 and N_2O_4.

C. Clinical Types of Toxic Reactions
1. SHOCK TYPE. Immediate death from asphyxia. There is generally no time for treatment of any kind.
2. IRRITANT GAS TYPE. Characterized by an immediate burning sensation in the mouth and throat, with violent nonproductive cough. A latent period up to 24 hours may follow, with secondary development of severe, frequently fatal, pulmonary edema (Topic 52). If the patient survives, pneumonia or pulmonary fibrosis is a frequent complication.
3. REVERSIBLE TYPE. Characterized by minimal respiratory irritation, but with nausea, vomiting, vertigo, severe dyspnea, cyanosis and syncope. These persons generally recover.
4. COMBINED TYPE. Various combinations of types 1, 2 and 3 above.

D. Treatment
1. In any case where a history of possible exposure is obtained, immediate transfer to a hospital by ambulance.
2. Symptomatic treatment (cleansing and assurance of the patency of the airway, administration of air or oxygen under pressure, supportive measures, etc.) if necessary before and during transfer.

49–427. **OXYGEN.** [Also see 49–503 (*Rocket Fuels*).]

In addition to retrolental fibroplasia in premature infants, high concentrations of oxygen can cause pulmonary hyaline membrane disease to develop shortly after birth in full-term infants. In adults, prolonged administration of concentrations of 60% or more can cause severe cough and acute chest pain associated with decreased vital capacity. In persons with chronic pulmonary disease, oxygen may cause a decrease in respiration by "washing out" of carbon dioxide.

Inhalation of oxygen at high pressures may cause severe poisoning in flyers and in professional and sport divers [Topic 26 (*Barotrauma*)].

A. Signs and Symptoms
1. Restlessness, nervousness, extreme hilarity.
2. Impaired cerebration, judgement and sensation.
3. Muscle fibrillation and spasm, followed by severe convulsions.

    4. Death from drowning, air embolism, and/or decompression sickness (Topic 26).

B. Treatment
    1. Rescue.
    2. Artificial respiration AT ONCE by mouth-to-mouth, mouth-to-nose or mechanical methods if cyanosis is present.
    3. Immediate transfer to a pressure chamber for recompression if the patient has become unconscious while diving with any type of gas-filled apparatus (Topic 26). Artificial respiration must be continued en route.

49–428.   OXYQUINOLINE DERIVATIVES

These drugs are used as amebicides in dysentery. Overdosage may cause acute symptoms which fortunately are practically never fatal, provided proper treatment is obtained.

A. Signs and Symptoms
    1. Nausea and vomiting associated with upper abdominal pain, sometimes severe enough to be mistaken for an acute surgical condition.
    2. Hepatitis with or without jaundice.

B. Treatment
    1. Stop administration of the drug at once.
    2. Give 5% dextrose in saline, 500 to 1000 ml., intravenously.
    3. Sedate by barbiturates as needed. Morphine sulfate may be given subcutaneously or, in small doses, slowly intravenously, if the pain is severe.
    4. Instruct the patient in use of a high carbohydrate diet.
    5. Arrange for follow-up care if evidence of hepatitis is present.
    6. Hospitalize severe cases.

49–429.   OZONE

Consumable electrode welding has resulted in an increase in the number of cases of acute ozone poisoning. In addition, ozone-producing equipment, allegedly of therapeutic benefit, may give toxic concentrations of ozone (more than 0.1 part per million of air).

A. Signs and Symptoms
    1. Headache, lethargy and generalized malaise.
    2. Persistent, usually nonproductive, cough, often associated with chest pain—sometimes severe enough to be mistaken for the pain caused by a myocardial or pulmonary infarct.
    3. Minimal clinical and x-ray findings in spite of acute discomfort.

B. Treatment
    1. Remove from exposure.
    2. Control restlessness and pain by administration of sedatives and anodynes orally. Severe cases may require subcutaneous injections of small doses of meperidine hydrochloride (Demerol) for relief of pain.
    3. Give oxygen inhalations by face mask and rebreathing bag if dyspnea is acute or accompanied by cyanosis.

4. Keep under observation with symptomatic care until acute symptoms have subsided. Severe cases require hospitalization since deferred pulmonary edema (Topic 52) may develop.

. . . . P . . . .

49–430. **PAINT.** See *Arsenic* (49–63); *Chromium* (49–145); *Lead Salts* (49–313); *Methyl Alcohol* (49–358); *Gasoline* (49–254); *Kerosene* (49–303); and *Turpentine* (49–633).

White lead (a basic carbonate) and red lead (the tetroxide) are the bases of many paints. Petroleum solvents give toxic symptoms and signs similar to gasoline and kerosene. Harmless titanium salts are the base of many inside house paints.

49–431. **PAINT REMOVERS.** See *Acetone* (49–14); *Benzene* (49–80); *Carbon Tetrachloride* (49–120); *Dichloroethane* (49–184); *Lye* (49–323); *Methyl Alcohol* (49–358); *Methylethylketone* (49–361); *Turpentine* (49–633).

49–432. **PAMAQUINE NAPHTHOATE**

Under the trade name of Plasmochin, this drug is used for specific antimalaria therapy. Excessive or prolonged dosage may cause dizziness and drowsiness, cyanosis and jaundice.

Treatment
1. Stop administration of the drug.
2. Give oxygen therapy under positive pressure for cyanosis.
3. Inject methylene blue, 50 ml. of a 1% solution in 1.8% sodium sulfate solution, intravenously.
4. Hospitalize severe cases. Permanent ill effects are rare.

49–433. **PAPER PRODUCTS**

Ornamental paper products, such as colored crepe, are often sucked or chewed by children. They are not toxic.

49–434. **PARACHLOROMETACRESOL** (PCMC)

Although ordinary commercial concentrations give no skin irritation, ingestion gives a toxic picture similar to that from phenol (49–450).

49–435.   **PARACHLOROMETAXYLENOL** (PCMX)

This complex insecticide can give an acute picture by penetration of the skin as well as by ingestion. For toxic symptoms and signs and treatment see *Phenol* (49–450).

49–436.   **PARADICHLOROBENZENE** (PDB)

This is the least toxic of the active agents used in moth repellent balls and flakes. Ingestion rarely causes acute toxicity, but prolonged exposure to fumes may be serious.

    Treatment. See *Naphthalene* (49–381).

49–437.   **PARALDEHYDE**

Although this very effective sedative has a relatively large margin of safety, some hypersensitive patients react unfavorably to even small doses. In addition, paraldehyde solutions deteriorate rapidly in the presence of light, with formation of toxic products.

    A. Signs and Symptoms
        1. Sudden onset of a rapid pulse.
        2. Accelerated respiration with cyanosis.
        3. Coma.
        4. Cardiac and respiratory failure.

    B. Treatment
        1. Universal antidote (49–10).
        2. Gastric lavage with 1:2000 potassium permanganate.
        3. Oxygen therapy by mask and rebreathing bag for cyanosis.
        4. Caffeine sodiobenzoate, 0.5 gm., intramuscularly.
        5. Saline cathartics.

49–438.   **PARATHION** (E605, Niran, Thiophos). See *Organic Phosphates* (49–421).

49–439.   **PAREGORIC** (Camphorated Tincture of Opium). See Topic 9 (*Narcotics*) and 49–370 (*Morphine*).

49–440.   **PARIS GREEN** (Copper Acetoarsenate, Schweinfurth Green). See *Arsenic* (49–63).

49–441.   **PCMC.** See *Parachlorometacresol* (49–434).

49–442.   **PCMX.** See *Parachlorometaxylenol* (49–435).

49–443. **PDB.** See *Paradichlorobenzene* (49–436).

49–444. **PENTOTHAL SODIUM**

This relatively safe and very effective intravenous anesthetic may cause cardiac arrest (Topic 29–2,A) in certain hypersensitive persons or if administered improperly or carelessly. It should never be used in children under 12 years of age.

Treatment
1. Stop administration of the anesthetic at once.
2. In moderately severe cases give respiratory and cardiac stimulants and oxygen under pressure. Complete recovery usually occurs.
3. In severe cases with cardiac arrest institute external cardiac massage immediately. For specific technique see Topic 17–2.

49–445. **PERFUMES**

The exact constituents of most perfumes are closely guarded professional secrets of the various manufacturers, but basically ambergris, volatile hydrocarbons, alcohols and natural or synthetic scents are used.

Treatment. If more than 4 ml. has been ingested, gastric lavage followed by symptomatic and supportive therapy.

49–446. **PERTHANE** (Q–137)

This insecticide is similar in action and toxicity to DDT, but without its ability to penetrate skin. For treatment see *DDT* (49–175).

49–447. **PETROLEUM DISTILLATES.** See *Benzene* (49–80), *Gasoline* (49–254), *Kerosene* (49–303), naphtha and its derivatives (49–380) and *Stoddard Solvent* (49–561).

49–448. **PEYOTE.** See *Mescal* (49–347) and *Hallucinogens* (49–261).

49–449. **PHENACETIN.** See *Acetanilid* (49–11).

49–450. PHENOL (Carbolic Acid)

A. Acute Toxic Signs and Symptoms may occur from:
1. Absorption through the skin.
2. Absorption through the mucous membrane of the rectum or vagina.
3. Ingestion by accident or with suicidal intent.

B. Signs and Symptoms Following Ingestion
1. Odor of phenol on the breath.
2. Burning in the mouth and throat with whitish discoloration of the tongue and mucous membrane of the throat.
3. Nausea and vomiting, with severe abdominal pain.
4. Slow, weak pulse; faintness, hypotension.
5. Coma.

C. Treatment
1. Removal as soon as possible by:
   a. Washing the skin or eyes with large amounts of cold water.
   b. Warm water enemas or douches.
   c. If ingested, gastric lavage with 10% alcohol or large quantities of warm water until the odor of phenol has disappeared.
2. Mineral or olive oil by mouth.
3. Normal salt solution, 500 to 1000 ml., intravenously.
4. Application of external heat.
5. Caffeine sodiobenzoate, 0.5 gm., intramuscularly.
6. Hospitalization as soon as the acute symptoms and signs have been treated.

49–451. PHENOLPHTHALEIN

This cathartic is the active ingredient in several popular "candy laxatives."

Signs and Symptoms

Although phenolphthalein is relatively nontoxic, large doses, especially in children, may cause severe enteritis and colitis, sometimes lasting for 3 to 4 days. Aside from treatment of any dehydration present, no specific therapy is usually required.

49–452. PHENOTHIAZINES. See Topic 59–53.

49–453. PHENYLENEDIAMINE

Used in eyelash dyes, this substance may give severe toxic reactions in certain hypersensitive individuals.

A. *Signs and Symptoms*
  1. LOCAL REACTIONS
      a. Severe smarting and pain in the eyes.
      b. Edema and lacrimation.
      c. Acute conjunctivitis with photophobia.
      d. Corneal ulcerations.
  2. SYSTEMIC REACTIONS
      a. Headache and sleepiness.
      b. Bizarre paresthesias.
      c. Nausea and epigastric pain.
      d. Edema of the face and neck, sometimes involving the glottis; asthmatic attacks, probably allergic type.
      e. Severe liver damage.

B. *Treatment*
  1. Immediate termination of exposure.
  2. Administration of pilocarpine nitrate, 5 mg., by mouth as a diaphoretic.
  3. Injection of epinephrine hydrochloride (Adrenalin) 1:1000 solution intramuscularly for asthmatic manifestations.
  4. Hospitalization if facial and/or cervical edema is marked or if there are signs of liver damage. All cases should be checked by an ophthalmologist, since permanent eye damage may result if prompt treatment is not given.

49–454. PHENYLHYDRAZINE

Accidental ingestion or therapeutic use in the treatment of polycythemia vera may cause rather severe toxic manifestations.

A. *Signs and Symptoms*
  1. Fatigue and headache; sometimes vertigo.
  2. Edema of the upper extremities, occasionally of the eyelids.
  3. Acute gastritis with or without diarrhea.
  4. Cyanosis secondary to blood destruction.
  5. Toxic hepatitis with severe anemia.

B. *Treatment*
  1. Mild cases will recover completely in a short time after drug is stopped.
  2. Severe cases require immediate hospitalization for blood transfusions after symptomatic and supportive therapy.

49–455. PHENYLMERCURIC SALTS

These are used as fungicides and break down to an ion which has less toxicity than the mercuric ion. For treatment see *Bichloride of Mercury* (49–87).

49–456. PHENYL SALICYLATE (Salol)

Mild toxicity is due to *phenol* (49–450), not to salicylates.

49–457.   **PHEOZUIN.** See *Cinchophen* (49–148).

49–458.   **PHOSGENE** (Carbonyl Chloride)

Although phosgene originally was used as a war gas [see *War Gases* (49–648)], toxic signs and symptoms from respiratory tract irritation occasionally occur in the chemical industry.

A. *Signs and Symptoms*
1. A foul taste in the mouth, with a "scratchy" feeling in the throat.
2. Anosmia after the first few whiffs so that large amounts of the gas may be inhaled without knowledge of its presence.
3. Dyspnea and severe cyanosis.
4. Bronchitis, emphysema and pulmonary edema (Topic 52). Bronchospasm may occur.
5. Acute cardiac failure.

B. *Treatment*
1. Removal from exposure. Contaminated clothes should be removed as soon as possible.
2. Absolute rest; local heat.
3. Oxygen under positive pressure by face mask and rebreathing bag.
4. Caffeine sodiobenzoate, 0.5 gm., intramuscularly.
5. Epinephrine hydrochloride (Adrenalin), 0.5 ml. of 1:1000 solution, subcutaneously for bronchospasm.
6. Hospitalization because of the danger of development of acute cardiac failure even after apparent recovery.

49–459.   **PHOSPHINE** (Phosphoretted Hydrogen)

Formed by the decomposition of phosphides in industry and in the manufacture of carbide, this foul-smelling gas in even low concentrations may be very toxic.

A. *Signs and Symptoms*
1. Headache and dizziness followed by restlessness, tremors and general fatigue.
2. Burning substernal pain.
3. Nausea and vomiting; sometimes diarrhea.
4. Bronchitis with fluorescent green sputum; acute dyspnea.
5. Pulmonary edema (Topic 52).
6. Death, usually preceded by tonic convulsions, which may occur suddenly after the patient has apparently completely recovered.

B. *Treatment*
1. Absolute rest.
2. Oxygen inhalations under positive pressure by face mask and rebreathing bag.

3. Dextrose, 5% in saline, 500 to 1000 ml., intravenously unless there is evidence of pulmonary edema (Topic 52).
4. Caffeine sodiobenzoate, 0.5 gm., intramuscularly.
5. Hospitalization, even though the patient has apparently recovered, because of the tendency of phosphine to cause delayed symptoms.

49–460. **PHOSPHORETTED HYDROGEN.** See *Phosphine* (49–459).

49–461. **PHOSPHORIC ACID**

For systemic effects see *Acids* (49–19) and *Phosphorus* (49–462). Locally, phosphoric acid burns require special emergency treatment.

Treatment
1. Flood with cold water and keep moist.
2. Compress with 2% sodium bicarbonate solution.
3. Wash with weak copper sulfate solution.
4. Treat as a third degree burn except that immediate debridement of damaged tissues should be done.

49–462. **PHOSPHORUS** (Yellow or White)

Acute poisoning may arise from ingestion of rat or roach poisons, certain types of fireworks, imported matches (especially from China and Japan) and old-fashioned "sulfur" matches. Severe, even terminal, effects have been caused by the ingestion of the heads of "strike anywhere" kitchen matches, and of the friction striking areas of "safety" book or box matches.

A. Signs and Symptoms
1. Garlicky taste in the mouth and odor on the breath.
2. Burning sensation in the mouth and throat.
3. Nausea and vomiting; the vomitus may be luminous in the dark.
4. Severe abdominal pain.
5. Slow, weak pulse.
6. Faintness and collapse.
7. Severe systemic damage manifested in 2 to 3 days after apparent complete recovery. Fatty enlargement of the liver, intense icterus and severe hemorrhage may occur.

B. Treatment
1. Immediate gastric lavage with 60 ml. of 1% copper sulfate solution, followed by large amounts of 1:1000 potassium permanganate solution. Both the patient and the attendants must be protected from contact with vomitus and gastric washings.
2. Administration of 100 ml. of liquid petrolatum by mouth or lavage tube.
3. Application of external heat.
4. Injection of 1000 ml. of 5% dextrose in saline intravenously.

5. Hospitalization for observation to ascertain possible liver damage.

49–463. PHYSOSTIGMINE

This is a powerful parasympathetic stimulator.
- **A. *Signs and Symptoms***
  1. Bradycardia.
  2. Intense salivation.
  3. Miosis.
  4. Twitching of skeletal muscles.
  5. Coma and collapse.
- **B. *Treatment*.** Administration of the physiologic antagonist, atropine sulfate, in large doses. Gastric lavage and administration of analeptics may be indicated if large amounts have been ingested.

49–464. PICRIC ACID

Used industrially in the manufacture of explosives and dyes and medicinally (usually as the picrate) as an antiseptic ointment, picric acid may cause acute toxic effects.
- **A. *Signs and Symptoms***
  1. Bright yellow color to the skin.
  2. Intense bitter taste.
  3. Nausea and vomiting; abdominal and epigastric tenderness and pain.
  4. Bladder tenesmus.
  5. Severe liver and kidney damage.
- **B. *Treatment***
  1. Administration of emetics followed by gastric lavage with 5% sodium bicarbonate solution. A saline cathartic should be left in the stomach.
  2. Administration of large amounts of fluid by mouth and/or intravenously (Topic 7).
  3. Hospitalization if there is evidence of kidney damage.

49–465. PICROTOXIN

Picrotoxin is the toxic ingredient of the bright red berries of an East Indian plant, commonly known as "fish eggs." Medicinally, it was formerly used as an analeptic, especially in barbiturate poisoning, but its use for this purpose is gradually becoming less prevalent.
- **A. *Signs and Symptoms***
  1. A burning sensation in the mouth.
  2. Pallor; cold perspiration.
  3. Nausea and vomiting.
  4. Shallow respiration.
  5. After ½ to 3 hours, confusion, stupor and unconsciousness. Clonic or tonic convulsions may occur, especially in children.

B. *Treatment*
1. If ingested, emetics followed by gastric lavage with 500 to 1000 ml. of 1:2000 potassium permanganate solution.
2. Control of convulsions by phenobarbital sodium, 0.1 to 0.2 gm., intravenously or paraldehyde, 5 ml., intramuscularly.
3. Administration of saline cathartics.

C. *Prognosis.* The mortality from ingestion is very low. Ill-advised injection in the treatment of coma may cause uncontrollable convulsions and death.

49–466. PILOCARPINE

Toxic manifestations and treatment are approximately the same as given for *Physostigmine* (49–463).

49–467. PINE OIL

Ingestion of even small amounts of this complex mixture of terpene alcohols may cause acute toxic effects, especially gastritis (sometimes hemorrhagic), decreased body temperature, central nervous system depression and respiratory failure. For treatment see *Turpentine* (49–633).

49–468. PLASTER OF PARIS (Anhydrous Calcium Sulfate or Dihydrate)

This has no toxic action, but if swallowed may harden and cause obstruction requiring surgical relief. Immediate ingestion of large amounts of water, gelatin or glycerin will sometimes delay setting long enough to allow removal by gastric lavage.

49–469. PLASTIC CEMENTS AND GLUES (Model Airplane Cement)

Sniffing of the fumes from the adhesive materials furnished in model airplane kits by children and adolescents has recently become fairly common. Transient exhilaration and euphoria result—probably due to the solvents employed, often amyl acetate (49–47). Habitual glue-sniffing may result in intoxication and coma. Whether or not permanent organic damage may result has not yet been determined, although a definite correlation with juvenile delinquency has been noted in several large cities. Similar effects have been reported from sniffing of paint thinner, lacquer and marking pencil fumes.

49–470. PLASTICS

Ever-widening uses of plastic materials have focused attention on three main types of toxic reactions:

A. Irritation of the skin and mucous membranes during manufacture. Often due to the solvents, plasticizers, dyes, etc.; rarely serious.

B. Polymer fume fever. Exact cause unknown. The toxic picture and treatment are similar to metal fumes (49–348).

C. Acute toxic signs and symptoms may be caused by decomposition products resulting from heating certain types of plastic materials used not only in industrial but also in medical and surgical therapy, i.e., fluorocarbons such as Teflon. Under certain conditions, extremely toxic substances including hydrocyanic acid [see *Cyanides* (49–170)], oxides of nitrogen (49–426), and tetrafluoroethylene may result from exposure to heat.

49–471. PMA (Phenyl Mercuric Acetate)

This fungicide is more toxic than mercuric chloride. For treatment see *Bichloride of Mercury* (49–87).

49–472. POISON IVY, OAK, SUMACH. See Topic 54–11.

49–473. POLYMER FUME FEVER. See *Plastics* (49–470).

49–474. POTASSIUM CHLORATE

This is used in many household toilet articles and medications, including cough mixtures, gargles, mouthwashes and toothpastes. Excessive ingestion may cause toxic effects.

A. *Signs and Symptoms*
1. Nausea, vomiting and severe epigastric pain.
2. Dyspnea and cyanosis.
3. Acute delirium.
4. Anuria.
5. Jaundice.

B. *Treatment*
1. Egg white or other demulcents by mouth.
2. Application of external heat.
3. Gastric lavage with salt solution.
4. Methylene blue, 50 ml. of a 1% solution in 1.8% sodium sulfate solution, intravenously.
5. Oxygen inhalations under positive pressure by face mask or endotracheal catheter and rebreathing bag.

6. Caffeine sodiobenzoate, 0.5 gm., intramuscularly or intravenously.
7. Careful follow-up medical care; severe degenerative nephritis may be a delayed result.

49–475. POTASSIUM OXALATE

Potassium oxalate is the active constituent of many popular household cleansing and bleaching agents.

A. *Acute Toxic, Even Fatal, Effects* may be caused by:
1. Ingestion, accidental or with suicidal intent.
2. Injection into the vagina or uterus in an attempt to produce an abortion.
3. Inhalation of fumes or steam from cleansing or bleaching solutions.

B. *Signs and Symptoms*
1. Burning sensation in the mouth and throat, with difficulty in swallowing.
2. Edema of the glottis.
3. Nausea, vomiting, often bloody, associated with severe epigastric pain.
4. Weak pulse, low blood pressure.
5. Muscular fibrillation and twitching.
6. Exaggerated reflexes with patellar clonus.
7. Uremic convulsions, coma and death from circulatory collapse.

C. *Treatment*
1. Chalk solution by mouth.
2. Gastric lavage with large amounts of lime water, followed by magnesium sulfate (Epsom salts).
3. Calcium gluconate, 10 ml. of 10% solution intravenously.
4. Large amounts of fluids by mouth and intravenously to prevent the formation of oxalate crystals in the kidneys.
5. Caffeine sodiobenzoate, 0.5 gm., intramuscularly or intravenously.
6. Hospitalization because of the tendency of potassium oxalate to cause severe kidney damage.

D. *Prognosis.* If the patient survives the initial acute period, complete recovery generally takes place. Stricture formation and visceral perforation are rare.

49–476. POTASSIUM PERMANGANATE

Crystals or solutions of potassium permanganate are common in many household medical cabinets and often are available to children. Ingestion of a few crystals usually does no harm, but larger amounts may be very dangerous. Severe mucous membrane burns, even perforation and peritonitis, have occurred following attempts at induction of an abortion by insertion of large amounts of the crystals into the vagina.

A. *Signs and Symptoms*
1. Film in the mouth or on other mucous membranes; may be violet or dark brown.
2. Stomatitis.

3. Nausea, vomiting, acute gastroenteritis with abdominal tenderness.
4. Shock from circulatory collapse—may be very severe and resistant to therapy.

B. *Treatment*
1. Administration of demulcents such as egg white.
2. Gastric lavage with large quantities of salt solution.
3. Treatment of shock (Topic 15–7).
4. Hospitalization if there is evidence of deep erosion or penetration of any mucous membrane.

C. *Prognosis.* Good unless a very concentrated solution (more than 3%) or a large amount of crystals have been swallowed, or perforation of a body cavity or viscus is present.

49–477. **PRIVINE** (Naphazoline Hydrochloride)

Ingestion, as well as local use, of this powerful vasoconstrictor may result in very disturbing and uncomfortable (but rarely dangerous) toxic effects. Many persons are hypersensitive to Privine and show extreme reactions after relatively small doses (Topic 24).

A. *Signs and Symptoms*
1. Severe headache; acute anxiety and excitement.
2. Cold perspiration.
3. Cyanosis, especially of lips and fingertips, followed by respiratory failure.

B. *Treatment*
1. If ingested, syrup of ipecac by mouth or, preferably, apomorphine hydrochloride, 5 mg., subcutaneously. Gastric lavage may be necessary.
2. Oxygen inhalations under positive pressure by face mask and rebreathing bag.
3. Caffeine sodiobenzoate, 0.5 gm., intramuscularly or intravenously.
4. Barbiturates intramuscularly for excitement or anxiety.

C. *Prognosis.* Complete recovery after 1 to 2 hours.

49–478. **PROCAINE** (Novocain). See *Anesthetics, Local* (49–52) and Topic 59–10.

49–479. **PROLAN**

Readily absorbable through the intact skin, this insecticide gives a toxic picture similar to DDT (49–175).

49–480. **PROPANONE.** See *Acetone* (49–14).

49–481. **PRUSSIC ACID**

Immediate treatment, especially oxygen under pressure (from a commercial tank if no other equipment is available) may be lifesaving if prussic acid (hydrocyanic acid, 2% in aqueous solution) has been swallowed. See *Cyanides* (49–170).

49–482. **PYRAMIDON** (Aminopyrine)

This is a very dangerous drug because of its tendency to produce malignant granulopenia and irreversible neurologic changes. See *Acetanilid* (49–11) and Topic 59–4.

49–483. **PYRETHRUM**

Many household and garden insecticides contain this relatively nontoxic compound, often combined with other more toxic insecticides, especially DDT. Pyrethrum sprays often have a kerosene or xylene base.
- **A.** *Signs and Symptoms* (after inhalation or ingestion of large amounts)
  1. Nausea, vomiting, and acute gastrointestinal pain followed by diarrhea.
  2. Burning and stinging around the anus.
- **B.** *Treatment.* Symptomatic only unless combined with more dangerous insecticides or suspended in harmful vehicles (distillate, kerosene, xylene, etc.). Pyrethrum alone never causes dangerous toxic effects.

49–484. **PYRIDINE**

Used commercially as a solvent and medicinally as an antiseptic and an antispasmodic, pyridine may cause acute but transient toxic reactions following inhalation of the fumes or by ingestion.
- **A.** *Signs and Symptoms*
  1. Headache, restlessness and insomnia.
  2. Vertigo, muscular incoordination.
  3. Disturbances in hearing.
  4. Severe peripheral neuritis.
- **B.** *Treatment*
  1. If inhaled, air or oxygen inhalations under positive pressure by face mask and rebreathing bag.
  2. If ingested, universal antidote (49–10) followed by emetics and/or gastric lavage with 1:2000 potassium permanganate solution.
  3. Control of restlessness by rapid-acting barbiturates.
  4. Intravenous administration of 5% dextrose in normal saline.

C. Prognosis. Complete recovery within a few hours.

49–485. PYROCATECHOL (Catechol)

This substance has, in general, the same actions as phenol but is much more toxic, especially in its tendency to cause convulsions. For treatment see *Phenol* (49–450).

49–486. PYROGALLOL (Pyrogallic Acid)

Pyrogallol is used commercially in hair dyes and proprietary ringworm "cures." Severe toxic signs and symptoms similar to those caused by phenol (49–450) may occur from absorption through the *intact skin* as well as by ingestion. In addition, renal damage, methemoglobinemia and red blood cell destruction similar to the effects of aniline (49–53) have been noted after prolonged use.

A. Signs and Symptoms
1. Sudden onset of collapse, convulsions and albuminuria due to severe toxic nephritis. This characteristically sudden onset may occur after use of a preparation containing pyrogallol for a long period without apparent previous ill effects.
2. Dyspnea, cyanosis and acute respiratory depression.

B. Treatment
1. Apomorphine hydrochloride hypodermically if the substance has been ingested by an adult; emetics should be used on children.
2. Caffeine sodiobenzoate, 0.5 gm., intramuscularly or intravenously.
3. Oxygen inhalations for dyspnea and cyanosis.
4. Purgation with magnesium sulfate (Epsom salts).
5. Hospitalization because of the characteristic severe blood and kidney damage.

49–487. PYROLAN

This is an insecticide, similar in action and toxicity to parathion. For treatment see *Organic Phosphates* (49–421).

. . . . Q . . . .

49–488. Q-137. See *Perthane* (49–446).

49–489. QUATERNARY AMMONIUM SALTS (QAC)

In 0.01 to 1% concentrations, many complex combinations of quaternary ammonium salts are used as antiseptics, deodorants and fungicides. Lauryl benzyl dimethyl ammonium chloride is used commonly in medicine under the U.S.P. name of benzalkonium chloride and the proprietary name of Zephiran.

Ingestion of large amounts of concentrated solutions, or absorption from a mucous membrane-lined cavity such as the vagina, may cause severe toxic effects.

A. Signs and Symptoms
1. Burning sensation in the mouth, throat and stomach if a concentrated solution has been ingested—may be very severe.
2. Restlessness and apprehension, dyspnea and cyanosis.
3. Generalized muscle weakness.
4. Death from respiratory failure, sometimes preceded by convulsions.

B. Treatment
1. Large amounts of demulcents (egg white, milk, soapsuds) by mouth, followed by gastric lavage with milk or soapy water.
2. Rapidly acting barbiturates for control of convulsions.
3. Oxygen under positive pressure by face mask or endotracheal catheter and rebreathing bag.
4. Hospitalization for supportive therapy if extreme muscle weakness or convulsions have been present.

49–490. QUICKLIME

Quicklime is *unslaked* lime, a very powerful and dangerous caustic alkali. For treatment see *Alkalies* (49–28) and *Lime* (49–317).

49–491. QUICKSILVER. See *Mercury* (49–343).

49–492. QUINACRINE (Atabrine)

Effective therapeutic doses in the treatment of malaria may cause severe toxic effects, as may overdosage. Individual tolerance varies markedly. Signs and symptoms of toxicity following excessive doses are similar to those given under *Chloroquine* (*Aralen*) (49–141).

49–493. QUININE AND QUINIDINE

A. Signs and Symptoms
1. Nausea and vomiting.
2. Tinnitus, dizziness—later deafness; disturbed vision—later blindness.
3. Delirium and coma.

B. Treatment
1. Gastric lavage with 1:1000 potassium permanganate solution or 1% tannic acid solution.
2. Caffeine sodiobenzoate, 0.5 gm., intramuscularly or intravenously.
3. Control of excitement by rapid-acting barbiturates.

49–494. **QUINOPHEN.** See *Cinchophen* (49–148).

. . . . R . . . .

49–495. **RAT KILLERS** (Rodenticides). See *Arsenic* (49–63);
Barium Compounds (49–77); *Cyanides* (49–170); *Fluorides* (49–242); *Red Squill* (49–498); *Strychnine* (49–565); *Thallium* (49–597); *Warfarin* (49–647); and *Zinc Phosphide* (49–669).

49–496. **RED LEAD.** See *Lead Salts* (49–313).

49–497. **RED PHOSPHORUS**

This form of phosphorus, in contrast to yellow and white phosphorus, is relatively nontoxic. Also see *Matches* (49–333) and *Phosphorus* (49–462).

49–498. **RED SQUILL**

Used as a rat poison. Ingestion of even small amounts of this drug causes a toxic picture similar to digitalis (49–191).

49–499. **REFRIGERATING AGENTS.** See *Ammonia* (49–42);
Methyl Bromide (49–359); *Methyl Chloride* (49–360); and *Sulfur Dioxide* (49–572).

49–500. **RESORCINOL**

Similar in many respects to phenol in its toxicity, resorcinol may give acute signs and symptoms from skin absorption as well as from ingestion. The toxic picture is generally not so severe as that caused by phenol, although the tendency toward convulsion is greater.

Hexylresorcinol (49–272) is slightly less toxic than resorcinol.

For treatment see *Phenol* (49–450).

49–501. **RHUBARB**

Ingestion of large amounts of rhubarb greens (leaves or blades) may be dangerous. For signs and symptoms of toxicity and treatment see *Oxalic Acid* (49–425).

49–502. **ROACH PASTE.** See *Arsenic* (49–63) and *Fluorides* (49–242).

49–503. **ROCKET FUELS**

None of the chemical substances now in use as rocket propellants are new; their properties and toxicities have been well known to chemists, laboratory workers and toxicologists for many years. What is new is the utilization of their peculiar physical and chemical properties in rocketry. Elaborate methods of protection from toxic effects of persons working with tremendous amounts of these very dangerous substances have been put in effect, so far successfully. Protection of the general public from transportation accidents, wind-blown fumes, explosions, etc., so far has been effective.

The following list contains some of the chemicals in use at the present time, with a notation regarding toxicity or other dangerous characteristics.

CHEMICAL	CHARACTERISTICS AND TOXICITY
Ammonia	Corrodes copper and brass; acutely toxic (49–42)
Anhydrous hydrazine	Explosive; fumes very toxic
Aniline	Acutely toxic (49–53)
Boron derivatives	Flammable; fumes acutely toxic; all exposed personnel required to wear special masks and protective clothing
Chlorine trifluoride	Reacts violently; toxic effects of both chlorine (49–133) and fluorides (49–242)
Decaborane	See Boron derivatives (above). In addition, boranes break into flame on contact with the atmosphere; therefore, special containers are necessary for transportation. Boron fires cannot be controlled by the usual methods
Diborane	See Decaborane (above)
Ethyl nitrate	Will explode when exposed to slight shock or temperature variations; fumes acutely toxic
Fluorine (liquid)	Will ignite spontaneously in the presence of another chemical (hypergolic); fumes very toxic

CHEMICAL	CHARACTERISTICS AND TOXICITY
Fuming nitric acid	Hypergolic; fumes very toxic (49–426); severe burns on contact.
Hydrazine	See Anhydrous hydrazine (above).
Hydrogen (liquid)	Very explosive. Exposure to air may result in severe burns before the presence of a fire is recognized since hydrogen burns with a completely nonluminous flame
Hydrogen peroxide (90%)	Very explosive; causes severe burns on contact; fumes very toxic
Isocyanates	Very toxic; see *Cyanides* (49–170)
LOX	See Oxygen (liquid), below
Mixed amines	Ignite spontaneously on contact with nitric acid (hypergolic)
Nitrogen tetraoxide	Must be kept absolutely dry, in presence of moisture forms nitric acid. See *Oxides of Nitrogen* (49–426)
Nitroglycerin	Very sensitive to percussion; see *Nitrites* (49–393)
Oxygen (liquid)	Acutely flammable; reacts violently with hydrocarbons and other combustible materials
Pentaborane	See Decaborane (above)
Perchlorates	Break down into hydrochloric acid and corrosive substances
UDMH (unsymmetrical dimethylhydrazine)	Highly explosive, flammable and very toxic. Based on experimental evidence, injection of pyridoxine hydrochloride, 25 mg. per kilogram of body weight, has been recommended

49–504. ROSEMARY

Oil of rosemary is used medicinally as a rubefacient but is very toxic if ingested.
A. Signs and Symptoms
1. Nausea and vomiting; severe gastric pain.
2. Rapid, weak pulse, with hyperactive reflexes.
3. Pulmonary edema (Topic 52).
4. Marked albuminuria.
5. Collapse and coma.
B. Treatment
1. Universal antidote (49–10).
2. Gastric lavage with 1:2000 potassium permanganate solution.
3. Caffeine sodiobenzoate, 0.5 gm., intramuscularly or intravenously.
4. Treatment of shock (Topic 15–7).
5. Hospitalization if treatment of pulmonary edema (Topic 52–3)

has been required or if evidence of renal irritation or marked leukocytosis is present.

49–505. **ROTENONE.** See *Pyrethrum* (49–483).

49–506. **RUBBING ALCOHOL.** See *Ethyl Alcohol* (49–227) and *Isopropyl Alcohol* (49–300).

The substances used to make rubbing alcohol unpotable are, in themselves, harmless even if ingested in large quantities. [See *"Waterfront Cocktails"* (49–651).]

. . . . S . . . .

49–507. **SACCHARIN** (Garantose, Glucide, Saccharinol, Sycose)

Commonly used as a sugar substitute in diabetic or reducing diets, this benzoic acid derivative may give toxic reactions in hypersensitive persons or if excessively large doses are ingested.

A. Signs and Symptoms
1. Loss of appetite.
2. Nausea and vomiting, gastric cramps and pain, sometimes diarrhea.
3. Acute myalgia, with muscular fibrillation and twitching.
4. Hallucinations (especially of hearing); delirium.

B. Treatment
1. Emptying of the stomach by emetics and gastric lavage.
2. Oral administration of saline laxatives.
3. Intravenous injection of 10 ml. of a 10% solution of calcium gluconate for muscle pain.
4. Hospitalization if large amounts have been ingested.

C. Prognosis. Complete recovery without residual ill effects after 2 or 3 days.

49–508. **SAFFRON**

Although oil of saffron is occasionally used as a flavoring and coloring agent, most of the cases of acute toxicity are caused by drinking strong teas or concentrated decoctions in attempts to induce abortions.

A. Signs and Symptoms
1. Vomiting, sometimes of bloodstained material; severe gastric pain with bloody diarrhea.
2. Rapid, weak pulse; hypotension.
3. Hematuria.
4. Convulsions and coma.

  B. Treatment
1. Universal antidote (49–10).
2. Gastric lavage with a 1:2000 solution of potassium permanganate.
3. Caffeine sodiobenzoate, 0.5 gm., intramuscularly.
4. Copious fluids intravenously and orally.
5. Hospitalization if bleeding from the gastrointestinal or urinary tracts is excessive or persistent.

  C. Prognosis. Good, although irritative symptoms referable to the stomach, intestines and kidneys may persist for several weeks.

49–509. **SAGE**

Oil of sage if ingested in even small amounts may be very toxic.

  A. Signs and Symptoms
1. Marked dyspnea.
2. Weak, rapid pulse; lowered blood pressure; shock.
3. Epileptiform convulsions.

  B. Treatment
1. Universal antidote (49–10) followed by gastric lavage with large amounts of water.
2. Treatment of shock (Topic 15–7).
3. Oxygen inhalations under positive pressure.
4. Barbiturates intramuscularly or intravenously for control of convulsions.
5. Hospitalization as soon as the patient's condition will permit.

49–510. **SALICYL ANILIDE** (Ansadol, Shirlan)

Used for mildew control and as a fungicide, salicyl anilide can cause both aniline and salicylate poisoning by inhalation or ingestion. For treatment see *Aniline* (49–53) and *Salicylates* (49–511).

49–511. **SALICYLATES** (*Aspirin*). [Also see *Methyl Salicylate* (49–363).]

Salicylic acid and all of the soluble salicylates may cause severe toxic signs and symptoms grouped under the heading of "salicylism" by skin absorption as well as by ingestion. The widespread use of oil of wintergreen (methyl salicylate) and candy-coated "baby aspirin" tablets makes therapeutic and accidental poisoning relatively common in children; the highest mortality is in the 1 to 4 age group. Any dosage above 65 mg. per year of age every 4 hours will produce acute toxic signs and symptoms in a child under 8 years old in a short time; if renal function is impaired even smaller doses may be dangerous. The minimal lethal dose of acetylsalicylic acid (aspirin) is usually considered to lie between 0.3 and 0.4 gm. per kilogram of body weight.

  A. Signs and Symptoms
1. Faintness; tinnitus, loss of hearing; disturbed vision.

2. Nausea, vomiting; gastrointestinal hemorrhage; dehydration.
3. Acetone odor on the breath (methyl salicylate only). Salicylism and diabetes (Topic 3–3) may give practically the same clinical picture.
4. Rapid hyperpneic ("panting dog") respiration (common in children) due to central action; cyanosis.
5. Acute edema of the larynx.
6. Convulsions (especially in children); delirium and coma.
7. Hemorrhage secondary to hypoprothrombinemia.
8. Circulatory and/or respiratory depression. Ingestion of massive doses causes death through complete irreversible respiratory collapse.

B. Treatment

1. Induction of vomiting as soon as possible.
2. Administration of large amounts of fluids orally and intravenously.
3. Gastric lavage with 1:2000 potassium permanganate solution. If aspirin has been ingested, its rapid absorption makes lavage of questionable value; if oil of wintergreen, lavage is indicated no matter how much time has elapsed. In either case, if hyperpnea ("panting dog" respiration) is established, lavage is valueless.
4. Application of external heat.
5. Injection of caffeine sodiobenzoate, 0.5 gm., intramuscularly in older children and adults—never in infants or children under 6 years of age. Intravenous injection of sodium bicarbonate solutions is of value in the younger age group.
6. Protection from injury during convulsions.
7. Control of excitement by barbiturates intramuscularly or intravenously. Paraldehyde intramuscularly may be indicated for convulsions. Both should be used very cautiously, since they tend to enhance the depressant action of the salicylate. Morphine sulfate and all of the synthetic narcotics are contraindicated.
8. Treatment of laryngeal edema by intramuscular injection of 1 ml. of epinephrine hydrochloride (Adrenalin) 1:1000 solution. Emergency tracheotomy (Topic 17–11,B) may be necessary.
9. Hospitalization in severe cases or when the amount ingested is not known even if evidences of toxicity are minimal. Careful balancing of fluid intake (Topic 7) and exchange transfusions may be necessary. The amount of blood used must be at least two times the patient's estimated blood volume.

49–512. SALT

Several series of severe poisoning in infants have been reported. See *Sodium Chloride* (49–537).

49–513. **SALTPETER** (Potassium Nitrate)

This is used in the manufacture of gunpowder and fireworks, as a fertilizer and in the chemical industry. Use as a food preservative and medicinally for suppression of sexual excitement is no longer common. Chile saltpeter is sodium nitrate.

For treatment of toxic effects see *Nitrates* (49–391).

49–514. **SAMARIUM CHLORIDE**

This is produced in the uranium industry and has about the same toxic effect as gadolinium chloride (49–252).

49–515. **SANOCHRYSINE** (Gold Sodium Thiosulfate). See *Gold Salts* (49–257).

49–516. **SAPROL**

Toxic effects are due to 40% cresols. For signs and symptoms of toxicity see *Phenol* (49–450).

49–517. **SCARLET RED** (Aminoazotoluene)

In ointment form this is used medicinally to promote epithelization. Its attractive color may result in ingestion by children, producing a toxic picture similar to that resulting from absorption from wound surfaces.

A. Signs and Symptoms
1. Nausea and vomiting, with severe abdominal pain; sometimes diarrhea.
2. Fever, general malaise.
3. Hypotension.

B. Treatment
1. Discontinue at once if used locally.
2. If ingested, gastric lavage with 1:2000 potassium permanganate solution.
3. Saline cathartics.
4. Administration of copious fluids, especially if diarrhea is marked.

49–518. **SCHEELE'S GREEN** (Copper Arsenite). See *Arsenic* (49–63).

49–519.   **SCHRADAN** (Octamethyl Pyrophosphoramide). See *Organic Phosphates* (49–421).

49–520.   **SCHWEINFURT GREEN.** See *Arsenic Color Pigments* (49–64) and *Arsenic* (49–63).

49–521.   **SELENIUM AND ITS SALTS**

The metal is dangerous only if vaporized; its salts, however, are acutely toxic by inhalation of dust or fumes, skin absorption or ingestion. The treatment is the same as given for arsenic (49–63) except that BAL should *not* be used.

49–522.   **SESAME OIL** (Benne, Teel, Gingilli Oil)

This is a mixture of glycerides which in large doses produce extreme catharsis. Acute dehydration may require fluid replacement (Topic 7).

49–523.   **SHEEP DIP.** See *Arsenic* (49–63) and *Phenol* (49–450).

49–524.   **SHELLAC**

White shellac contains rosin; other colors contain arsenic trisulfide. All varieties are dissolved in ethyl or methyl alcohol to which various aliphatic hydrocarbons and ketones have been added in small amounts. For treatment see *Arsenic* (49–63) and *Methyl Alcohol* (49–358).

49–525.   **SHOE CLEANERS.** Usually contain a small amount of trisodium phosphate with isopropyl alcohol (49–300).

49–526.   **SHOE DYES.** See *Aniline Dyes* (49–54), *Isopropyl Alcohol* (49–300) and *Nitrobenzene* (49–394).

49–527.   **SHOE POLISH.** See *Aniline Dyes* (49–54) and *Nitrobenzene* (49–394).

49–528.   **SILICOFLUORIDES.** See *Fluorosilicates* (49–244) and
            Fluorides (49–242).

49–529.   **SILVER POLISH.** See *Cyanides* (49–170).

49–530.   **SILVER SALTS AND COMPOUNDS**

Silver acetate and nitrate are available in many households and are
acutely toxic if ingested. Silver nitrate caustic pencils may be broken up
and eaten by children. Less than 2 gm. (½ drachm) is generally harmless;
larger amounts may cause severe symptoms and signs.

    A. Signs and Symptoms
1. Burning of the throat and epigastrium.
2. Black vomitus with violent abdominal pain.
3. In severe cases, convulsions and coma which may be terminal.

    B. Treatment
1. Sodium chloride, 15 gm., well diluted, by mouth.
2. Gastric lavage with large amounts of warm water.
3. Codeine sulfate or morphine sulfate for pain.
4. Magnesium sulfate (Epsom salts) by mouth as a purgative.
5. Caffeine sodiobenzoate, 0.5 gm., intramuscularly.
6. Hospitalization if more than 2 gm. have been swallowed or if
   convulsions or coma have been present.

    C. Prognosis. Good with small amounts. Ingestion of 2 to 10 gm. may
be fatal; over 10 gm. almost always causes death.

49–531.   **SLAKED LIME.** See *Lime* (49–317).

49–532.   **SNAIL BAITS.** See *Metaldehyde* (49–349). Older pro-
            prietary products may contain arsenic (49–
            63).

49–533.   **SNUFF.** See *Nicotine* (49–389).

49–534.   **SOAPS AND DETERGENTS**

White, unperfumed household soaps are harmless even in large quantities; addition of coloring or perfume may cause nausea, vomiting and mild
gastrointestinal irritation. Some laundry soaps contain enough caustic
alkalies to cause severe mucous membrane damage and require treatment as outlined under alkalies (49–28) together with fluid replacement

(Topic 7) if vomiting has been prolonged enough to have caused dehydration.

Detergents are divided into 3 classes, depending on the purpose for which they are designed.

Class 1 Light-duty, high sudsing: For dishes, baby clothes, etc.—slightly toxic.

Class 2 All-purpose, high sudsing: For laundry and general use—moderately toxic.

Class 3 Washday, low sudsing: Made for use in automatic washers—relatively high toxicity. Deaths from ingestion have been reported.

  A. Treatment for Class 1 and 2
1. Immediate dilution with large amounts of water, milk, olive oil or other demulcents.
2. Induction of vomiting if large amounts have been swallowed and vomiting has not already occurred.
3. Calcium gluconate, 10 ml. of 10% solution, intravenously to prevent development of hypocalcemia.

  B. Treatment for Class 3
1. Dilution; administration of demulcent.
2. Gastric lavage with a small bore tube if mucous membrane erosion is not extreme.
3. Control of pain. Small doses of narcotic may be required.
4. Air or oxygen by face mask and rebreathing bag for dyspnea and cyanosis.
5. Tracheotomy (Topic 17–11,B) for laryngeal edema.
6. Recognition and treatment of pulmonary edema (Topic 52).
7. Hospitalization for prolonged observation, supportive and symptomatic treatment. Permanent strictures of the esophagus may occur.

49–535. **SODIUM ARSENATE AND ARSENITE**

These contain about 50 and 75% arsenic (49–63), respectively.

49–536. **SODIUM AUROTHIOMALATE.** See *Gold Salts* (49–257).

49–537. **SODIUM CHLORIDE** (Salt)

Common table salt in excess can cause severe, often fatal, toxic effects in infants and small children, characterized by nausea, vomiting, excitement, hypertonicity, extensor spasticity, convulsions and eventual coma.

  Treatment
1. Control of hypertonicity and convulsions by sedatives.
2. Prevention of dehydration and potassium depletion (Topic 7).
3. Removal of salt by repeated 50 ml. of peritoneal dialyses using 5% dextrose in water per kilogram of body weight as the dialysate. For technique see Topic 17–9.

49–538. **SODIUM CYANIDE**

Inhalation or ingestion of even minute amounts is usually fatal. See *Cyanides* (49–170).

49–539. **SODIUM FLUORIDE.** See *Fluorides* (49–242).

49–540. **SODIUM FLUOROACETATE.** See *Fluoroacetates* (49–243).

49–541. **SODIUM FLUOROSILICATE.** See *Fluorosilicates* (49–244).

49–542. **SODIUM HYDROXIDE** (Caustic Soda). See *Alkalies* (49–28).

49–543. **SODIUM MONOFLUOROACETATE** (Compound 1080)

This is a delayed convulsant and has little, if any, fluoride action. See *Fluoroacetates* (49–243).

49–544. **SODIUM NITRITE.** See *Nitrites* (49–393).

49–545. **SODIUM OXALATE.** See *Oxalic Acid* (49–425).

49–546. **SODIUM PENTOTHAL.** See *Pentothal Sodium* (49–444).

49–547. **SODIUM PERBORATE.** See *Borates, Boric Acid* and *Boron* (49–96).

49–548. **SODIUM RHODANATE** (Sodium Thiocyanate). See *Thiocyanates* (49–600).

49–549.   **SODIUM SELENATE.** See *Selenium and Its Salts* (49–521).

49–550.   **SODIUM SULFIDE**

Usually mixed with barium sulfide or thallium salts, sodium sulfide is the main active agent in many depilatories (hair removers). Toxic effects following ingestion are due partly to local corrosive action on the mucous membrane and partly to the formation of hydrogen sulfide.

A. *Signs and Symptoms*
1. Foul breath from the odor of hydrogen sulfide.
2. A burning sensation in the mouth, throat and stomach.
3. Rapid onset of pulmonary irritation and edema (Topic 52).
4. Convulsions and coma, followed by death from respiratory paralysis.

B. *Treatment*
1. IMMEDIATE emptying of stomach by emetics or lavage.
2. Oxygen inhalations under positive pressure by face mask or endotracheal catheter and rebreathing bag, continued as long as there is any evidence of heart action.
3. Caffeine sodiobenzoate, 0.5 gm., intramuscularly or intravenously.
4. Hospitalization for observation for at least 24 hours after control of the acute signs and symptoms.

49–551.   **SODIUM SULFOCYANATES.** See *Thiocyanates* (49–600).

49–552.   **SOIL FUMIGANTS.** See *DD Compounds* (49–173) and *Vapam* (49–637).

49–553.   **SOLANINE**

A mixture of very toxic glucosides, including solanine, is present in several species of plants. Among these are:
1. BITTERSWEET. In the leaves, berries and seeds. The green berries contain large amounts of solanine; the ripe berries, very little.
2. JERUSALEM CHERRY. The fruit contains a large amount of solanine and is very poisonous.
3. NIGHTSHADE. The green, unripened berries and the leaves of this plant are very toxic; the ripe berries are relatively nontoxic.
4. POTATO. In the sprouts, leaves, berries and seeds.
5. TOMATO. In the leaves and stems.

A. *Signs and Symptoms* (usually delayed for 1 to 3 hours after ingestion)
1. Cold, clammy skin.
2. Nausea and vomiting; multiple soft stools.
3. Mental confusion, sometimes delirium; muscular twitching.
4. Mydriasis.
5. Respiratory and cardiac depression, often acute.

B. *Treatment*
1. Universal antidote (49–10) followed by emetics and/or gastric lavage with potassium permanganate (1:2000 solution).
2. Sedation by parenteral administration of rapid-acting barbiturates if muscular twitching is extreme.
3. Administration of saline cathartics by mouth or through the lavage tube.
4. Observation for at least 6 hours after ingestion because of the tendency of solanine to cause delayed toxic effects.

49–554. **SOMNIFEN**

This is a very potent sedative and hypnotic. For toxic signs and symptoms and treatment see *Barbiturates* (49–76).

49–555. **"SPEED-BALLS"**

Two well-known preparations have recently been substituted by ingeniously minded individuals—often narcotic addicts—for more difficult-to-obtain heroin, morphine and meperidine. These are:
1. PERCODAN. A proprietary preparation containing dihydrocodeinone, homatropine, acetylsalicylic acid, acetophenetidin and caffeine in a nonsterile tablet for oral use.
2. METHAMPHETAMINE HYDROCHLORIDE (Methedrine). Usually 15 or 30 mg. sterile solution in ampules, suitable for intravenous injection.

One Percodan tablet is usually dissolved in one ampule of Methedrine to produce a "speed-ball" which is injected intravenously with an effect similar to powerful opiates [see *Morphine* (49–370)] but of much shorter duration.

Since the Percodan tablets are not sterile, habitual users may show evidences of multiple abscesses in different stages of healing at the sites of injections.

49–556. **SPIRITS OF NITRE.** See *Nitrites* (49–393).

49–557. **SQUILL** (Sea Onion)

White squill is used medicinally as a diuretic and cardiac agent; red squill is used as a rat poison. The toxicity and treatment are practically the same as outlined under digitalis (49–191).

49–558. SQUIRREL POISONS. Usually contain thallium (49–597).

49–559. STANNIC AND STANNOUS (TIN) SALTS

In certain instances these may cause nausea, vomiting, diarrhea and encephalitis. No specific treatment is effective, although BAL (49–74) probably should be tried.

49–560. STILBESTROL. See *Diethylstilbestrol* (49–190).

49–561. STODDARD SOLVENT

This is a petroleum distillate which has about the same toxicity as kerosene. For treatment see *Kerosene* (49–303).

49–562. STRAMONIUM

This is found in common plants (Jimson weed, stinkweed, thorn apple, etc.) in many localities. The toxicity and treatment are the same as outlined for atropine sulfate (49–71).

49–563. STROBANE. Slightly toxic. See *Toxaphene* (49–615).

49–564. STROPHANTHUS. See *Digitalis* (49–191).

49–565. STRYCHNINE

This is a powerful poison which formerly had a wide use medicinally as a tonic and respiratory stimulant and commercially as a rodenticide. A household hazard for children is often present in patent medicines (usually laxatives and tonics) which may contain appreciable quantities. Strychnine acts by increasing the reflex excitement of the spinal cord and the medullary center. The toxic picture can be confused with acute *tetanus* (Topic 32–31).

A. Signs and Symptoms

1. Dyspnea and cyanosis, often associated with a feeling of suffocation.
2. Profuse perspiration.
3. Opisthotonos and tetanic convulsions. No matter how acute the poisoning, the patient is always fully conscious.

B. Treatment

1. Absolute rest in a quiet, darkened room to prevent initiation of tetanic convulsions by external stimuli.
2. Pentobarbital sodium, 0.12 to 0.3 gm., intravenously for control of convulsions.
3. Ether, very light inhalations, to relax the tightness of the diaphragm and allow respiration.
4. Assistance with respiration by mechanical methods if necessary.
5. Hospitalization as soon as the patient's condition permits. Relapses are common even after several hours.
6. DO NOT USE
   a. *Emetics* of any type. Choking, strangling and aspiration of vomitus may result.
   b. *Gastric Lavage,* unless
      (1) Within 10 minutes of ingestion.
      (2) The patient is in narcosis.
         If the stomach is washed, 1:2000 potassium permanganate solution should be used.
   c. *Caffeine.* It increases the strychnine effect.
   d. *Bromides.* Their action is too slow.
   e. *Opiates or Synthetic Narcotics.* They react synergistically with strychnine and may result in acute respiratory depression.
   f. *Cathartics, Purgatives or Diuretics.* They are of no value.

49–566. **SULFIDES.** See *Hydrogen Sulfide* (49–280).

49–567. **SULFOCYANATES.** See *Thiocyanates* (49–600).

49–568. **SULFONAL.** See *Barbiturates* (49–76).

49–569. **SULFONAMIDES**

The sulfonamides most commonly used medicinally are

Sulfadiazine	Sulfapyridine
Sulfaguanidine	Sulfathalidine
Sulfanilamide	Sulfathiazole

All may give acute toxic reactions following overdosage or accidental ingestion of large amounts. Some persons may demonstrate hypersensitivity even to very small doses (Topic 59–68).

Toxic signs and symptoms vary markedly with the offending drugs but, in general, the treatment is the same.

Treatment

1. Stop the administration of the medication at once.
2. Give emetics and/or gastric lavage if large amounts have been ingested.
3. Give copious amounts of fluids by mouth and intravenously.

4. Hospitalize for determination of the blood level and for further treatment.

49–570. SULFUR

This has a relatively low toxicity. Toxic signs and symptoms may develop after ingestion of large amounts which break down in the large intestine to hydrogen sulfide (49–280).

49–571. SULFUR CHLORIDE

Sulfur chloride is a commonly used insecticide which in the presence of moisture breaks down into hydrochloric acid and sulfur dioxide. For treatment see *Acids* (49–19) and *Sulfur Dioxide* (49–572).

49–572. SULFUR DIOXIDE

This is used as an insecticide and as a food preservative. Supposedly it is one of the most toxic components of the "smog" common in highly industrialized areas.

A. Signs and Symptoms
1. Irritation of the upper respiratory tract (choking, coughing, sneezing). Even moderate concentrations can cause dyspnea, cyanosis and pulmonary edema (Topic 52).
2. Acidosis (Topic 44–1).
3. Convulsions with terminal reflex respiratory arrest.

B. Treatment
1. Removal at once from exposure to fumes.
2. Insurance of a clear airway.
3. Immediate oxygen inhalations under positive pressure preferably by face mask and rebreathing bag.
4. Application of external heat.
5. Intravenous injection of 500 to 1000 ml. of normal salt solution.
6. Control of bronchospasm by subcutaneous injection of 0.5 to 1.0 ml. of 1:1000 solution of epinephrine hydrochloride (Adrenalin).

49–573. SULFURIC ACID (Oil of Vitriol). See *Acids* (49–19).

49–574. SUN TAN CREAMS AND LOTIONS

These cosmetic preparations are used as "sun screens" to absorb ultraviolet rays and to prevent sunburn and usually contain Dicumarol and amyl salicylate. Toxic effects from skin absorption never develop except in allergic individuals. If ingested, severe toxic effects may develop due to the Dicumarol (49–187) and the salicylate (49–511) content.

. . . . T . . . .

49–575. **TALCUM POWDER**

Talc (magnesium silicate) is harmless unless large amounts are aspirated, but some popular brands of talcum powder contain a considerable amount of boric acid (49–96) and zinc stearate (49–670).

49–576. **TANNIC ACID** (Tannin)

By ingestion this powerful astringent will cause uncomfortable but never fatal symptoms and signs—nausea, vomiting, gastritis and lower bowel disturbances.

In contrast, by injection it is a deadly poison and may cause severe convulsions, circulatory and/or respiratory collapse, and death from hepatic necrosis.

49–577. **TAR**

All types and derivatives of tar are toxic if ingested because of their cresol content. For signs and symptoms of toxicity and treatment see *Phenol* (49–450).

49–578. **TARTAR EMETIC** (Antimony and Potassium Tartrate). See *Antimony* (49–57).

49–579. **TARTARIC ACID**

Although relatively nontoxic, large doses of tartaric acid may cause very severe signs and symptoms. Fatalities have been reported.

    A. Signs and Symptoms
        1. Nausea and vomiting, severe abdominal cramping and diarrhea.
        2. Circulatory collapse.

    B. Treatment
        1. Emptying of the stomach as soon as possible by emetics and/or gastric lavage with large quantities of warm water.
        2. Large amounts of fluids by mouth and/or intravenously.
        3. Administration of saline cathartics by mouth or through the lavage tube.

49–580. **TCA** (Trichloracetic Acid)

This is a powerful caustic but has no systemic toxic actions. See *Acids* (49–19).

49–581. TCE (Tetrachlorethane)

This is similar in action to, but more dangerous than, carbon tetrachloride. For treatment see *Carbon Tetrachloride* (49–120).

49–582. TDE (Tetrachlorodiphenylethane)

Used as an insecticide, this substance is much safer than most of the others used for the same purpose. Symptoms and signs of toxicity following inhalation or ingestion (general malaise, prostration and collapse) are usually relatively mild, with recovery in 2 to 4 days without residual ill effects. The treatment is similar to that outlined for DDT (49–175).

49–583. **TEETHING POWDERS**

These usually contain calomel (49–110) with talc or chalk. Some brands contain small amounts of boric acids, borates (49–96) and bromides (49–100).

49–584. **TEFLON.** See *Plastics* (49–470).

49–585. **TEPP** (Tetraethyl pyrophosphate, TEP). See *Organic Phosphates* (49–421).

49–586. **TERPINEOL** (Lilacin)

This very toxic substance occurs in pine oil and because of its attractive lilac odor is a constituent of many perfumes and cosmetics. Ingestion of preparations containing terpineol in even very small amounts may cause ill effects.
  A. *Signs and Symptoms*
      1. Acute gastritis—sometimes hemorrhagic.
      2. General malaise and weakness; decreased body temperature.
      3. Vertigo, excitement or drowsiness, together with convulsions and other signs of central nervous system disturbances.
      4. Respiratory depression.
  B. *Treatment.* See *Turpentine* (49–633).

49–587. **TERPIN HYDRATE**

This commonly used expectorant has approximately the same toxicity as turpentine. For signs and symptoms from overdosage and treatment, see *Turpentine* (49–633).

49–588. **TETRACHLORODIPHENYLETHANE** (DDD)

This insecticide has the same action as, but less toxicity than, DDT (49–175).

49–589. **TETRACHLOROETHYLENE.** See *Carbon Tetrachloride* (49–120).

49–590. **TETRAETHYL LEAD.** See *Ethyl Gasoline* (49–229).

49–591. **TETRAETHYL DITHIOPYROPHOSPHATE.** (Sulfotepp). See *Organic Phosphates* (49–421).

49–592. **TETRAETHYL PYROPHOSPHATE** (TEPP, Tetrin). See *Organic Phosphates* (49–421).

49–593. **TETRAFLUOROETHYLENE.** See *Plastics* (49–470).

49–594. **TETRAHYDRONAPHTHALENE** (Tetralin)

The effects of ingestion of this drug are not known. Inhalation of fumes causes:
   1. Severe headaches; acute conjunctivitis and nasotracheobronchitis.
   2. Nephritic irritation with grass-green urine.
Treatment
   1. Removal from exposure.
   2. Administration of oxygen under positive pressure by face mask and rebreathing bag.
   3. Prescription of sedative cough mixtures.
   4. Reference for follow-up care. The toxic nephritis usually clears in 7 to 10 days.

49–595. **TETRAMETHYLTHIURAM DISULFIDE.** See *Thiram* (49–602).

49–596. **TETRIN** (TEPP, Tetraethyl pyrophosphate). See *Organic Phosphates* (49–421).

49–597. **THALLIUM**

With or without the sulfides of barium (49–77) and sodium, thallium acetate is used in depilatories (hair removers) in spite of the fact that it is only slightly less toxic than *arsenic* (49–63). Thallium sulfate is the active toxic ingredient in some brands of rodenticides and ant poisons.

Toxic signs and symptoms usually develop 1 to 2 hours after ingestion, but they may be delayed for as long as 36 hours if thallium has been administered medicinally.

A. Signs and Symptoms

1. Nausea and vomiting with severe abdominal pain and bloody diarrhea.
2. Marked ulcerative stomatitis.
3. Bizarre paresthesias.
4. Ptosis, strabismus and mydriasis; facial palsies.
5. Superficial ecchymoses and petechiae.
6. Convulsions; sometimes delirium.
7. Respiratory failure.

B. Treatment

1. Mouth-to-mouth artificial respiration followed if necessary by oxygen inhalations under positive pressure.
2. Gastric lavage with 1% sodium or potassium iodide.
3. Control of convulsions by intravenous barbiturates or intramuscular paraldehyde.
4. Catharsis by castor oil or magnesium sulfate (Epsom salts) by mouth.
5. Application of external heat.
6. Intravenous injection of 1000 ml. of 5% dextrose in normal salt solution. Ephedrine sulfate, arterenol bitartrate (Levophed) or metaraminol bitartrate (Aramine) to counteract circulatory collapse may be necessary.
7. Hospitalization for extensive, and sometimes prolonged, symptomatic and supportive treatment. Permanent neurologic damage may occur.

49–598. **THANATE.** See *Thiocyanates* [Organic (Aliphatic) (49–600,B)].

49–599. **THINNER INTOXICATION**

Use of paint thinner as an intoxicating agent has been reported among teen-agers. Ordinary paint thinner made up of benzene, butyl acetate, butyl alcohol, ethyl acetate, ethyl alcohol and toluene is used to saturate a handkerchief which is held over the nose. Another method is to spray the thinner into the nose with an ordinary atomizer. All degrees of intoxication can be obtained.

Treatment is the same as for alcoholic intoxication. See *Ethyl Alcohol* (49–227). Also see *Gasoline* (49–254) and *Plastic Glues and Cements* (49–469).

49–600. THIOCYANATES (Sulfocyanates, Rhodanates)

A. **Inorganic Salts** (ammonium, potassium, sodium, etc.) present a completely different toxic picture from that given by the more complex organic (aliphatic) thiocyanates.

Sodium thiocyanate is sometimes used in the treatment of hypertension.

1. AVERAGE THERAPEUTIC DOSES in certain individuals may cause:
   a. Nausea, vomiting, acute gastric pain and diarrhea.
   b. Acute depression and exhaustion.
   c. Edema of the glottis or larynx.
   d. Signs of hypothyroidism.
2. LARGER DOSES (with a thiocyanate level above 12 mg. per 100 ml.) may cause:
   a. High fever.
   b. Angina.
   c. Gastric hemorrhage; purpura.
   d. Enlargement of the thyroid.
   e. Hyperactive reflexes, muscular twitching and convulsions.
   f. Hallucinations.
   g. Motor paralysis of the lower extremities.
   h. Toxic hepatitis.
   i. Coma and collapse.

Treatment
1. Stop the medication at once.
2. Force fluids by mouth and intravenously.
3. Hospitalize as soon as possible.

B. **Organic (Aliphatic) Derivatives**

These substances are used almost exclusively as contact insecticides, usually in kerosene or toluene bases. Not only does their toxicity differ from that of inorganic thiocyanates, but also the various members of the aliphatic group have different toxic characteristics.

1. Ethyl, isopropyl and methyl thiocyanates.
TREATMENT. As outlined under cyanides (49–170).
2. All other derivatives (lauryl, Lethane, Thanite, etc.).
TREATMENT
   a. Empty the stomach by lavage with large amounts of water, followed by lavage with at least 100 ml. of mineral oil, leaving a small amount of oil, together with 30 gm. of magnesium sulfate (Epsom salts) in the stomach.
   b. Combat convulsions by intravenous injection of rapid-acting barbiturates.
   c. Administer oxygen under positive pressure by face mask and rebreathing bag.
   d. Give caffeine sodiobenzoate, 0.5 gm., intramuscularly or intravenously.

e. Hospitalize for continued supportive therapy and for evaluation and treatment of liver damage.

49–601. **THIOGLYCOLLATES**

These salts are the active ingredients of several "cold-wave" preparations. On the skin and scalp they may cause acute dermatitis with extreme
edema and, occasionally, bleeding. If ingested they have only a mild caustic action. Treatment consists of stopping use of the cold-wave preparation.

49–602. **THIRAM** (Tetramethylthiuram Disulfide)

This substance is used extensively as a fungicide and in the rubber industry. It is the methyl analogue of disulfiram (Antabuse) and has almost
exactly the same toxic action. For signs and symptoms of toxicity and
treatment following ingestion of small amounts see Topic 59–11. If large
amounts have been ingested, gastric lavage with large amounts of water
should be done. Ingestion of fats, oils and/or ethyl alcohol should be avoided
for at least a week.

49–603. **THORIUM OXIDE**

This extraordinarily insoluble salt is a by-product of the uranium industry. Inhalation of dust causes deposits of radioactive particles in the lungs
and pulmonary lymph nodes which are, for practical purposes, permanent.

No toxic effects from inhalation of thorium oxide particles have been
reported as yet, although a preparation of thorium dioxide (Thorotrast)
which was used by intravenous injection as a roentgenolographic contrast
medium about 10 years ago is known to have been responsible for several
radiation-induced cancers of the liver cells.

49–604. **THORN APPLE**

These plants contain stramonium. The signs and symptoms of toxicity
and treatment are the same as for atropine sulfate (49–71).

49–605. **THUJA** (Arbor Vitae, Yellow Cedar). See *Arbor Vitae* (49–677).

49–606. **THYMOL**

A. Uses
1. As an oral antiseptic, deodorant gargle and mouthwash.
2. As a deodorant in dirty, draining wounds.
3. As a specific against hookworm.

B. Signs and Symptoms
1. A sensation of warmth in the stomach, followed by nausea, vomiting and severe epigastric pain.
2. Dizziness and ataxia; acute excitement.
3. Subnormal temperature; rapid, soft pulse.
4. Marked generalized weakness.
5. Collapse with cyanosis.

C. Treatment
1. Emetics and/or gastric lavage with 1:2000 potassium permanganate solution. Oily substances and alcohol increase absorption and should be avoided.
2. Oxygen therapy if cyanosis is marked.
3. Magnesium sulfate (Epsom salts) by mouth or through the lavage tube for purgation.
4. Caffeine sodiobenzoate, 0.5 gm., intramuscularly.
5. Hospitalization if evidences of toxicity are still present after the treatment outlined above.

49–607. TIN COMPOUNDS. See *Stannic and Stannous Salts* (49–559).

49–608. TITANIUM TETRACHLORIDE

This substance is highly corrosive to soft tissues on contact and its fumes extremely irritating if inhaled. Severe chemical bronchitis and pneumonia, followed by pulmonary edema (Topic 52), may be caused by inhalation of a heavy concentration of fumes.

A. Treatment Following Inhalation
1. Remove from exposure at once.
2. Give artificial respiration at once, followed as soon as possible by oxygen inhalation under positive pressure.

B. Treatment Following Splashes on Skin or in Eyes
DO NOT WASH OR IRRIGATE. Addition of water causes production of extreme heat. Instead, wipe the affected parts (including the eyes) with a soft cloth until they are absolutely dry; wait several minutes and then irrigate with copious amounts of water. All eye cases should be referred to an ophthalmologist as soon as possible.

49–609. TNT. See *Trinitrotoluene* (49–628).

49–610. TOADSTOOLS. See *Muscarine* (49–372) and *Mushroom Poisoning* (49–373).

49–611. **TOBACCO**. [Also see *Cigarettes and Cigars* (49–147) and *Nicotine* (49–389).]

Commercial tobacco contains 1 to 2½% nicotine. A cigarette contains about 25 mg. Except for the fact that tobacco causes vomiting, ingestion of 2 or 3 cigarettes could well be fatal to an adult unaccustomed to tobacco. Fatalities have been reported in small children from ingestion of one-half of one cigarette. For treatment of toxic effects see *Nicotine* (49–389).

49–612. **TOLUENE AND TOLUOL**. See *Benzene and Its Derivatives* (49–80).

49–613. **TOLUIDINE**

Toluidine is similar in action but more toxic than aniline and causes more renal damage. For treatment see *Aniline* (49–53).

49–614. **TOOTHPASTES AND POWDERS**. See *Potassium Chlorate* (49–474).

49–615. **TOXAPHENE** (Octochlorocamphene)

This is an insecticide which is moderately toxic. Signs and symptoms from inhalation and ingestion are of about equal intensity. It has only a slight irritant effect on the skin and mucous membranes, but inhalation or ingestion may cause dizziness, involuntary muscle tremors and epileptiform convulsions.

Treatment
1. If inhaled, symptomatic treatment only is indicated. Rapid recovery usually occurs.
2. If ingested, emetics or gastric lavage, followed by symptomatic treatment, usually will result in complete recovery within 4 to 6 hours.

49–616. **TREMETOL**

This is an unsaturated alcohol occurring in many native uncultivated plants in many parts of the United States. It is the cause of "trembles" in cattle and of "milk sickness" in humans resulting from ingestion of milk of animals who have eaten the leaves or shoots. Plants which contain tremetol include the deerwort, rayless goldenrod, witchweed, squaw weed and white snake root.

A. Signs and Symptoms
1. Slow onset of toxic effects beginning with weakness, fatigue, anorexia and subnormal temperature.
2. Acetone-like odor on the breath.
3. Constipation.
4. Severe vomiting and abdominal pain developing 24 to 36 hours after ingestion.
5. Coma and collapse.

B. Treatment
1. Sodium bicarbonate by mouth in large amounts, as much as 10 gm., followed by gastric lavage with large quantities of water.
2. Magnesium sulfate (Epsom salts), 30 gm., by mouth or through the lavage tube.
3. Dextrose, 5% in saline, 500 to 1000 ml., intravenously.
4. Hospitalization as soon as the patient's condition will allow. Supportive therapy over a lengthy period may be necessary.

C. Prognosis. The mortality from tremetol poisoning is about 50%. If the patient survives the acute stage, it is usually many months before he regains full strength and endurance.

49–617. **TRIALKYL THIOPHOSPHATE** (Parathion). See *Organic Phosphates* (49–421).

49–618. **TRICHLOROACETIC ACID** (TCA). See *TCA* (49–580) and *Acids* (49–19).

49–619. **TRICHLOROBENZENE**

Used in termite control, trichlorobenzene fumes may cause mild irritation of the eyes, nose and throat. For treatment see *Naphthalene* (49–381).

49–620. **TRICHLOROETHYLENE** (Ethylene Tricholoride, Trilene)

A. Uses
1. As a solvent for fats and greases in industry. It is rapidly replacing carbon tetrachloride because inhalation of its fumes does not cause hepatic and renal damage.
2. Medicinally as an anesthetic (Topic 59–8).

B. Signs and Symptoms
1. Following ingestion:
   a. Severe burning in mouth, throat, esophagus and stomach; nausea and vomiting.
   b. Acute excitement followed by depression.
   c. Hyperactive reflexes; muscular tremors; in severe cases, rigor.
   d. Respiratory and/or cardiac collapse.
   e. Serious liver damage.

2. Following inhalation of excessive or narcotic concentrations:
   a. Pallor, profuse perspiration.
   b. Dyspnea and cyanosis.
   c. Bradycardia and hypotension.
   d. Unconsciousness with death from respiratory and/or cardiac failure.

C. Treatment
   1. Following inhalation of concentrations not sufficient to cause immediate death from cardiorespiratory failure, recovery generally takes place as soon as exposure is stopped; in severe cases, oxygen therapy and analeptic drugs may be indicated. Analeptics, however, should be used with extreme caution because of their tendency to cause cardiac irregularities. For detailed treatment see *Anesthetics, Inhalation* (Topic 59–8).
   2. If trichloroethylene has been ingested the following measures are in order:
      a. Administration of demulcents by mouth.
      b. Emptying the stomach by means of emetics or gastric lavage.
      c. Purgation by magnesium sulfate (Epsom salts), 30 gm., by mouth or through the lavage tube.
      d. Hospitalization for observation for at least 48 hours.

49–621. **TRICHLORONITROMETHANE** (Chloropicrin). See *War Gases* (49–648).

49–622. **2, 4, 5-TRICHLOROPHENOXY ACETIC ACID** (2-4-5-T)

Used as a weed and shrub killer. Same toxic effects as 2-4-D (49–185).

49–623. **TRICRESOL.** See *Phenol* (49–450).

49–624. **o-TRICRESYL PHOSPHATE.** See *Triorthocresyl Phosphate* (49–630).

49–625. **TRIETHYLENE GLYCOL.** See *Ethylene Glycol* (49–231).

49–626. **TRIIODOMETHANE.** See *Iodoform* (49–293).

49–627. **TRINITROBENZENE**

The symptoms and signs of toxicity and treatment are approximately the same as for dinitrobenzene (49–199).

49–628. **TRINITROTOLUENE** (TNT)

Inhalation of the fumes and/or dust of TNT may cause a very serious toxic picture.

  A. *Signs and Symptoms*
   1. Loss of appetite.
   2. Nausea and vomiting; acute diarrhea.
   3. Cyanosis, especially of the fingertips, ears and lips.
   4. Delirium and convulsions.
   5. Hepatitis and jaundice.
   6. Aplastic anemia.
  B. *Treatment*
   1. Immediate removal from exposure.
   2. Oxygen therapy under positive pressure by face mask and re-breathing bag.
   3. Sedation by rapidly acting barbiturates.
   4. Intravenous administration of 500 to 1,000 ml. of 5% dextrose in saline.
   5. Hospitalization.

49–629. **TRIONAL.** See *Barbiturates* (49–76).

49–630. **TRIORTHOCRESYL PHOSPHATE** (o-Tricresyl Phosphate)

This substance is the toxic agent in so-called "jake poisoning," caused by drinking extract of ginger or ingestion of parsley extract (apiol).

  A. *Signs and Symptoms*
   1. Nausea, vomiting and gastrointestinal irritation lasting for 2 to 3 days.
   2. After an interval of 5 days to 3 weeks (usually about 10 days) development of footdrop and/or wristdrop. Other muscle groups may be involved.
  B. *Treatment*
   1. Emptying of the stomach by emetics and/or gastric lavage if ingested within past 24 hours.
   2. Administration of saline cathartics by mouth.
   3. Hospitalization.
  C. *Prognosis.* Poor—muscle weaknesses and paralysis may be permanent.

49–631. **TTD** (Disulfiram, Antabuse). See Topic 59–11, and *Thiram* (49–602).

49–632. **TUNG OIL** (Chinawood Oil) **AND NUTS**

Tung oil is nontoxic, but ingestion of the Brazil-nut-like nuts may cause an acute toxic picture.

A. Signs and Symptoms
1. Severe gastric pain with vomiting and profuse diarrhea.
2. Painful muscle cramping.
3. Complete prostration from shock and respiratory depression.

B. Treatment
1. Gastric lavage with 1:3000 potassium permanganate solution.
2. Oxygen inhalations by face mask and rebreathing bag if dyspnea or cyanosis are severe.
3. Dextrose (5%) in salt solution, 1000 to 1500 ml., intravenously. If shock is severe, 4 ml. of 0.2% arterenol bitartrate (Levophed) should be given slowly in the dextrose solution with the rate of injection controlled by frequent blood pressure checks. Metaraminol bitartrate (Aramine) may be used in place of Levophed.
4. Calcium gluconate, 10 ml. of 10% solution, intravenously.
5. Magnesium sulfate (Epsom salts), 30 gm., by mouth.

C. Prognosis. Complete recovery without residual ill effects.

49–633. **TURPENTINE** (Gum Turpentine, Oil of Turpentine, Spirits of Turpentine)

Varying combinations of terpenes, especially α-pinene, are responsible for the toxicity of this common solvent and medication. Although ingestion is more common, inhalation of high concentrations of fumes and absorption through the skin also can cause acute toxicity.

A. Signs and Symptoms
1. Characteristic odor on the breath.
2. A sensation of burning in the mouth, throat, esophagus and stomach followed by nausea, vomiting, diarrhea and very severe abdominal pain.
3. Ataxia, delirium and acute excitement, often followed by convulsions.
4. Painful urination with a violet-like odor of the urine; later, hematuria and albuminuria.
5. Coma; death from respiratory failure.

B. Treatment
1. Liquid petrolatum, 120 ml., by mouth.
2. Gastric lavage with warm water or weak sodium bicarbonate solution even after the lapse of many hours since ingestion.
3. Oxygen therapy by face mask or endotracheal catheter using positive pressure.
4. Rapidly acting barbiturates intravenously for control of acute excitement and convulsions.
5. Magnesium sulfate (Epsom salts), 30 gm., by mouth.

6. Camphorated tincture of opium (paregoric), 4 ml., by mouth for colic.
7. Caffeine sodiobenzoate, 0.5 gm., intramuscularly or intravenously.
8. Application of external heat.
9. Large amounts of fluids intravenously and by mouth.
10. Hospitalization if large amounts have been ingested, if a lengthy period has elapsed since ingestion or if convulsions have developed.

49–634. TWO-FOUR-D (2-4-D). See 2,4-Dichlorophenoxyacetic Acid (49–185).

.... U ....

49–635. URANIUM SALTS

Inhalation of dust of this very insoluble radioactive oxide results in accumulation in the lungs and pulmonary lymph nodes; it is slowly, but never completely eliminated after termination of exposure.

To date, no cases of acute or chronic toxicity caused by uranium salts have been reported.

.... V ....

49–636. VANADIUM

Vanadium poisoning is usually caused by the pentoxide and occurs in persons working around oil-burning furnaces and oil refineries, in the manufacture of vanadium steel, and in the dyeing industry.

A. Signs and Symptoms
1. Greenish-black discoloration of the tongue.
2. Dry nonproductive cough, often lasting 2 to 3 weeks.
3. Headaches, very severe, resistant to all therapy.
4. Disturbances in vision, sometimes blindness.
5. Hemoptysis.
6. Nervousness; sometimes psychic derangement.
7. Gastrointestinal and urinary disturbances which persist for 2 to 3 weeks.

B. Treatment
1. Removal from exposure.
2. Intravenous fluids if dehydration is acute.
3. Sedative cough mixtures.
4. Ascorbic acid by mouth in large doses—up to 1 gm. per day.
5. Hospitalization because of the persistence of headaches, cough and uncomfortable gastrointestinal complaints.

C. Prognosis. Good in acute cases; chronic cases may show permanent renal damage.

49–637. **VAPAM** (Sodium n-Methyl Dithiocarbamate Dihydrate)

This soil fumigant if ingested acts much like disulfiram (antabuse). For signs of toxicity and treatment see *Antabuse* (Topic 59–11).

49–638. **VARNISH AND VARNISH REMOVERS.** See *Acetone* (49–14), *Benzene* (49–80), *Carbon Tetrachloride* (49–120), *Ethyl Alcohol* (49–227), *Gasoline* (49–254), *Lead* (49–313), *Methyl Alcohol* (49–358), *Methyl Chloride* (49–360), *Methylethylketone* (49–361), *Naphtha* (49–380), *Sodium Hydroxide* (49–542), Toluene [*Benzene* (49–80)], *Tung Oil* (49–632), and *Turpentine* (49–633).

49–639. **VERATRINE** (Cevadine)

This is a complicated mixture of alkaloids sometimes used in the treatment of pediculosis capitis and certain types of neuralgia. It is also found in the "death camas" (*Zygadenus*) plant common in the grazing lands of the western United States. Ingestion may cause ill effects.

A. *Signs and Symptoms*
   1. Burning in the mouth and stomach, salivation and nausea and vomiting, followed by acute abdominal pain and diarrhea.
   2. Acute anxiety; headache and vertigo.
   3. Slow and feeble pulse; extreme hypotension.
   4. Dilated pupils.
   5. Muscular twitching.
   6. Respiratory and circulatory collapse. In spite of the severity of the symptoms the patient is conscious at all times.

B. *Treatment*
   1. Universal antidote (49–10).
   2. Gastric lavage with 1:2000 potassium permanganate solution.
   3. Magnesium sulfate (Epsom salts), 30 gm., by mouth or through the lavage tube as a saline purgative.
   4. Normal salt solution, 1000 ml., intravenously.
   5. Caffeine sodiobenzoate, 0.5 gm., intramuscularly or intravenously as a stimulant and diuretic. Ephedrine sulfate, arterenol bitartrate (Levophed) or metaraminol bitartrate (Aramine) may be necessary for support of the circulation.
   6. Oxygen therapy under positive pressure if the respiratory depression is profound.
   7. Hospitalization, since the toxic substances are excreted very

slowly (probably through the kidneys), and a relapse may occur after apparent improvement.

C. Prognosis. Fair only, because of the profound respiratory and cardiac depression.

49–640.   **VERATRUM VIRIDE** (Green Hellebore)

Acute toxic signs and symptoms may occur following ingestion of the roots, drinking of "herb teas," or through confusion with certain other tinctures used medicinally, especially tincture of valeriana. The toxic action is due mainly to the alkaloid *protoveratrine* which should not be confused with *cevadine,* the toxic agent in veratrine (49–639).

Although veratrum is a reliable cardiac depressant, medicinal use is now unusual. Most cases of poisoning occur from accidental ingestion of the powder, which is used as an insecticide.

A. Signs and Symptoms
1. Burning in the throat and stomach; pain on swallowing.
2. Vomiting, often extreme and persistent, followed by diarrhea.
3. Bradycardia and hypotension.
4. Muscular cramping.
5. Convulsions, generally light, with or without loss of sphincter control.

B. Treatment
1. Universal antidote (49–10).
2. Gastric lavage with large quantities of warm water even though profuse vomiting has occurred.
3. Caffeine sodiobenzoate, 0.5 gm., intramuscularly.
4. Purgation with magnesium sulfate (Epsom salts).
5. Calcium gluconate, 10 ml. of a 10% solution, intravenously for muscle twitching and myalgia.

C. Prognosis. Most cases of veratrum viride poisoning recover in a short time because of its immediate emetic action.

49–641.   **VERONAL** (Barbital). See *Barbiturates* (49–76).

49–642.   **VINYL CHLORIDE**

Similar in action to, but weaker than, ethyl chloride, this substance is used as a refrigerant and occasionally as an inhalation anesthetic. Its toxic effects are transient and require no treatment.

49–643.   **VIOFORM.** See *Oxyquinoline Derivatives* (49–428).

49–644.   **VIOSTEROL** (Vitamin D, Vitamin D_3)

Although commonly and indiscriminately used medicinally in the treatment of many conditions (rickets, osteomalacia, arthritis, etc.) viosterol is a dangerous substance. Large doses (150,000 to 600,000 units per day) may result in serious, sometimes fatal, toxic reactions from hypercalcemia.

A. Signs and Symptoms
1. Nausea and vomiting associated with abdominal cramping and pain, with or without diarrhea. The abdominal pain may be severe enough to be mistaken for an acute surgical abdomen.
2. Severe headache and general lassitude.
3. Dyspnea.
4. Neuralgia and myalgia.
5. Signs of urinary tract irritation (polyuria, nocturia, albuminuria).
6. Urticaria; asthma; and congestive heart failure.

B. Treatment
1. In mild cases, decrease in the dosage of vitamin D will result in complete recovery.
2. Severe cases may require
   a. Oxygen therapy for dyspnea.
   b. Epinephrine hydrochloride (Adrenalin), 0.5 to 1.0 ml., subcutaneously for urticaria and asthma.
   c. Codeine sulfate or morphine sulfate subcutaneously if muscular pain is severe.
   d. Hospitalization if signs and symptoms of severe hypercalcemia are present, for correction of fluid-electrolyte imbalance (Topic 7) and for corticosteroid therapy.

49–645.   **VITRIOLIC ACID** (Sulfuric Acid). See *Acids* (49–19).

49–646.   **VOLATILE OILS.** See *Oil, Essential* (49–407).

. . . . W . . . .

49–647.   **WARFARIN**

This powerful anticoagulant, often used in powder form as a rodenticide, is very toxic if ingested; it is not absorbed through the skin.

For signs and symptoms of toxicity and treatment, see *Dicumarol* (49–187).

49–648. WAR GASES

A. Lacrimators (chloroacetophenone and brombenzylcyanide)

    1. Signs and symptoms. Profuse lacrimation, smarting and burning of eyes, blurred vision and temporary blindness. The effect is panic-inducing but transient and not dangerous.

    2. Treatment

        a. Irrigate the eyes thoroughly with 2% sodium bicarbonate solution.

        b. Protect the eyes with dark glasses. DO NOT BANDAGE.

B. Pulmonary Irritants (chlorine, phosgene, palite, chloropicrin)

    All of these gases have an insidious onset and are very dangerous.

    1. Signs and symptoms. Bronchospasm, dyspnea, pulmonary edema, intense cyanosis, nausea and vomiting, coma and collapse.

    2. Treatment

        a. Bed rest, warmth.

        b. Insurance of an adequate airway.

        c. Oxygen therapy under positive pressure by face mask and re-breathing bag. An endotracheal catheter may be necessary.

        d. Caffeine sodiobenzoate, 0.5 gm., intramuscularly.

        e. Epinephrine hydrochloride (Adrenalin), 0.5 to 1.0 ml., intramuscularly for bronchospasm.

C. Irritant Smokes (diphenylaminechlorarsine and diphenylchlorarsine)

    1. Signs and symptoms. Violent sneezing, nausea and vomiting, coughing, dyspnea, pulmonary edema. Dangerous only if very severe.

    2. Treatment

        a. Wash the nose and mouth with water or 2% sodium bicarbonate solution.

        b. Rest.

        c. Oxygen inhalations.

D. Vesicants [mustard gas (dichloroethylsulfide) and lewisite (chlorvinyldichlorarsine)]

    1. Signs and symptoms

        a. Itching, blistering.

        b. Blurred vision, sneezing, blindness, collapse from severe shock.

        c. Delayed arsenic poisoning (49–63) (from lewisite).

    2. Treatment for mustard gas in the eyes

        a. Wash the eyes with large amounts of water or 2% sodium bicarbonate solution.

        b. Instill tetracaine (Pontocaine) into the eyes to relieve pain.

    3. Treatment for mustard gas on the skin

        a. Wash the contaminated areas with 2% sodium bicarbonate solution followed by soap and water.

        b. Spot sponge with alcohol or gasoline; avoid spreading.

        c. If available, rub in a paste of chlorinated lime or wipe with sodium hypochlorite solution.

    4. TREATMENT FOR LEWISITE ON THE SKIN
      a. Wipe with sodium hypochlorite solution and alcohol; then wash with soap and water.
      b. Neutralize with BAL by local and systemic administration [see *BAL* (49–74)]. The intravenous dosage should be as given under *Antimony* (49–57).
      c. Treat the blisters as second degree burns (Topic 28–2,B).
      d. Give caffeine sodiobenzoate, 0.5 gm., intramuscularly.
      e. Treat for collapse and shock (Topic 15–7).

49–649. **WATER HEMLOCK**

The roots of this plant (also called spotted cowbane and musquash root) are very toxic if ingested.

    A. Signs and Symptoms
      1. Nausea and vomiting.
      2. Fixed, nonreactive pupils.
      3. Trismus and opisthotonus.
      4. Labored respiration, frothing at the mouth.
      5. Convulsions.
      6. Circulatory collapse.

    B. Treatment
      1. Universal antidote (49–10).
      2. Gastric lavage with 1:2000 solution of potassium permanganate.
      3. Caffeine sodiobenzoate, 0.5 gm., intramuscularly.
      4. Oxygen inhalations by face mask.
      5. Hospitalization because of the danger of delayed circulatory collapse.

49–650. **WATER PURIFIERS.** See *Hypochlorites* (49–284).

49–651. **"WATERFRONT COCKTAILS"**

For a small amount of money, persons who cannot afford the usual alcoholic beverages can obtain about 50 ml. of *rubbing alcohol* (49–506) and 100 ml. of white (nonethyl containing) gasoline. This mixture, when ingested, results in acute intoxication, terminated in 2 to 3 hours by vomiting, triggered by the substances added to the alcohol to make it unpotable.

49–652. **WHITE ARSENIC** (Arsenic Trioxide). See *Arsenic* (49–63).

49–653. **WHITE HELLEBORE.** See *Veratrum Viride* (49–640).

49–654. **WHITE VITRIOL.** See *Zinc Sulfate* (49–671).

49–655. **WILD PEPPER.** See *Daphne* (49–703).

49–656. **WINTERGREEN OIL.** See *Methyl Salicylate* (49–363).

49–657. **WOOD**

In addition to skin reactions commonly caused by many different types of wood, several tropical woods used in cabinetmaking may give rise to acute toxic symptoms, apparently resulting from absorption through the intact skin or from inhalation of dust or fumes.

    A. Signs and Symptoms
        1. Swelling and stiffness of the hands and fingers, associated with a heavy feeling in the arms.
        2. Severe headaches, often with visual disturbances.
        3. Dyspnea; rapid pulse.
        4. Dysphagia.
        5. Watery diarrhea with dehydration.

    B. Treatment
        1. Removal from exposure.
        2. Treatment of dyspnea by oxygen inhalations.
        3. Administration of large amounts of fluids by mouth or intravenously.

    C. Prognosis. Complete recovery is the rule although some fatalities have been reported. Desensitization to certain tropical woods has been successful.

49–658. **WOOD ALCOHOL** (Methanol). See *Methyl Alcohol* (49–358).

49–659. **WORMSEED.** See *Chenopodium* (49–126).

. . . . X . . . .

49–660. **XYLENE** (Xylol). See *Benzene and Its Derivatives* (49–80).

. . . . Y . . . .

49–661. **YATREN.** See *Oxyquinoline Derivatives* (49–428).

49–662. **YELLOW CEDAR.** See *Arbor Vitae* (49–677).

. . . . Z . . . .

49–663. **ZEPHIRAN** (Benzalkonium Chloride)

The 1% aqueous or alcohol solution of Zephiran has been used extensively for cold sterilization of surgical instruments and supplies. See *Quaternary Ammonium Salts* (49–489).

49–664. **ZERLATE** (Zinc Dimethyldithiocarbamate)

Combined with an oily base this substance is an effective insecticide with toxic properties similar to those of disulfiram.

For signs and symptoms of toxicity and treatment see Topic 59–11 (*Antabuse*).

49–665. **ZINC ARSENATE AND ARSENITE**

Arsenic, not zinc, is the toxic ingredient in these salts. For treatment see *Arsenic* (49–63).

49–666. **ZINC CHLORIDE**

A. *Uses*
   1. Medicinally as an escharotic and astringent; sometimes as a deodorant and disinfectant.
   2. Commercially in zinc plating and in alloys.
B. *Methods of Absorption*
   Inhalation of fumes (common) and ingestion (rare) may cause acute toxic signs and symptoms; about 50% of ingestion cases are fatal. Inhalation cases generally recover, although there is a tendency toward development of severe pneumonia.
C. *Signs and Symptoms Following Inhalation of Fumes*
   1. Hoarseness, loss of voice.
   2. Chest pain.
   3. Rapid pulse and respiration.
   4. Tracheobronchitis; sometimes severe and even fatal pneumonia.
Treatment
   1. Removal from exposure.
   2. Oxygen inhalations by face mask and rebreathing bag.
   3. Immediate hospitalization. Antibiotic therapy to minimize the chances of development of a severe respiratory tract infection is indicated if hospitalization must be delayed.

D. *Signs and Symptoms Following Ingestion*
   1. Severe gastric and substernal pain.
   2. Swollen lips, edema of the glottis.
   3. Severe vomiting, with or without bloody diarrhea.
   4. Cold skin, low blood pressure.
   5. Dyspnea.
   6. Collapse with the picture of acute shock.
   7. Perforation of a viscus may occur.

Treatment
   1. Universal antidote (49–10) or demulcents by mouth.
   2. Gastric lavage with 1:2000 potassium permanganate solution.
   3. Oxygen inhalations by face mask and rebreathing bag.
   4. Shock therapy (Topic 15–7).
   5. Immediate hospitalization. If edema of the glottis is marked, tracheotomy (Topic 17–11) should be done before transfer.

49–667. **ZINC CYANIDE**

This is used as an insecticide. For signs and symptoms of toxicity and treatment see *Cyanides* (49–170).

49–668. **ZINC OXIDE**

Inhalation may cause metal fume fever. [See *Metal Fumes* (49–348).] Ingestion causes toxic symptoms and signs from formation of zinc chloride in the stomach. The treatment is the same as outlined for *Zinc Chloride* (49–666).

49–669. **ZINC PHOSPHIDE**

Decomposition of this zinc salt by water and acids results in the formation of phosphine. If inhaled, the treatment given under *Phosphine* (49–459) should be followed; if ingested, this treatment should be preceded by gastric lavage with 1:2000 potassium permanganate solution.

49–670. **ZINC STEARATE**

Inhalation of the fine dust from zinc stearate talcum powder by infants may result in pneumonia with a mortality of over 20%. Hospitalization is indicated in all cases.

49–671. **ZINC SULFATE** (White Vitriol)

A. *Signs and Symptoms*
   1. Violent vomiting with severe abdominal pain and bloody diarrhea.
   2. Sudden collapse.

B. Treatment
1. Demulcents by mouth followed by gastric lavage with a 1:2000 solution of potassium permanganate.
2. Control of pain with opiates.
3. Hospitalization for observation for at least 48 hours because of the possibility of severe delayed kidney damage.

49–672. **ZIRAM.** See *Zerlate* (49–664).

49–673. **ZYGADENUS** (Death Camas). See *Veratrine* (49–639).

POISONOUS CULTIVATED OR GARDEN PLANTS

The flowers, plants and shrubs listed in the following section are some of those, planted in gardens for their decorative effect, which may cause acute toxic symptoms following ingestion. Fatalities, usually in children, have been reported from ingestion of varying amounts of each of the plants listed below.

49–674.   **AKEE**. After apparent recovery from acute gastrointestinal irritation from eating the saponin-containing fruit, convulsions, hypertension and coma may develop.

49–675.   **ALOES**. All species of aloes contain aloin, which may cause violent gastrointestinal symptoms. The treatment consists of gastric lavage, saline cathartics and sedation. Unless large amounts have been ingested, the symptoms and signs are more uncomfortable than dangerous.

49–676.   **ANGEL'S TRUMPET**. Toxic signs and symptoms from ingestion are due to depression of the parasympathetic mechanism and to stimulation of the central nervous system. For toxic effects and treatment see *Atropine Sulfate* (49–71).

49–677.   **ARBOR VITAE** (*Thuja, Red Cedar, Yellow Cedar*). The twigs and leaves may cause severe toxic symptoms if chewed. Decoctions of the young twigs have been used in attempts to induce abortions.
   A. Signs and Symptoms
   1. Severe abdominal pain with diarrhea.
   2. Frothing at the mouth; difficult respiration, sometimes pulmonary edema (Topic 52).
   3. Convulsions, tonic or clonic.
   4. Circulatory failure.
   B. Treatment
   1. Universal antidote (49–10) or demulcents by mouth.
   2. Emetics and/or gastric lavage.
   3. Oxygen therapy under positive pressure using a face mask and rebreathing bag.
   4. Caffeine sodiobenzoate, 0.5 gm., intramuscularly.
   5. Treatment of pulmonary edema (Topic 52–3) if present.
   6. Hospitalization in even mild cases because of the tendency of thuja to cause delayed cystitis, necrosis of the bladder and abortion.

49–678.   **AUTUMN CROCUS.** The signs and symptoms of toxicity and treatment are similar to those for *Colchicine* (49–154).

49–679.   **AZALEA.** Andromedotoxin, the poisonous substance contained in these plants, is similar to aconite in many respects; in addition, it has a curare-like effect on voluntary muscles and a depressant action on the heart. See *Aconite* (49–20) and *Curare* (49–168).

49–680.   **BELLADONNA.** See *Atropine Sulfate* (49–71).

49–681.   **BITTERSWEET.** Ingestion of the green berries or leaves may cause acute signs and symptoms due to solanine (49–553). The ripe berries are harmless.

49–682.   **BLACK LAUREL.** All parts of this shrub contain andromedotoxin [see under *Azalea* (49–679)].

49–683.   **BLACK LOCUST.** The bark and leaves of this shrub or tree contain a very dangerous toxalbumin. The signs and symptoms of toxicity and treatment are the same as given under castor bean (49–694).

49–684.   **BLOODROOT.** All parts of the plant contain a toxic substance (sanguinarine) which on ingestion causes nausea, vomiting, diarrhea and collapse. Treatment consists of emptying the stomach by emetics and/or gastric lavage and purgation by saline cathartics.

49–685.   **BLUEBERRY LEAVES** contain myrtillin, an antiglycemic agent which may cause severe and permanent liver damage.
   Treatment
   1. Universal antidote (49–10), followed by emetics and gastric lavage with 1:2000 solution of potassium permanganate.
   2. Saline cathartics.
   3. Close observation for several weeks for possible liver damage.

49–686.   **BLUE LUPINE.** The symptoms and treatment following ingestion of the flowers, leaves or stalks of this flowering plant are given under coniine (49–156).

49–687. **BOXWOOD** contains an alkaloid, buxine—a powerful intestinal irritant and central nervous system depressant. For treatment see *Alkaloids* (49–29).

49–688. **BRIONIA** is a strong irritant poison and may cause very severe gastrointestinal irritation, followed by severe shock. Treatment consists of gastric lavage and supportive therapy.

49–689. **BROOM TOP** (Scoporius). This plant contains an alkaloid, sparteine, similar in action to nicotine (49–389) and coniine (49–156).

49–690. **BURNING BUSH.** See *Euonymin* (49–236).

49–691. **BUTTERCUPS.** These plants, which belong to the crowfoot family, if ingested cause severe nausea, vomiting, restlessness, excitement, burning and tingling of the skin, convulsions and coma. Treatment consists of emptying the stomach, oxygen therapy and injection of atropine sulfate parenterally in large doses.

49–692. **CALLA LILIES.** Ingestion causes severe irritation of the mouth and throat with acute gastrointestinal irritation. Swelling of the G.I. tract is pronounced and may lead to ulceration. Large amounts may cause severe shock and death.

    Treatment consists of removal by mouthwashes, emetics and gastric lavage, followed by a saline cathartic. Supportive measures may be necessary.

49–693. **CAMELLIA.** The seeds contain a glucoside which acts like digitalis (49–191).

49–694. **CASTOR BEAN** (*Ricinus communis*). The large red seeds of this shrub are very attractive and dangerous to children since they contain a very deadly poison, ricin. Ingestion of 4 or 5 seeds is usually fatal to a child; the mortality in recorded cases in all age groups is about 6%.

  A. *Signs and Symptoms* (usually do not come on for 1 to 3 days after ingestion)
    1. Severe headache with nausea, persistent vomiting and gastroenteritis, often with bloody diarrhea. Jaundice may be present.
    2. Convulsions.

3. Death in 6 to 10 days from convulsions or exhaustion.

B. *Treatment*
1. Immediate emptying of the stomach, even if ingestion is only suspected.
2. Hospitalization for observation for at least 3 days.

For toxic reactions during commercial processing see 49–123.

49–695. **CEDAR (RED).** See *Arbor Vitae* (49–677).

49–696. **CHERRY.** The bark, leaves and pits of certain cherry trees, especially the wild black cherry (*Prunus serotina*), are toxic owing to the presence of amygdalin which breaks down into hydrocyanic acid. Also see *Chokecherry* (49–144).

49–697. **CHRISTMAS ROSE.** The roots contain a toxic glucoside, helleborein. Ingestion of even small amounts causes a very severe intractable diarrhea but generally no other systemic effect. See *Helleborein* (49–263).

49–698. **CLEMATIS.** This gastrointestinal irritant gives a toxic picture similar to that from aloes (49–675).

49–699. **COLUMBINE.** Like aloes (49–675) this climbing plant contains a substance in the stalks and leaves which causes intense gastrointestinal distress and sometimes a shock-like state following ingestion of even a small amount.

49–700. **CRYBABY TREE.** Ingestion of the leaves, bark or shoots may cause a paralysis similar to that caused by curare (49–168).

49–701. **CYCLAMEN.** The stalks and leaves contain a saponin which causes intense gastrointestinal symptoms without nausea or vomiting. Ingestion of large amounts may cause convulsions or coma. Gastric lavage followed by saline cathartics and supportive therapy is indicated.

49–702. **DAFFODIL.** The bulbs contain a substance which if ingested causes nausea, vomiting and diarrhea, which is uncomfortable but not dangerous. See *Grape Hyacinth* (49–712).

49–703.   DAPHNE

The attractive red berries and the bark of this shrub are sometimes ingested by children, with a fatality rate of about 20%. Even contact of the juice with the skin may cause severe and even fatal symptoms, although recovery following this method of absorption usually occurs.

Treatment
1. Immediate gastric lavage with a 1:5000 solution of potassium permanganate.
2. Magnesium sulfate (Epsom salts), 30 gm., by mouth.
3. Caffeine sodiobenzoate, 0.5 gm., intramuscularly.
4. Large amounts of fluids by mouth and intravenously.
5. Hospitalization because of the danger of severe kidney damage.

49–704.   DEADLY NIGHTSHADE. The leaves and berries contain several very toxic glucosides, especially solanine (49–553).

49–705.   DELPHINIUM (Larkspur)

A. Signs and Symptoms
1. Burning and dryness of the mucous membranes of the mouth and throat with stiffness of the facial muscles.
2. Nausea and vomiting.
3. Loss of urinary and rectal sphincter control.
4. Extreme hypotension.
5. Respiratory depression.

B. Treatment
1. Gastric lavage with large quantities of warm water.
2. Emptying of the bowel by enemas or saline cathartics.

49–706.   DOG PARSLEY

Transient toxic signs and symptoms, very uncomfortable but never fatal, have followed accidental ingestion in place of edible parsley. Signs and symptoms are caused by irritation of the gastrointestinal tract and disappear rapidly.

Treatment
1. Emptying of the stomach by emetics or gastric lavage.
2. Administration of saline cathartics, followed by enemas.

49–707.   ELEPHANT'S-EAR. These plants contain in the leaves, stalks and roots an unidentified substance which upon ingestion causes a prickly burning sensation on the tongue and in the throat, followed by very severe gastroenteritis, shock, and sometimes death. Treatment consists of gastric lavage and supportive measures.

49–708. FINGER CHERRY

The fruit of this flowering shrub, common in Australia, if ingested may cause sudden onset of complete and permanent blindness from optic nerve damage. Signs and symptoms of toxicity usually do not develop until 18 to 24 hours after ingestion; hence, only symptomatic treatment can be given.

49–709. **FOUR-O'CLOCK.** The roots and seeds contain a mildly narcotic gastrointestinal irritant.

49–710. **FOXGLOVE.** See *Digitalis* (49–191).

49–711. **GLORIOSA.** The toxic action is similar to that of colchicine (49–154).

49–712. **GRAPE HYACINTH.** Although this plant is a strong irritant, its action is mostly on the gastric mucosa; hence, vomiting with removal of the toxic substances usually results before much absorption has taken place. Treatment consists of gastric lavage even if the patient has vomited. This applies to bulbs in general. Tulips (49–755) are the main exception.

49–713. **HEATHER.** Andromedotoxin is the active toxic agent in all varieties of heather. See *Aconite* (49–20) and *Curare* (49–168).

49–714. **HENBANE.** See *Hyoscyamus* (49–283).

49–715. **IRIS.** All members of this family contain solanine (49–553), contained mostly in the underground stems.

49–716. **JASMINE, YELLOW.** See *Gelsemium* (49–255).

49–717. **JET BERRY BUSH.** The berries contain amygdalin (49–46).

49–718. **JONQUIL.** See *Grape Hyacinth* (49–712).

49–719.   **LABURNUM.** This ornamental tree contains in its shoots, leaves and flowers a toxic alkaloid, cytisine, similar in its actions to nicotine (49–389).

49–720.   **LARKSPUR.** See *Delphinium* (49–705).

49–721.   **LAUREL.** All varieties of laurel contain andromedotoxin. See *Aconite* (49–20) and *Curare* (49–168).

49–722.   **LILY OF THE VALLEY.** The flowers, leaves, stalks and roots contain the glucoside convallamarin, similar to digitalis (49–191) in action and toxicity.

49–723.   **LOBELIA** (Indian Tobacco). Plants of this species contain alkaloids that act like nicotine (49–389).

49–724.   **LOCUST.** The seeds of certain varieties of these common ornamental trees contain a very toxic substance similar to that found in castor beans (49–694). Signs and symptoms are usually less severe than in castor bean poisoning and the mortality less. The treatment is the same.

49–725.   **LUPINE.** All parts of this flowering plant contain lupinine, an alkaloid which causes respiratory and circulatory depression, paralysis and convulsions if ingested in even very small amounts.

Treatment
1. Immediate emptying of the stomach by emetics and/or gastric lavage.
2. Oxygen by face mask and rebreathing bag.
3. Support of the circulation by caffeine sodiobenzoate, ephedrine sulfate or, in severe cases, arterenol bitartrate (Levophed) or metaraminol bitartrate (Aramine).
4. Control of convulsions by rapidly acting barbiturates.
5. Hospitalization as soon as possible.

49–726.   **MAGNOLIA.** The seeds of all of the numerous varieties of magnolias contain a substance similar in action and toxicity to picrotoxin (49–465).

49–727. **MEADOW SAFFRON.** See *Colchicine* (49–154).

49–728. **MILKWEED** contains a resin which is highly irritant to the gastro-intestinal tract. Treatment consists of emptying the stomach by emetics and gastric lavage.

49–729. **MIMOSA.** This saponin-containing plant has the same effect as given for cyclamen (49–701).

49–730. **MISTLETOE.** All parts, but especially the berries, contain a toxic substance similar in action to digitalis (49–191).

49–731. **MOCK ORANGE.** See *Akee* (49–674).

49–732. **MONKSHOOD.** Aconite (49–20) is the toxic principle. It is found only in the root.

49–733. **MOUNTAIN LAUREL** contains andromedotoxin similar in toxicity to aconite (49–20) and curare (49–168).

49–734. **NARCISSUS** (Daffodil, Jonquil). The toxic action of these bulbs is similar to that given above under grape hyacinth (49–712).

49–735. **NIGHT BLOOMING CEREUS** contains a toxic active principle similar to digitalis (49–191).

49–736. **OLEANDER**

Chewing the leaves, flowers or bark of this common ornamental shrub may result in fatal poisoning. Cases have been reported from eating food roasted while spitted on oleander sticks. There is usually a time lag of 2 to 5 hours before the onset of the toxic picture.

    A. Signs and Symptoms
        1. Nausea and vomiting associated with very severe abdominal pain.
        2. Localized cyanosis of the ears, lips and fingertips.
        3. Cold perspiration.
        4. Respiration shallow and weak; temperature subnormal; hypotension.
        5. Pupils pinpoint—do not react to distance or light.
        6. Increasing sleepiness followed by coma.

7. Collapse, with death from acute respiratory paralysis.

B. Treatment
1. Universal antidote (49–10).
2. Gastric lavage with 1:2000 potassium permanganate solution.
3. Magnesium sulfate (Epsom salts) by mouth.
4. Oxygen inhalations under positive pressure, preferably by face mask or catheter and rebreathing bag.
5. Caffeine sodiobenzoate, 0.5 gm., intramuscularly or intravenously.
6. Dextrose, 5% in saline, 500 to 1000 ml., intravenously. If hypotension is extreme, arterenol bitartrate (Levophed) or metaraminol bitartrate (Aramine) should be added to the dextrose in saline and given slowly, with the blood pressure being checked at frequent intervals.
7. Hospitalization in all cases.

49–737. **PANSY.** The rhizomes contain a very toxic alkaloid, violine. For treatment see *Alkaloids* (49–29).

49–738. **PINKS.** The seeds are the only toxic parts of the plant. Ingestion may cause intense gastrointestinal irritation—rarely fatal because of the emetic action.

49–739. **POMEGRANATE BARK.** The bark and stems of most of the species of pomegranate contain a mixture of alkaloids called pelleterine.

A. Ingestion of Moderate Amounts may cause:
1. Mydriasis, sometimes partial blindness.
2. Severe headache, vertigo.
3. Vomiting and diarrhea.
4. Convulsions.

B. Treatment
1. Universal antidote (49–10).
2. Tincture of iodine, 1 ml. in 100 ml. (15 drops in ½ glass of water), by mouth.
3. Gastric lavage with large amounts of water.
4. Aspirin for headache.
5. Barbiturates for control of convulsions, given intravenously if necessary.

49–740. **POPPIES.** California and Oriental poppies contain a mixture of alkaloids with a depressant action on heart muscle. For treatment see *Alkaloids* (49–29). Also see *Morphine* (49–370) and *Narcotics* (Topic 9).

49–741. **POTATOES.** Seeds, sprouts, leaves and berries contain toxic glucosides. See *Solanine* (49–553).

49–742.   **PRIVET.** The leaves and berries of this hedge shrub have a toxic action similar to that of aloes (49–675) in addition to the effect of andromedotoxin. [See *Aconite* (49–20) and *Curare* (49–168).]

49–743.   **PYROCANTHA.** (Fire Thorn, Fire Bush). Ingestion of the berries causes a picture similar to belladonna. [See *Atropine Sulfate* (49–71).]

49–744.   **RAGWORT,** if ingested, causes a very severe type of liver damage without any other toxic effects.

49–745.   **RAYLESS GOLDENROD.** See *Tremetol* (49–616).

49–746.   **RHODODENDRON.** The foliage and shoots of these flowering plants contain andromedotoxin; the signs and symptoms of toxicity and treatment are similar to those for aconite (49–20) and curare (49–168).

49–747.   **SCOTCH BROOM.** See *Broom Top* (49–689).

49–748.   **SPANISH BAYONET** (Yucca). Plants of this family contain a toxic saponin which produces irritation of the gastrointestinal tract. See *Cyclamen* (49–701).

49–749.   **SPIDER LILY.** The bulbs contain an alkaloid (lycocine). Fatalities are rare because of its irritant action on the stomach.

49–750.   **SPINDLE TREE.** See *Euonymin* (49–236).

49–751.   **STAGGERBUSH** contains andromedotoxin which may cause symptoms which may be mistaken for acute alcoholic intoxication. The action is primarily a peripheral paralysis of the vagus and depression of the brain associated with a voluntary muscle effect similar to that from curare (49–168).

49–752.   **STAR ANISE.** This plant belongs to the magnolia family. Ingestion of its seeds may result in toxic symptoms similar to those of poisoning by picrotoxin (49–465).

49–753.   **STAR OF BETHLEHEM** contains a toxic resin similar to that described under milkweed (49–728).

49–754.   **SWEET PEAS.** The stalks or stems of sweet peas, as well as of ordinary peas, contain active toxic alkaloids. Ingestion of large amounts has been known to cause cerebral motor paralysis and acute cardiac depression. The clinical syndrome from ingestion resembles that of curare (49–168) and is known as lathyrism.

   Treatment
   1. Universal antidote (49–10).
   2. Tincture of iodine, 1 ml. in 100 ml. (15 drops in ½ glass of water), by mouth.
   3. Gastric lavage.

49–755.   **TULIPS.** A toxic alkaloid, tulipine, contained in the bulbs may cause a very severe reaction if ingested in even small amounts. The action and treatment are similar to that for colchicine (49–154).

49–756.   **VIOLETS.** The rhizomes contain violine, a very toxic alkaloid. See *Alkaloids* (49–29).

49–757.   **WATER HEMLOCK.** See 49–649.

49–758.   **YEW.** The leaves and berries of both the Japanese and English varieties contain the toxic alkaloid, taxine. For treatment see *Alkaloids* (49–29).

50. PREGNANCY

Many conditions during pregnancy may require emergency care.

PRIOR TO TERM

50–1. **Abortions.** (For definitions see Topic 66–5.)

    A. Suspected Early or Threatened. These patients should be hospitalized at once if bleeding is excessive—by ambulance if necessary. Sedation by barbiturates and control of pain and uterine contractions by opiates or meperidine hydrochloride (Demerol) are in order. Intravenous administration of plasma volume expanders may be necessary before transfer if the patient is in shock (Topic 15).

        Patients who show only slight spotting can be sent home for bed rest and given stilbestrol, 25 mg. by mouth daily. Progesterone (progestin) in the form of 10 mg. buccal tablets dissolved under the tongue four times a day or ethisterone (Pranone), 10 mg., orally every 2 hours (3 doses only) may control the bleeding. All patients should be instructed to obtain further medical care if spotting persists or if clots are passed.

    B. Incomplete. Hospitalization as soon as possible is essential. If a delay in arranging hospitalization is anticipated, small doses of morphine sulfate subcutaneously may be necessary to control restlessness and anxiety. Excessive bleeding can sometimes be controlled by ergonovine maleate (Ergotrate), 0.2 mg., intramuscularly. Shock therapy (Topic 15–7) should be given before transfer if blood loss has been excessive.

    C. Complete. If the attending physician is sure that no membranes have been retained and that bleeding has been controlled, home or office treatment may be feasible after antibiotics have been given.

      D. Any case in which the history or physical examination suggests the possibility of a criminally induced abortion must be reported at once to the proper authorities.

50–2.   **Eclampsia.** See 50–10 below.

50–3.   **Ectopic pregnancy.** Ruptured ectopic pregnancy is an acute surgical emergency requiring immediate hospitalization for operative treatment after treatment of shock (Topic 15–7).

50–4.   **Miscarriage.** See Topic 50–1, above (*Abortions*).

50–5.   **Premature separation of the placenta**

    A. Signs and Symptoms

      1. Sudden onset during the latter months of pregnancy of sharp abdominal pain associated with a hard firm uterus.

      2. Evidence of fetal distress.

      3. Signs of acute blood loss and shock (Topic 15).

    B. Treatment

      1. Control of pain by small doses of morphine sulfate or dihydromorphinone hydrochloride (Dilaudid) subcutaneously or intravenously.

      2. Immediate shock therapy (Topic 15–7).

      3. Transfer by ambulance for hospitalization as soon as shock has been controlled. Pelvic or rectal examination should not be done.

50–6.   **Toxemias of Pregnancy**

50–7.   **True toxemia of pregnancy**

    A. This serious condition is characterized by:

      1. Lassitude and general malaise; severe headaches.

      2. Generalized edema; albuminuric retinitis.

      3. Increasing hypertension, with convulsions and coma.

    B. Treatment

      1. Mild cases without convulsions or coma need no special emergency treatment but require careful prenatal care.

      2. Severe cases with convulsions and coma require immediate hospitalization after symptomatic supportive therapy.

50–8.   **Acute yellow atrophy of the liver**

    A. Signs and Symptoms

      1. Acute headache, usually with a subnormal temperature.

      2. Nausea, vomiting and diarrhea.

    3. Acute onset of severe convulsions which may be mistaken for eclampsia (50–9, below) or acute poisoning (Topic 49).

    4. Jaundice, mild or pronounced.

    5. Decreased urinary output with high specific gravity. Albumin and casts of all types may be present.

B. Treatment

    1. Protection from injury during convulsions. The use of a folded handkerchief or padded stick between the teeth to prevent tongue biting is very important.

    2. Insurance of an adequate airway.

    3. Control of convulsions by intravenous injection of rapid-acting barbiturates in large doses or intragluteal injections of paraldehyde.

    4. Intravenous administration of 500 ml. of 5% dextrose in saline.

    5. Immediate hospitalization for probable emptying of the uterus.

50–9. Eclampsia. Limited almost exclusively to the second half of pregnancy, an eclamptic convulsion coming on without premonitory signs or symptoms may require emergency care. Generally, however, signs and symptoms of a pre-eclamptic toxemia can be elicited on careful questioning and examination.

Treatment

    1. Insurance of an adequate airway.

    2. Protection against injury, especially tongue biting and musculoskeletal damage.

    3. Immediate subcutaneous injection of meperidine hydrochloride (Demerol), 50 to 100 mg.

    4. Administration of oxygen under positive pressure, preferably by means of a face mask or endotracheal tube and rebreathing bag.

    5. Transportation to a hospital at once, with an attendant in the ambulance if possible. Inhalations of ether to control convulsions, or of oxygen to combat cyanosis, may be necessary en route.

50–10. Pre-eclamptic toxemia should be suspected whenever a patient in the second half of pregnancy complains of headache, lassitude or edema, or whenever examination shows an elevated blood pressure with diminished urine containing albumin. In severe cases epigastric pain, impaired vision and hallucinations may be present.

Treatment

    1. Mild cases need no emergency treatment but should be referred to an obstetrician. Bed rest, sedation and a milk diet may be prescribed in the interim.

    2. Severe cases require the same treatment as eclampsia (50–9, above).

50–11. **Pernicious vomiting of pregnancy** may be either neurotic or toxemic in origin. Either type may result in extreme dehydration, malnutrition, and cachexia—even death—unless controlled.

    A. Treatment of Mild Cases. Administration of sedatives and/or antispasmodics and reference to an obstetrician for care. Any of the following drugs may be tried:

    1. Atropine sulfate, 0.5 to 1.0 mg., by mouth three times a day.

    2. Amphetamine sulfate (Benzedrine), 10 mg., three or four times daily by mouth.

    3. Adiphenine hydrochloride (Trasentine), 30 mg., orally three or four times a day.

    4. Dimenhydrinate (Dramamine), 50 to 100 mg., by mouth every 6 hours.

    5. Meclizine hydrochloride (Bonamine or Bonine) orally either in the form of tablets or medicated chewing gum.

    6. Pyridoxine hydrochloride (Vitamin B_6), 25 to 50 mg.

    7. Chlorpromazine hydrochloride (Thorazine), 25 to 50 mg., orally or intramuscularly. The patient should lie down for at least ½ hour after a dose of Thorazine because transient drowsiness, hypotension, tachycardia and syncope may occur. Promazine hydrochloride (Sparine) or prochlorperazine (Compazine) may be substituted for Thorazine.

    8. Perphenazine (Trilafon), 4 mg., orally three times a day.

    B. Treatment of Severe Cases

    1. Control of acute dehydration by intravenous administration of 500 to 1000 ml. of 5% dextrose in

saline. Correction of electrolyte imbalance (Topic 7) may be necessary.
2. Hospitalization for definitive care.

50–12.   **Peripheral neuritis** is sometimes associated with vomiting of pregnancy. The pain from this condition may be severe enough to cause the patient to seek emergency care.

Palliative symptomatic treatment by sedation and anodynes, occasionally opiates, is indicated, with reference for thorough investigation to an obstetrician or internist.

AT TERM
50–13.   **Decisions to be made by emergency physician**
  A. Is the Patient in True Labor? This can generally be determined by consideration of the following criteria:
    1. History regarding months of gestation. (If a prenatal chart is available, this should be reviewed.)
    2. Type, duration, strength and frequency of uterine contractures.
    3. Bloody show.
    4. Rupture of the membranes.
    5. Position of the presenting part and dilation of the cervix by rectal or vaginal examination. If a vaginal examination is done, the patient should be warned in advance of the possibility of slight bleeding.
  B. Is There Time for Transportation to a Hospital for Delivery?
    1. PRIMIPARAS. It is generally safe to transport primiparas in labor to a hospital for delivery unless:
      a. The cervix is fully dilated.
      b. The presenting part lies on the perineum.
    2. MULTIPARAS
      a. In many cases women who have had children are able to tell when delivery is near. Before arranging for transportation to a hospital the physician should question the patient regarding previous precipitate labors and, if possible, review the prenatal record. Rectal or vaginal examination is essential but can often be misleading. In making his decision regarding transfer, the physician should be guided more by the time since onset of pains, the frequency,

strength and length of uterine contractions, and the patient's opinion regarding the time available before delivery than by his examination.

b. All patients should be instructed to breathe through the mouth and warned against bearing down during transportation to the hospital. However, if delivery en route becomes imperative, it is much better for both the mother and the baby to avoid all delaying procedures.

c. Narcotic drugs, natural or synthetic, should never be given under emergency conditions in an attempt to stop or slow up delivery. Their effect is just the opposite; in addition, their use may result in marked depression of the child's respiratory center.

C. Is Emergency Delivery Necessary? If, in the opinion of the attending physician, sufficient time for transfer to a hospital for delivery is not available, delivery should be effected using the best possible technique that time and circumstances will allow.

51. PSYCHIATRIC EMERGENCIES

51–1. **Abnormal mental reactions** which may require emergency care are of two main types.

A. Organic Psychosis caused by
  1. Abnormalities in circulation, innervation, metabolism or nutrition.
  2. Infection or injury.
  3. Intoxication (alcohol, drugs, etc.).
  4. Neoplasms.

Signs and Symptoms
  1. Personality changes.
  2. Progressive loss of brain functions, especially of the higher centers.
     a. Loss of calculating ability and specialized knowledge.
     b. Poor judgement and memory.
     c. Faulty orientation.

3. Delirium and acute excitement states (Topic 36) characterized by:
   a. Confusion, disorientation, anxiety and hallucinations.
   b. Ataxia and tremors.
   c. Slurred speech.

Treatment

1. Prevention of self-injury and injury to others by gentle physical restraint if necessary. If forcible restraint is required, sedation is indicated.
2. Sedation by one of the following drugs:
   a. Sodium amobarbital (Amytal), 100 to 250 mg., intramuscularly or slowly intravenously.
   b. Chloral hydrate orally, 1.0 gm., repeated if necessary at hourly intervals.
   c. Chlorpromazine hydrochloride (Thorazine), 50 to 100 mg., orally or intramuscularly.
   d. Paraldehyde, 10 to 15 ml., orally or intramuscularly.
   e. Prochlorperazine (Compazine), 10 to 15 mg., orally or intramuscularly.
   f. Pentothal sodium intravenously, administered if possible by an anesthesiologist.
3. Hospitalization for treatment of the underlying cause.

B. Psychogenic Psychoses. (See also Topic 36, *Excitement States.*)

Recognition of these conditions so that early arrangements for psychiatric care can be made is one of the chief responsibilities of the emergency physician.

1. MANIC-DEPRESSIVE PSYCHOSES
   a. Marked changes in behavior and personality with fluctuation between acute excitement (Topic 36–8) and acute depression.
   b. Complete lack of comprehension by the patient of his condition.
2. PARANOIA. Characterized by intense feelings of guilt and failure, these patients are potentially homicidal and suicidal (Topic 16).
3. POSTPARTUM PSYCHOSES
4. SCHIZOPHRENIA. Inability to distinguish between actual environment and a fantasy world is the

chief distinguishing characteristic of an acute schizophrenic.

5. SUICIDAL TENDENCIES. (See also Topic 16, *Suicide*.)

Physical Signs and Symptoms
1. Decrease in appetite; weight loss.
2. Insomnia.
3. Disturbances in bowel function.
4. Menstrual abnormalities; impotency.
5. Abnormal activity, ranging from catatonia to mania.

Psychologic Signs
1. Deep depression.
2. Disorientation and disorganization.
3. Hallucinations.
4. Delusions.
5. Responses to 3 and 4.

Treatment
1. Tactful handling of the patient WITH AN ABLE-BODIED ATTENDANT PRESENT AT ALL TIMES.
2. Sedation as needed, with avoidance if possible of physical restraint.
3. Arrangement for hospitalization for psychiatric evaluation and treatment either in a private hospital equipped for care of mentally disturbed patients or in an institution designated by local law enforcement authorities.

51–2. **Delirium tremens.** See Topic 36–3.

51–3. **Fainting (vasodepressor syncope).** See 51–9, below.

51–4. **Hyperventilation.** See Topic 36–6.

51–5. **Hysteria.** (See also 51–9, below.) Emotional or physical strain in certain individuals may cause bizarre hysterical symptoms severe enough to require emergency care.

A. Common Manifestations of Hysteria
1. COMA. See *Unconsciousness, Episodic,* (51–9, below).
2. GLOBUS. A subjective sensation of a lump in the throat, sometimes so severe that the patient is convinced that he is unable to swallow.
3. HYPERVENTILATION (Topic 36–6; and 51–9,C, below).
4. PARALYSIS. Transient, partial or complete, usually

not corresponding to any motor nerve distribution.

5. SENSORY ABNORMALITIES. Usually hypesthesia or paresthesia, often of stocking or glove distribution. Gag and corneal reflexes may be absent.

B. Treatment

1. Sedation by barbiturates, chlorpromazine hydrochloride (Thorazine) or reserpine (Serpasil).
2. Explanation of the condition in simple terms.
3. Reference for psychiatric evaluation if the condition is severe, persistent or recurrent.

51–6. **Insomnia.** Persons who request emergency care for sleeplessness usually complain of:

1. Difficulty in getting to sleep.
2. Inability to stay asleep long enough to become rested.
3. Inability to sleep soundly enough to become rested.

Except in those instances where severe emotional trauma is a factor, most cases of insomnia are chronic and require emergency therapy only because previous medical and psychiatric care and lack of rest have resulted in extreme exhaustion.

After emphasizing to the patient or members of the family that only emergency treatment is being given, one of the following drugs may be administered:

DRUG	DOSE	METHOD
Chloral hydrate	0.6 to 2.0 gm.	Orally, diluted with water or milk
Paraldehyde	2 to 8 ml.	Orally, with fruit juice or cracked ice
	or 5 to 10 ml.	Intramuscularly, deep in the glutei
Phenobarbital sodium	0.06 to 0.2 gm.	Subcutaneously

All patients should be advised to make arrangements for further care and told that treatment on an urgent emergency basis will not be repeated. Large quantities of barbiturates, bromides, "tranquilizers" or sedatives of any type should not be prescribed for home use. Under no circumstances should opiates or synthetic narcotics be administered or prescribed.

51–7.   Manic-depressive psychoses. See Topic 36–8; and 51–1, B, above.

51–8.   Schizophrenia. See 51–1,B, above.

51–9.   Unconsciousness, episodic

    A. Common Causes. Between 90 and 95% of the cases of transient and recurrent loss of consciousness are due to epilepsy (Topic 33), hysteria (51–5, above), hyperventilation (Topic 36–6), and vasodepressor syncope (fainting).

    B. Rare Causes of episodic loss of consciousness (complete or partial)

        1. CAROTID SINUS SYNCOPE. These attacks generally follow twisting the neck in a certain way or pressure (tight collar, etc.) over the junction of the external and internal carotid arteries at the level of the upper border of the thyroid cartilage. The diagnosis can be confirmed by applying pressure OVER ONE SIDE ONLY with the patient lying down. This test is not without danger and should not be done unless facilities for combatting cardiac arrest (Topic 29–2) are immediately available.

        2. CARDIAC ARRYTHMIAS AND STANDSTILL. (See Topic 29.)

          a. Complete heart block (Adams-Stokes syncope) Topic 29–3.

          b. Aortic stenosis.

          c. Paroxysmal auricular tachycardia.

          d. Ventricular fibrillation.

        3. INTERMITTENT CEREBRAL ISCHEMIA.

        4. SURREPTITIOUS INTAKE OF CAUSATIVE DRUGS. See Topic 16 (*Suicide*).

        5. ORTHOSTATIC HYPOTENSION. Persons with this condition lose consciousness IN THE UPRIGHT POSITION ONLY. No emergency treatment (except for injuries sustained in falls) is indicated.

    C. Differential Diagnosis between the four common causes requires a careful history, especially in regard to previous episodes and onset of symptoms. The most important points are summarized in the following table.

DIFFERENTIAL DIAGNOSIS OF EPISODIC UNCONSCIOUSNESS

	Epilepsy (Grand Mal) (See Topic 33, Convulsive Seizures)	Hyperventilation (See Topic 36-6, Excitement States)	Hysteria (See 51-5, above)	Vasodepressor Syncope (Fainting) (See Topic 60-4)
Onset	Rapid; may be prodromal symptoms	Gradual—vertigo first	Slow or rapid, depending upon surrounding attention	Rapid, often preceded by stretching and yawning
Duration of symptoms	Usually 5–10 minutes; may be longer	Not over 2–5 minutes	Often prolonged	2–3 minutes
Type, results of fall	Sudden; may result in severe injury	Gradual and slow; generally no injury	Careful; practically never any injury	Sudden; may result in injury
Unconsciousness	Total; no response to stimuli	Usually partial, brief	Partial or complete; usually respond to pain	Complete but very brief
Time or place of onset	Anywhere, even when asleep	In the presence of any situation causing anxiety	In the presence of potential sympathizers	In the presence of real or imagined severe suffering
Muscular movements	Rhythmical	Spasmodic twitching	Inconstant, irregular and bizarre	None
Recovery	Slow; confused, disoriented for 10–30 minutes	Gradual but complete	Complete at once	Usually complete in a few moments

DIFFERENTIAL DIAGNOSIS OF EPISODIC UNCONSCIOUS

	Epilepsy (Grand Mal) (See Topic 33, Convulsive Seizures)	Hyperventilation (See Topic 36–6, Excitement States)	Hysteria (See 51–5, above)	Vasodepressor Syncope (Fainting) (See Topic 60–4)
Skin	Cyanotic from apnea	Usually normal	Normal	Pallor and sweating
Pulse	Normal	Rapid	Normal	Slow
Blood pressure	Slightly elevated during episode	Lower than normal	Normal	Marked transient hypotension
Neurologic changes	None except loss of response to pain; occasionally positive Babinski	Signs of tetany (Topic 44–23)	Decreased corneal and gag reflexes	None
Treatment	1. Prevention of injury if possible 2. Gentle restraint 3. Treatment of injuries 4. Long-term care	1. Rebreathing (paper bag method) 2. Sedation by barbiturates 3. Investigation and treatment of cause	1. Sedation by barbiturates if necessary 2. Psychiatric care	1. Supine position 2. Aromatic spirits of ammonia 3. Treatment of injuries
Prognosis	Good for recovery from immediate attack	Complete recovery	Guarded; complete psychiatric evaluation indicated	Excellent for complete recovery

52. PULMONARY EDEMA

52–1. Causes

A. Paroxysmal Cardiac Dyspnea (cardiac asthma, acute left ventricular failure (Topic 29)

B. Acute Poisoning from absorption, ingestion or inhalation of many toxic substances. Among these toxic substances (see Topic 49) are:

Aconite (49–20)   Hydrogen sulfide (49–280)
Acrolein (49–21)   Iodine (49–292)
Barbiturates (49–76)   Kerosene (49–303)
Cadmium salts (49–106)   Methyl bromide (49–359)
Carbon monoxide (49–119)   Morphine (49–370)
Chlorates (49–130)   Phosgene (49–458)
Cyanides (49–170)   Pyrogallol (49–486)
Dinitrophenol (49–201)   Salicylates (49–511)
Epinephrine hydrochloride   Sulfur dioxide (49–572)
   (49–214)   Thallium (49–597)
Ethylene [under *Anesthetics,*   Thuja [under *Arbor Vitae*
   Inhalation (59–8)]   (49–677)]

C. Barotrauma. See Topic 26–5,A,4 (*Thoracic Squeeze*).

52–2. Signs and symptoms

A. Acute apprehension, sometimes apparent several hours before other signs and symptoms develop.

B. Choking sensation.

C. Violent cough; frothy, sometimes blood-stained, sputum.

D. Gradually developing dyspnea and cyanosis.

Any or all of these signs and symptoms may develop within a short time or, following acute poisoning, may not appear for as much as 15 hours after apparent complete recovery.

52–3. Treatment

A. Position of maximum comfort. Usually the patient prefers a semi-Fowler position or insists on sitting on the edge of the bed with his legs hanging down.

B. Oxygen inhalations under positive pressure by face mask and rebreathing bag. Ethyl alcohol vapor added to the oxygen may be beneficial.

C. Morphine sulfate, 10 to 20 mg., subcutaneously or slowly intravenously according to the urgency of the situation. Minimal doses only should be used in patients with kidney disease, chronic pulmonary pathology or hypothyroidism. Opiates and synthetic narcotics are contraindicated in the presence of pulmonary insufficiency.

D. Atropine sulfate, 0.4 to 0.6 mg., subcutaneously if tachycardia is not a prominent feature.

E. Application of tourniquets serially to all four extremities with periods of release, one at a time.

F. Aminophylline (theophylline ethylenediamine), 0.25 gm., intravenously very slowly (Topic 59–3).

G. Rapid intravenous digitalization by lanatoside C (Cedilanid); initial dose, 0.8 mg., intravenously, followed by 0.8 mg. intravenously in 1 hour.

H. Hospitalization as soon as condition will permit. Relapses after apparently complete recovery are common.

53. RESPIRATORY TRACT CONDITIONS

A large number of persons who request emergency care have signs and symptoms referable to the respiratory tract which are more uncomfortable than serious. Some of the acute respiratory conditions which, if severe, may warrant emergency care are listed below.

53–1.   **Asthma.** [Also see Topic 48–6 (*Asthma in Children*).] Wheezing due to bronchospasm may be caused by:

1. Allergic reactions (Topic 24).
2. Foreign bodies in the upper respiratory tract (Topic 38–4).
3. Infections.
4. Left heart failure.

Treatment

Acute Severe Bronchospasm

1. Elimination of foreign bodies as causative factors by history and examination.
2. Hydration by intravenous injection of 1000 ml. of 5% dextrose in water.
3. Bronchodilation by:

    a. Epinephrine hydrochloride (Adrenalin), 0.25 to 0.5 ml. of 1:1000 solution, subcutaneously; repeat in 20 minutes if bronchospasm has not decreased.

    b. Aminophylline (theophylline ethylenediamine), 0.25 gm. in 10 ml. of sterile water, SLOWLY intravenously (Topic 59–3).

4. Control of dyspnea and cyanosis by administration of air or oxygen under positive pressure using a face mask and rebreathing bag. Mechanical devices which deliver a gradually increasing volume are superior to those which deliver a sudden spurt of oxygen or air. Aerosols are of value when used in conjunction with positive pressure. Discontinue oxygen therapy at once if breathing becomes more difficult or cyanosis increases; either is an indication that stimulation of the respiratory center by alveolar carbon dioxide is keeping the patient alive—washing it out may be fatal.

5. Sedation as required. The most effective sedative drugs in treatment of asthma are the barbiturates, chloral hydrate, and chlorpromazine hydrochloride (Thorazine). Oversedation should be avoided.

6. Hydrocortisone sodium succinate, 100 mg., intravenously, may give relief in severe cases.

7. Hospitalization as soon as acute bronchospasm has been controlled.

Slight or Moderate Asthmatic Attacks

1. Hydration by:

    a. Large amounts of fluids by mouth (Topic 7).

    b. Dextrose 5% in water, 500 to 1000 ml., intravenously.

2. Bronchodilation by:

    a. Ephedrine sulfate, 25 mg., orally every 4 hours.

    b. Epinephrine hydrochloride (Adrenalin), 1:100 solution by nebulizer or, in severer cases, 0.25 to 0.5 ml. of 1:1000 solution subcutaneously.

    c. Aminophylline (theophylline ethylenediamine) rectally or, in severer cases, very slowly intravenously.

  d. Sedation by barbiturates or chlorpromazine hydro-
     chloride (Thorazine) in the smallest possible
     effective doses.
  e. Thinning of bronchial secretions by oral iodides.
3. Administration of oxygen by face mask and rebreathing bag.
4. Arrangement for detailed medical supervision on an
   ambulatory basis. The need for further care
   should be stressed most emphatically since many
   patients after relief from an acute attack will
   postpone medical care until another acute episode occurs.

DO NOT

1. Administer opiates or synthetic narcotics in any
   form; any of these drugs may cause:
   a. Depression of the respiratory center.
   b. Decrease of the cough reflex.
   c. Addiction.
2. Oversedate.
3. Allow use of stramonium fume inhalations.
4. Permit excessive use of tobacco. On the other hand,
   attempting to cure the tobacco habit is not a
   part of the emergency therapy of asthma.
5. Prescribe or administer corticosteroids of any type
   as emergency therapy until after hospitalization
   or supervised ambulatory care is in effect.
6. Encourage the patient to cough very forcibly to raise
   tenacious sputum.
7. Prescribe or administer antibiotics unless infection
   is a proved causative factor.
8. Recommend a climate change.

53–2. **Bronchitis.** See also Topic 48–44,A (*Bronchitis in Chil-*
dren).

Treatment

1. Sulfathiazole, 2 gm. by mouth; then 1 gm. every 4
   hours.
2. Cough mixtures containing codeine sulfate, dihydrocodeinone bitartrate (Hycodan) and ammonium
   chloride.
3. Aerosol inhalations if tenacious mucus is present.
4. Bed rest with large amounts of fluids by mouth.

53–3. **Coryza.** (See also Topic 63–3.) No satisfactory treatment for "colds" except bed rest and copious fluids is known. The following measures may give symptomatic relief:

1. Sedative cough mixture containing codeine sulfate and dihydrocodeinone (Hycodan) mixtures will usually relieve persistent coughs. Ammonium chloride is useful if tenacious mucus is present.
2. Codeine sulfate and acetylsalicylic acid (aspirin) by mouth every 4 to 6 hours.
3. Fluids in large amounts by mouth.
4. Phenylephrine hydrochloride (Neo-Synephrine) nose drops (0.25%) may give symptomatic relief. Naphazoline hydrochloride (Privine) should not be used or prescribed because of the relatively high percentage of allergic reactions [see Topic 49–477 (*Privine*)].

53–4. **Croup.** See Topic 48–15.

53–5. **Deafness.** See Topic 34–5.

53–6. **Epiglottitis.** Acute swelling of the epiglottis is often overlooked as a cause for respiratory obstruction in children. Its development is very rapid and fatalities have been reported, especially in preschool children. Diagnosis is based on direct inspection of the swollen epiglottis. A single lateral inspiratory x-ray may show characteristic changes (ballooned hypopharynx, thickening of the epiglottis, widening of the aryepiglottic fold).

   Treatment
1. Immediate tracheotomy (Topic 17–11). Attempts at intubation should be avoided.
2. Treatment of the causative infection.

53–7. **Hiccups** (Singultus)

   A. *In Infancy,* this condition is often caused by overdistention of the stomach by food or swallowed air. Pressure over the upper abdomen usually gives relief. A teaspoonful of weak sodium bicarbonate solution or lemon juice may be tried.

   B. *In Adults,* hiccups may be idiopathic, but also may occur with gastric distention, posterior myocardial infarction and uremia.

   C. *Mild Attacks* can sometimes be controlled by one or more of a long list of "household cures". Among these are:

1. Pressing on, or application of ice to, the back of the neck.
2. Holding the breath as long as possible.
3. Swallowing finely cracked ice.
4. Pressing on the eyeballs (not too hard!).
5. Pulling on the tongue.
6. Cervical traction and manipulation.
7. Drinking a glass of water while holding a pencil crossways between the teeth.
8. Manipulation of single long hairs in the external auditory canal with a cotton applicator.

D. Severe Attacks sometimes yield to some of the following measures:
1. Rebreathing using a paper bag or face mask.
2. Inhalations of Carbogen or ether.
3. Gastric lavage.
4. Extreme sedation by chloral hydrate, paraldehyde or barbiturates.
5. Chlorpromazine hydrochloride (Thorazine), 25 to 50 mg., intramuscularly; repeat in 3 hours if necessary.
6. Hyoscine hydrobromide, 0.4 to 0.6 mg., subcutaneously.
7. Opiates, especially apomorphine hydrochloride, 5 mg., subcutaneously.
8. Amphetamine sulfate (Benzedrine), 10 to 20 mg., subcutaneously or slowly intravenously.
9. Adiphenine hydrochloride (Trasentine), 75 mg., subcutaneously (one dose), or every 4 hours by mouth.
10. Atropine sulfate, 1 mg., subcutaneously.
11. Calcium gluconate, 10 ml. of 10% solution, intravenously.

E. Prolonged intractable cases require hospitalization for replacement fluids (Topic 7) and for treatment of extreme exhaustion which may be terminal.

53–8. **Hyperventilation.** See Topic 36–6.

53–9. **Laryngitis.** The emergency treatment is the same as outlined for bronchitis (53–2, above).

53–10. **Mastoiditis.** See Topic 34–10.

53–11. **Metal fume fever.** See Topic 49–348 (*Metal Fumes*).

53–12. **Otitis media.** See Topic 34–12,B.

53–13. **Pleurisy**
   Treatment
   1. If possible, identify and give symptomatic treatment for the underlying pulmonary or cardiac condition, with arrangements for follow-up care by an internist.
   2. If pain is very severe, limit respiratory excursion as much as possible by strapping or application of a binder. However, partial immobilization should be avoided as a routine measure; adequate aeration is necessary to lessen the chance of development of intrapleural pathology.
   3. Give codeine sulfate and acetylsalicylic acid (aspirin) by mouth as needed.
   4. Hospitalize if the pain is very severe or if there is evidence of fluid by clinical or x-ray examination.

53–14. **Pneumonia.** (See also Topic 48–41; and Topic 63–11.)

The patient's general condition should be the deciding factor in the management of cases of suspected or proved pneumonia. Many patients with extensive lung involvement can be treated satisfactorily at home by bed rest, antibiotics, sulfonamides, analgesics and good nursing care. Penicillin in adequate doses is often all that is necessary for control, but chlortetracycline (Aureomycin), chloramphenicol (Chloromycetin), oxytetracycline (Terramycin) and other antibiotics may be more effective if a mixed infection or a penicillin-resistant organism is present.

Severe pain on respiration, dyspnea and cyanosis, plus the physical findings of pneumonia, establish the diagnosis, but laboratory studies and x-rays may be necessary to determine the extent of involvement, causative organism and disposition of the case. Lobar pneumonia almost invariably, bronchopneumonia often, and viral pneumonia rarely, require hospitalization.

53–15. **Pneumonitis**
   Causes
   1. Viral or bacterial infection.
   2. Trauma to the chest (Topic 31), especially severe crushing injuries. In some instances the findings may be on the opposite side of the chest from the external site of injury.

3. Inhalation or respiration of toxic substances: e.g., gasoline (Topic 49–254).

Treatment

1. Limited activity; bed rest in severe cases.
2. Sedative cough mixtures.
3. Penicillin, 600,000 units, intramuscularly and/or chlortetracycline (Aureomycin) and oxytetracycline (Terramycin) in large doses by mouth, depending on the sensitivity of the causative organism.
4. Hospitalization if the condition is extensive or severe, if it is associated with severe injury to the bony thorax, or if other types of acute or chronic chest pathology are present.

53–16.   **Pneumothorax.** (See also Topic 48–42.)

A. Spontaneous Pneumothorax. Usually a benign process, spontaneous rupture of an air-containing vesicle or of an alveolus may result in the passage of air into the pleural cavity or mediastinum. X-rays are useful not only in establishing the diagnosis but in disclosing underlying causative diseases. Symptomatic treatment is generally all that is required. Oxygen inhalations under positive pressure for cyanosis and dyspnea may be needed, followed by sedation and bed rest, preferably in a hospital, for a few days. Underlying disease processes should be recognized and arrangements made for proper care.

B. Tension Pneumothorax. See Topic 31–5; and Topic 48–42.

C. Traumatic Pneumothorax. See Topic 31–4; and Topic 48–42.

D. Therapeutic Pneumothorax. Emergency care may be indicated for bleeding following therapeutic injection of air.

Treatment

1. Sedation by intramuscular or intravenous barbiturates.
2. Slow (1 ml. per minute) intravenous injection of Pituitrin, 1 ml. in 10 ml. of normal saline.
3. Hospitalization if bleeding is severe or persistent.

53–17.   **Pulmonary embolism.** See Topic 60–3,B.

53–18.   **Pulmonary hemorrhage.** See Topic 8–3,P.

53–19. **Pulmonary edema.** See Topic 52.

53–20. **Rhinorrhea.** Drainage of spinal fluid, usually mixed with blood, from the nose indicates a basal fracture of the skull (Topic 43–16) whether or not x-rays show bony injury.

53–21. **Sinusitis**

Treatment

1. Penicillin, 600,000 units, intramuscularly, or chlortetracycline (Aureomycin), 250 mg., by mouth every 4 to 6 hours.
2. Phenylephrine hydrochloride (Neo-Synephrine) nose drops (0.25%) to shrink the engorged mucous membranes and promote drainage. Postural drainage also may be effective.
3. Application of local heat.
4. Bed rest; copious fluids.
5. Codeine sulfate and acetylsalicylic acid (aspirin) by mouth for pain and headache.
6. Referral to an otolaryngologist for further treatment if symptoms persist.

53–22. **Tonsillitis.** Acute tonsillitis requires the same treatment as bronchitis (53–2, above). In addition, an ice collar to the neck may give relief.

53–23. **Virus infections.** See Topic 63.

54. SKIN AND MUCOUS MEMBRANE CONDITIONS

The skin surface area of an average-sized adult (70 kg., 154 lb.) is about 1.72 square meters (18½ square feet)—most of it under the frequent narcissistic inspection and palpation stressed by present-day advertising, radio commercials and television. The same applies to a lesser degree to inspectable and palpable areas of mucous membrane. This self-inspection probably is a definite contributory factor in the increasing number of persons requesting immediate treatment for alleged dermatologic and mucous membrane emergencies—supposed variations from the usual in color, temperature, texture, shape or sensation of some part of the body.

Although the majority of dermatologic conditions do not require urgent therapy as a means of saving life or function, many of them do cause acute discomfort which can be relieved by prompt and appropriate therapy.

54–1. Allergic reactions. See Topic 24.

54–2. Angioedema. See Topic 24–2; and Topic 48–4 (*Angioedema in Children*).

54–3. Bites. See Topic 27; and Topic 62 (*Venoms*).

54–4. Burns. See Topic 28; Topic 48–10 (*Burns in Children*); and Topic 64–4 (*Thermal Effects of a Nuclear Blast*).

54–5. Contagious diseases. See Topic 32.

54–6. Dermatitis

    A. Contact. Many of these cases are caused by exposure to irritating substances at work. [See Topic 76 (*Workmen's Compensation Cases*).] Removal from exposure is the most important part of treatment. [Also see 54–11, below (*Poison Oak, Ivy and Sumach*).]

    B. Exfoliative. This very serious condition is most frequently the result of drug therapy and involves not only the skin but also mucous membranes. Arsenic preparations are notorious offenders; very severe cases have been reported following prolonged phenylbutazone (Butazolidin) therapy (Topic 59–54).

    Treatment

      1. Discontinuance of the offending drug.

      2. Sedation as required.

      3. Control of intense pruritus by cold compresses. Trimeprazine tartrate (Temaril), 2.5 mg., orally every 4 to 6 hours may give subjective relief.

54–7. Drug reactions

Practically every drug in use can cause acute edema, angioedema, pruritus and urticaria in sensitive individuals, sometimes severe enough to require emergency care. See under Topic 49 (*Poisoning, Acute*); and under Topic 59 (*Toxic Reactions to Average Doses of Common Drugs*).

54–8. Eczema

Acute itching, weeping areas occasionally bring sufferers for emergency care; more commonly, however, acute secondary infection superimposed on chronic eczematous areas due to circulatory stasis require bed rest, elevation and antibiotic therapy.

54–9. **Hives.** See 54–16, below.

54–10. **Paresthesias**

Disturbances in normal skin sensation are very disturbing and, fortunately, often result in an emergency visit early enough in a serious cerebrovascular or other potentially catastrophic condition so that neurologic evaluation can be done and preventive therapy begun.

54–11. **Poison oak, ivy and sumach**

The lesions caused by these plants are caused by a fixed non-volatile oil, toxicodendrol, and, contrary to general belief, are not contagious and do not spread.

Treatment

1. Washing of exposed parts with nonmedicated soap and hot water as soon as possible after exposure. Sponging with a fat solvent such as equal parts of ether and acetone may be helpful.
2. Local application of soothing lotions or of sodium bicarbonate paste. Preparations containing phenol (carbolic acid) should not be used.
3. Administration of sedatives and analgesics to control itching and burning.
4. Hospitalization if there is generalized skin involvement, especially of the face or genitals, if secondary infection is present, or if the pain, itching and burning are severe and intractable.
5. Administration of cortisone by mouth in full doses for 2 days, then gradually decreasing doses for 5 days. Poison oak or ivy antigens should not be administered during the acute state. Their use may result in serious aggravation or complications.

54–12. **Pruritus ani**

Itching in and around the anus and rectum may be so persistent and severe that it is practically unbearable. Persons suffering from this condition may scratch so forcibly that they tear off strips of skin, subcutaneous tissue and mucous membrane with their fingernails. Antipruritic medications may give some relief; those most commonly used are as follows:

1. Ergotamine tartrate, 0.5 mg., subcutaneously.
2. Thiamine chloride, 50 to 100 mg., subcutaneously.

3. Epinephrine hydrochloride (Adrenalin), 0.5 to 1 ml. 1:1000 solution, subcutaneously.
4. Tripelennamine hydrochloride (Pyribenzamine), 50 to 100 mg., by mouth three times a day.
5. Trimeprazine tartrate (Temaril), 2.5 mg., by mouth every 4 to 6 hours.

Common causes of pruritus ani are:

A. Fissure-in-Ano. See Topic 39–6,B.

B. Food Allergy

Treatment

1. Give sedatives and antihistaminics by mouth.
2. Treat secondary infection from scratching by sitz baths and application of bacitracin (Parentracin) ointment.
3. For local application prescribe one of the following:
   a. Dibucaine hydrochloride (Nupercaine) ointment (1%).
   b. Fluorohydrocortisone acetate (Florinef) cream (0.2%).
   c. Pramoxine hydrochloride (Tronothane) cream (1%).
   d. Tripelennamine hydrochloride (Pyribenzamine) cream (1%).
4. Arrange for further medical care, preferably by an allergist.

C. Fungous Infection

Treatment

1. Prescribe sedatives by mouth.
2. Treat secondary infection from scratching by hot sitz baths and bacitracin (Parentracin) ointment.
3. Give symptomatic relief, if possible, by local application of:
   a. Dibucaine hydrochloride (Nupercaine) ointment (1%).
   b. Fluorohydrocortisone acetate (Florinef) ointment (0.2%).
   c. Pramoxine hydrochloride (Tronothane) cream (1%).
   d. Resorcinol lotion.
   e. Whitfield's ointment.
4. Refer to a dermatologist for definitive therapy.

D. Hemorrhoids. See Topic 39–6,C.

E. Medications
The wide use of antibiotics, especially the tetracyclines, has resulted in a very stubborn type of pruritus ani resulting from suppression of the normal intestinal organisms.
Treatment
1. Discontinuance of the offending medication.
2. Local application of dibucaine hydrochloride (Nupercaine) ointment (1%).
3. Prescription of vitamin B complex in large doses, orally or parenterally.
4. Inclusion of buttermilk and/or cottage cheese in the daily diet.
5. Assurance of the patient that the condition will clear completely with time.

F. Pinworms (oxyuriasis) are frequently the cause of anal itching in children; occasionally, in adults.
Treatment
1. Pyrvinium pamoate orally, 5 mg. per kilogram of body weight, should be given to the patient and all members of the family or other close contacts. Tablets should be swallowed whole to avoid staining the teeth.
2. Personal care to prevent contamination and reinfection through hands, fingernails, etc.
3. Sanitary measures.
   a. Boil all bed linen, underclothes, washcloths, towels, etc., daily.
   b. Scrub toilet seats daily.
   c. Sterilize metallic objects used by patient by baking in a hot oven for at least 10 minutes.

54–13. **Pruritis vulvae.** See Topic 41–11.
54–14. **Stings.** See Topic 56.
54–15. **Sunburn.** See Topic 28–27.
54–16. **Urticaria.** [See also Topic 24 (*Allergic Reactions*).]
Characterized by the appearance in the skin and mucous membranes of pruritic reddened or whitish swellings of various sizes and shapes called wheals, acute urticaria may be caused either exogenously or endogenously, usually the former.

A. Exogenous Causes
1. Food—especially berries, chocolate, fish, nuts and spices.
2. Drugs.

3. Commercial chemicals such as DDT (Topic 49–175).
4. Animal serums used in injections.
5. Animal dander.
6. Feathers.
7. Perfumes and cosmetics.
8. Physical factors—heat, cold, light of different wave lengths.

B. Endogenous Causes
1. Microorganisms.
2. Parasites.
3. Secretion from endocrine glands.
4. Products of altered metabolism.
5. Psychogenic stimuli.

Treatment
1. Epinephrine hydrochloride (Adrenalin), 0.5 to 1.0 ml. of 1:1000 solution, intramuscularly, or in severe cases, intravenously.
2. Immediate tracheotomy (Topic 17–11) if the wheals involve the mucous membrane of the throat [see Topic 24–2; and Topic 48–4 (*Angioedema in Children*)].
3. Antihistamines by mouth.
4. Vasoconstrictors such as ephedrine.
5. Corticosteroid therapy.
6. Hospitalization if response to the measures given above is not satisfactory or if a tracheotomy has been done.

54–17. **Varicose eczema and ulcers.** See 54–8, above.
54–18. **Vincent's angina.** (Ulcerative Stomatitis, Trench Mouth).

This acutely contagious ulcer-forming inflammation of mucous membranes is caused by a fusiform bacillus and a coarsely coiled spirochete, both of which can usually be easily identified in smears. The gums and the mucous membranes of the mouth and throat are most commonly involved but the external ear, internal nares, female genitalia and glans penis are occasionally the sites of infection.

A. Signs and Symptoms
1. Reddened painful mucosa; later covered with a grayish white adherent membrane which on removal leaves punctate bleeding areas. Laboratory studies may be necessary to differentiate it from diph-

theria (Topic 32–4) and from infectious mono-
nucleosis.
2. General malaise and chills and fever, especially in
children. Some adults show no systemic reaction
although extensive mucous membrane involvement is present.
3. Pain on swallowing if the oral cavity is involved.
4. Marked swelling; subacute cases show a boggy
edema.
5. Blood-stained oral or mucous membrane secretion if
the membrane is disturbed.
6. Leukopenia.

B. Treatment
1. Isolation and sterilization of all dishes, eating utensils, washcloths, towels, etc.
2. Close attention to oral and other personal hygiene.
3. Removal of crusts and cleansing of sloughs with
hydrogen peroxide.
4. Application to the gums or other affected areas of
sodium perborate paste.
5. Administration of 600,000 units of penicillin intramuscularly daily for 3 or 4 days. Tetracycline
should be substituted if the patient gives a history of sensitivity to penicillin.
6. Referral for specialist care if the systemic reaction
is severe, or if the condition is extensive or extending. Permanent damage to the gums and
mucous membranes may occur without proper
and prolonged treatment.

54–19. **X-ray (radiation) burns.** See Topic 28–31.

55. SOFT TISSUE INJURIES

Soft tissue injuries of varying degrees of severity make up
the bulk of cases treated on any emergency service.

55–1. **Abdominal injuries.** [See also Topic 22 (*Abdominal
Pain*).]
A. Nonpenetrating injuries caused by direct blunt trauma
to the abdominal wall are far more common than

penetrating or perforating injuries and may be so severe that hemorrhage and shock cause death before any treatment can be given, or so slight that no treatment is required. Between these two extremes lies the intermediate field in which accurate diagnosis and prompt and proper treatment can influence the degree of recovery.

1. The severity of the trauma inflicted on an underlying viscus by a blunt object depends upon:
   a. The force exerted.
   b. The size and shape of the striking object.
   c. The location of impact.
   d. The ability of the person struck to give way with the blow, or to tighten his muscles in preparation for it.
   e. The strength of the abdominal musculature.
   f. Concomitant injuries elsewhere in the body.
2. NONPENETRATING ABDOMINAL INJURIES IN ORDER OF FREQUENCY.

STRUCTURE INVOLVED	PER CENT (*Approximate*)
Spleen	26.0
Kidneys	24.0
Intestines	16.5
Liver	15.5
Abdominal wall	4.5
Retroperitoneal hemorrhage	3.5
Mesentery	3.0
Pancreas	1.5
Diaphragm	1.0
Other	4.5

More than 80% of abdominal injuries from blunt trauma are the result of automobile accidents; industrial accidents (Topic 76) account for another 10%. The mortality from nonpenetrating abdominal injuries is about three and one-half times that for penetrating injuries, probably due in great part to the difficulty in making an accurate diagnosis.

For treatment, see under the organ involved.

   3. Absolute indications for laparotomy, no matter what
       viscus is suspected, are as follows:
       a. Pneumoperitoneum demonstrable by x-rays.
       b. Abdominal paracentesis which yields blood [must
           be associated with clinical signs of active
           bleeding or evidence of contamination from
           contents of a hollow viscus (stomach contents,
           bile, feces, urine)].
       c. Secondary collapse following recovery from pri-
           mary posttraumatic shock.

B. Penetrating Abdominal Injuries
Treatment
   1. Shock therapy (Topic 15–7).
   2. Application of a sterile dressing to the external
       wound.
   3. Immediate hospitalization for close observation and
       probable laparotomy.

C. Perforating Abdominal Injuries are usually bullet
       wounds (55–6, below).
Treatment
   1. Shock therapy (Topic 15–7).
   2. Application of sterile dressings to entrance and exit
       wounds.
   3. Hospitalization for definitive care. Any observations
       which might be of value to law enforcement
       agencies (powder marks on clothing, powder
       burns on skin, course of wound tract, etc.)
       should be recorded on the emergency chart.

55–2.   Abrasions. (For corneal abrasions see Topic 37–32.)
   Treatment
   1. Thorough scrubbing with soap and water for removal
       of embedded foreign material is essential. If
       necessary, a narcotic can be given, topical anes-
       thetic applied, or procaine or lidocaine (Xylo-
       caine) block anesthesia used before the cleansing
       process to control pain. If removal of all em-
       bedded foreign bodies and devitalized tissue from
       the skin or subcutaneous structures cannot be
       accomplished under topical or local anesthetic,
       hospitalization for administration of general
       anesthesia is necessary to prevent permanent
       and disfiguring tattooing.

2. Extensive abrasions should be dressed with petrolatum gauze. As a rule nitrofurazone (Furacin) or bismuth tribromophenate (Xeroform) gauze should not be used unless definite infection is present. Collodion dressings should not be used routinely because they are very difficult to remove and because they promote anaerobic growth. Application of tincture of benzoin compound to the surrounding skin followed by sterile gauze and Elastoplast under slight tension makes a much more satisfactory dressing.

3. All patients who have sustained extensive pavement or gravel burns should receive tetanus antitoxin and/or tetanus toxoid (Topic 19).

55–3.   Bites. (See Topic 27.)

55–4.   Bladder injuries. (See Topic 40–2.)

55–5.   Brain injuries. See Topic 43, and Topic 48–8 (*Brain Injuries in Children*).

55–6.   Bullet wounds

Whenever possible the exact site of entry, the course of the bullet, and the point of exit should be described in detail in the patient's record. The presence or absence of powder burns or marks on the skin and clothing should be noted. If the bullet is recovered it should be turned over to the proper law enforcement officers. For treatment see 55–1,C, above, and the discussion of the body area involved. All cases require protection against tetanus (Topic 19).

55–7.   Burns. See Topic 28, and Topic 48–10 (*Burns in Children*).

55–8.   Cardiac injuries. See Topic 29–4.

55–9.   Chest injuries. See Topic 31.

55–10.   Contusions. (Also see 55–1, above.)

A. *Mild Contusions.* Ordinary contusions (provided fracture has been ruled out) need only symptomatic emergency treatment to reduce pain and swelling. The patient should be instructed to limit use of an extremity, given crutches or a splint if indicated, and instructed regarding application of hot or cold compresses at home. As a general rule, cold is more effective for the first day; after 24 hours, hot compresses or contrast baths may be used. Marked relief, especially of throbbing fingers and toes, may be obtained by gentle inunction of the injured part for 10 to 15 minutes every 3 or 4 hours with a 2.5% ointment of hydrocortisone acetate in neomycin sulfate (Neo-Cortef).

B. Severe Contusions, especially of the extremities, may require elevation and snug elastic bandages to prevent and control intramuscular bleeding. Hyaluronidase, 500 TRU in 1 ml. of normal saline solution, injected directly into a hematoma may be of benefit.

55–11. **Crush injuries**

A. Crushing Injuries to the Chest may cause serious damage without external evidence of trauma.

1. Alveolar rupture and hemorrhage, especially in children (Topic 31–3).
2. Cardiac contusion with or without severe symptoms, such as hemopericardium (Topic 29–4) and cardiac arrest (Topic 29–2). Milder contusions may result in ECG changes (RST and T-wave flattening) which persist for lengthy periods.
3. Diaphragmatic damage (Topic 31–6).
4. Fractured ribs and sternum (Topic 31–2).
5. Mediastinal hemorrhage (Topic 31–1).
6. Tension pneumothorax (Topic 31–5).

B. Crushing Injuries to the Extremities may cause severe damage not apparent on initial examination. X-rays are indicated in all cases. Also see Topic 48–61 (*Wringer Injuries*).

C. Crushing Injuries to the Low Back or Flanks may cause severe kidney damage (Topic 40–3). Hematuria, gross or microscopic, is present in 75 to 80% of cases.

55–12. **Diaphragmatic injuries.** See Topic 31–6.

55–13. **Duodenal rupture**

Severe blunt nonpenetrating trauma to the upper abdomen or back may cause retroperitoneal rupture of the duodenum. X-ray studies are the only preoperative method of diagnosis. Suspicion of duodenal rupture requires immediate exploratory laparotomy.

55–14. **Ear injuries.** See Topic 34–4.

55–15. **Eye injuries.** See Topic 37–29 to 37 (inclusive).

55–16. **Foreign bodies.** See Topic 38–6.

55–17. Gallbladder and bile duct injuries

Because of its sheltered location, the gallbladder and its duct system are rarely injured by blunt trauma unless there is also extensive liver damage (55–21, below). It may, however, be injured by penetration or perforation. Suspicion or evidence (usually by abdominal paracentesis) calls for immediate exploratory laparotomy.

55–18. Grease gun injuries

Severe injuries, usually to the hand, may result from injection through a small puncture wound in the skin of lubricating grease under as much as 600 lbs. per square inch pressure. Following the tracts of least resistance (fascial compartments, intermuscular septa, tendon and nerve sheaths, etc.), the grease may dissect for considerable distance in the brief moment of contact. Even with extensive damage, immediate pain is unusual but becomes agonizing within a few hours due to tissue ischemia.

Treatment

1. Anodynes or narcotics for control of pain.
2. Release of tension and removal of the contaminant as an urgent emergency procedure. Wide surgical exposure with painstaking debridement, usually under regional nerve block, must be done to minimize permanent disability.
3. Intensive and prolonged antibiotic therapy.

55–19. Intestinal injuries

Rupture or perforation of any portion of the bowel calls for immediate surgical exploration and repair. A history of possible trauma, with some immediate severe abdominal pain followed by a brief pain-free period, is typical. Demonstration by x-ray of free air under the diaphragm is conclusive, but absence of air does not rule out perforation.

55–20. Lacerations

Before treatment of any laceration the presence or absence of damage to nerves, tendons and other deep structures should be determined by tests of function.

A. Preparation for Repair

1. Shave the area around the wound for at least 2 inches. This includes the scalp and eyebrows unless the laceration is minute and nongaping.
2. Give preliminary sedatives, anodynes or narcotics as needed to control pain, apprehension and rest-

lessness except in infants and small children (Topic 5).

3. Cover the wound with sterile gauze; cleanse the surrounding skin with a mild detergent such as pHisoHex and with soap and water. Irrigate thoroughly with saline.

4. Remove the gauze and scrub the laceration with bland nonmedicated soap and water, loosening and removing foreign bodies; follow with copious irrigations with sterile saline, using a bulb syringe or gravity apparatus. Remove any excess saline with sterile gauze; then paint with tincture of quaternary ammonium chloride (QAC), tincture of thimerosal (Merthiolate) or tincture of iodine (¼ strength).

5. If tetanus antitoxin is indicated (Topic 19) as a time-saving measure the intracutaneous sensitivity test (Topic 14) may be given before the patient is taken to surgery. In apprehensive, excited or undisciplined children, all injections (with the exception of local anesthesia) should be postponed until after surgical repair.

6. If cleansing the wound is extremely painful, it should be performed under 1 or 2% procaine or lidocaine (Xylocaine) infiltration or block anesthesia.

B. Principles of Treatment

1. Repair (debridement, control of hemorrhage, primary closure) is safe within SIX hours of injury. This time may be extended at the discretion of the physician if the wound is not grossly contaminated or obviously infected. In certain instances delay in repair may be necessary while a valid operative permit is being obtained (Topic 70–14).

2. Small lacerations may be closed by adhesive butterflies and pressure dressings after irrigation and ruling out of the presence of foreign bodies. X-rays (Topic 21) should be taken if the history suggests the possibility of the presence of any radiopaque foreign material.

3. STERILE OPERATING ROOM TECHNIQUE is essential in all cases. All persons in the operating room, IN-

CLUDING THE PATIENT (unless a face screen is in use or the laceration involves the face or head), should be capped and masked. The surgeon must wear a cap, mask and sterile gloves, and the surgery nurse should confine her hair. A sterile operating gown should be worn if a lengthy or extensive repair is necessary.

4. A tourniquet should be used to insure a bloodless field whenever the location of the laceration will allow. Strips of rubber dam or heavy rubber bands clamped with a hemostat make excellent finger tourniquets. A blood pressure cuff inflated to 20 mm. of mercury above systolic pressure works very well on the forearm or lower leg. In lengthy procedures the tourniquet should be relaxed for a few seconds every hour. At the conclusion of the procedure, the patient should be examined carefully for loss of temperature and light touch perception indicative of blocking of conduction through the peripheral nerves by the localized pressure of the tourniquet ("tourniquet paralysis").

5. ANESTHESIA
   a. Infiltration or local block with 1 or 2% procaine or lidocaine (Xylocaine) is the method of choice for emergency use.
   b. IF ANOTHER PHYSICIAN OR AN ANESTHETIST IS PRESENT, short light inhalation anesthesia [nitrous oxide, ether, vinyl ether (Vinethene) or ethyl chloride] or intravenous Pentothal Sodium may be given (not in children). Because of the danger of aspiration of stomach contents and subsequent development of pneumonia, general anesthesia should never be started until at least 6 hours after the last meal. If a general anesthetic is used, THE PATIENT MUST BE WATCHED AT ALL TIMES UNTIL FULLY CONSCIOUS.
   c. Brachial plexus blocks, sciatic blocks and spinal anesthesia should not be attempted as emergency procedures unless under the direction

of an anesthesiologist or physician experienced in their use.

d. Nerve blocks of the ulnar, radial and medium nerves at the wrist, or of the nerves above the ankle, are very satisfactory if the physician is familiar with the technique.

e. Anesthesia (preferably local) should be used while repairing lacerations requiring suturing unless:

   (1) The patient is comatose or in such condition that he does not feel pain.

   (2) Satisfactory closure of the laceration can be obtained with one or two sutures.

   (3) Acute sensitivity to local anesthetic agents is present (Topic 59–10).

   (4) The patient requests repair without anesthesia on religious or other grounds.

   (5) Cooperation of the patient cannot be obtained.

6. EXAMINATION OF THE WOUND UNDER ANESTHESIA FOR:

   a. Foreign bodies, superficial or embedded.

   b. Severance of muscles, tendons, blood vessels or nerves.

   c. Fractures or dislocations.

   d. Hematomas.

   e. Any openings into joints, tendon sheaths or fascial spaces which might cause contamination. If examination under anesthesia shows such severe or extensive damage that emergency repair would be difficult or very lengthy, a sterile bandage should be applied, the patient given a sedative and hospitalization for repair arranged. The physician to whom the patient is being sent should, if possible, be contacted by telephone and full details given. A brief summary of findings and treatment should be sent with the patient.

7. DEBRIDEMENT. The object of debridement is to convert a wound lined with damaged and potentially infected tissue into a surgically clean wound. Therefore, starting with the skin and working toward the depths of the wound, all damaged tissues should be removed by sharp dissection,

sparing nerves, tendons, blood vessels, joint capsules and articular surfaces. Hematomas should be evacuated and bleeding vessels clamped and tied, using No. 000 plain catgut, fine silk, or No. 40 or 50 cotton. Buried sutures should be kept to an absolute minimum. No disinfectants, antiseptics or medications of any type should be painted, sprinkled, sprayed or insufflated into the wound.

Debridement should be limited in certain areas. The most important of these are:

a. The eyelids. Lacerations in this region should be thoroughly cleansed and closed with fine Dermalin to prevent ectropion (Topic 37–8) or entropion (Topic 37–11).

b. The hand and fingers (Topic 42–5,A,8).

c. The face.

d. The lips, especially in the region of the vermillion line.

e. The penis (Topic 40–5,F). In these areas little if any tissue should be removed unless gross contamination or maceration is present. Skin edges should be approximated without tension and sutured loosely without inverting or overlapping.

8. CLOSURE

a. Obliteration of dead spaces by mattress sutures of No. 000 plain catgut, fine silk, or No. 40 or 50 cotton. Buried sutures should be kept to a minimum.

b. Careful approximation of skin edges without undue tension, using interrupted sutures of No. 40 or 50 cotton or fine Dermalin. All external knots should be placed away from the approximated skin edges.

c. Essential structures (tendons, nerves, blood vessels, joints and bone) MUST be covered. If necessary a pedicle graft (with the base proximally) can be swung from the immediate neighborhood and the resultant defect covered with a split graft.

d. Completely severed soft tissue, if small and not

not macerated (fingertips, nose, ear, etc.), may be cleansed, kept moist in normal solution, and sutured back in place as full thickness grafts.

9. DRESSINGS

a. A petrolatum gauze or a Telfa nonadherent dressing should be applied over the sutures, covered with sterile gauze and the surrounding area painted with tincture of benzoin. When this has dried enough to be "tacky," an elastic pressure bandage should be applied. On any portion of an extremity, care should be taken to allow for postoperative edema. Circular bandages completely around an extremity should never be applied.

b. Nitrofurazone (Furacin) and bismuth tribromophenate (Xeroform) gauze should not be used for the original dressing unless evidence of gross infection has been noted.

c. Collodion dressings should never be applied directly over the wound, but collodion is useful for anchoring the edges of dressings, especially on the face.

10. IMMOBILIZATION. In some areas of the body, motion may interfere with healing. Limited activity, splinting, use of a sling or Velpeau bandage, plaster of Paris immobilization or crutches may be indicated. Elevation of an injured extremity will help to control swelling, throbbing and pain.

11. POSTOPERATIVE CARE

a. Specific instructions must be given to the patient regarding recheck examination (see Topic 65 for suggested recheck examination form).

(1) All grossly contaminated or severely crushed or contused injuries. These must be rechecked in 24 hours. So should injuries in which debridement only, without closure, has been done as late treatment.

(2) All finger, hand, wrist or elbow injuries. These should be seen by a physician on the day following surgical repair.

(3) Minor lacerations, except as specified in (2)

above. Inspection in not more than 3 days is indicated.

b. Tetanus antitoxin or tetanus toxoid. One or both (Topic 19) should be given routinely unless:

   (1) The condition is minimal or of a type which, in the opinion of the attending physician, does not require this protection.

   (2) Some definite contraindication such as acute sensitivity to horse serum is present (Topic 14).

c. Antibiotics. Penicillin and/or broad spectrum antibiotics may be indicated if:

   (1) Gross contamination or infection has been noted.

   (2) Repair has been delayed more than 6 hours after injury.

d. Sedatives and anodynes. Only enough to last until the next scheduled recheck visit should be prescribed or furnished.

55–21. **Liver injuries**

If severe blunt trauma (usually the result of vehicular or industrial injury) without external evidence of injury has occurred and deep shock not explainable by other injuries is present, damage to the liver should always be suspected. Usually, however, hepatic damage is associated with other injuries (fractured ribs, fractured pelvis, ruptured diaphragm, mediastinal hemorrhage, etc.) and is signaled by upper abdominal pain, tenderness and spasm. Shoulder pain may be present, often only on deep inspiration.

    Treatment. Shock therapy (Topic 15–7) before and during transfer for laparotomy.

55–22. **Nasal injuries.** See Topic 46–6 and 55–20, above.

55–23. **Nerve injuries.** See Topic 42–6 (*Nerve Injuries in the Hand*); and Topic 47–4.

55–24. **Pancreatic injuries**

Blunt trauma to the abdomen, usually from automobile accidents, and usually associated with other serious injuries, is a common cause of traumatic pancreatitis. Injury limited to the gland is usually the result of bullet or stab wounds. Serum amylase levels are of value in diagnosis.

Treatment consists of wide exposure at laparotomy, with opening of the lesser omental sac to allow inspection of the complete gland for ecchymoses, edema, fat necrosis, tears of the capsule and parenchyma, and retroperitoneal hematomas.

55–25. Penetrating wounds. [Also see Topic 29–4 (*Hemopericardium*); Topic 31–9 to 12 (*Penetrating Chest Wounds*); Topic 37–29 to 37 (*Eye Injuries*); and 55–27, below (*Puncture Wounds*).]

This general category covers all types of injuries, usually but not necessarily caused by small pointed objects, in which there is a wound of entrance but none of exit. Diagnosis is apparent and treatment well-standardized; therefore, the mortality is much less than in injuries resulting from blunt force.

55–26. Perforating wounds

Through-and-through wounds with unmistakable skin defects at the points of entrance and exit are usually caused by bullets. The mortality is less than for contusions caused by blunt force or for penetrating wounds because surgical exploration without delay is more frequently and promptly carried out.

55–27. Puncture wounds. (Also see 55–25 and 26, above.)

A. Conservative Treatment. Superficial cleansing, bandaging, protection against tetanus by administration of tetanus antitoxin or toxoid (Topic 19) and prophylactic antibiotics if indicated are all that is required in the majority of cases. Large, deep or grossly contaminated puncture wounds should be handled in the same manner as lacerations (55–20, above).

B. Puncture Wounds Requiring Special Treatment

1. BITES. See Topic 27.
2. CHEST INJURIES INVOLVING THE PLEURA (Topic 31–10) OR PERICARDIUM (Topic 29–4).
3. EYE INJURIES. See Topic 37–29 to 37 (inclusive).
4. FOREIGN BODIES. See Topic 38.
5. GUNSHOT WOUNDS. Treatment varies with the caliber and type of bullet (hard or soft nosed), and the tract of the projectile into or through the body. Protection against tetanus (Topic 19) is always indicated.
6. HEMORRHAGING PUNCTURE WOUNDS usually can be controlled by pressure or, if on an extremity, by a properly applied tourniquet. Extension of the wound under local anesthesia with evacuation of hematomas and identification and ligation of the bleeding vessels may be necessary.

7. PERITONEAL OR VISCERAL PUNCTURE. If perforation or penetration of the peritoneum or of solid or hollow abdominal viscus is known or suspected, immediate hospitalization is mandatory. Pre-transportation shock therapy (Topic 15–7) is essential.

8. STAB WOUNDS. See 55–32, below.

9. STINGS. See Topic 56.

55–28. **Scalp wounds.** See Topic 43–22.

55–29. **Spinal cord injuries.** See Topic 45–11; and Topic 47–7.

55–30. **Splenic injuries**

Injuries to the spleen represent the largest group (approximately 26%) in most statistical series concerned with the effects of blunt trauma. Automobile injuries represent the largest part of this group. Rupture of the spleen is often associated with rib fractures and other chest and abdominal traumatic pathology.

Signs and Symptoms

1. Upper abdominal pain which may vary markedly in intensity.

2. Tenderness and muscle spasm of the right upper quadrant, sometimes extending below the level of the umbilicus.

3. Left shoulder pain (in about 50% of cases) elicited by manual pressure over the left upper quadrant and by deep inspiration.

4. Evidence of shock (Topic 15–6). Bleeding may be temporarily tamponaded by perisplenic hematomas, with irreversible circulatory collapse when capsular rupture occurs—sometimes several weeks after injury.

Treatment. Splenectomy as soon as the condition is recognized. If the diagnosis is in doubt, or conservative measures are used for any reason, cross-matched blood should be available for immediate use.

55–31. **Sprains and strains.** See Topic 45–11,B; and Topic 47–4,K.

55–32. **Stab wounds**

The treatment of stab wounds depends upon the injury tract, the structures involved, and the length of time since injury. Close observation for several hours may be required to determine the true extent of injury, particularly if the weapon used has produced a very small entrance wound (hat-pins, ice picks, thin knife blades, etc.).

55–33. **Stings.** See Topic 56.

55–34. **Stomach injuries**
Penetrating wounds of the stomach are usually associated with other abdominal damage and require immediate surgical repair. Blunt trauma may cause rupture of the stomach wall, particularly if scarring from old ulceration is present.

55–35. **Stud gun injuries**
A modern stud driving device used in the construction industry utilizes .22 or .32 caliber powder charges for propulsion of rivets and studs. As a result, it offers two sets of hazards:

1. The bullet-like effect of the stud or rivet. For treatment see 55–6, above (*Bullet Wounds*).
2. The gunpowder danger from the charge. Any break in the skin is an indication for protection against tetanus (Topic 19) after skin testing for sensitivity (Topic 14).

55–36. **Tracheobronchial injuries**
Rupture of the trachea or of the main bronchi can be caused by direct trauma such as steering wheel impact, by heavy glancing blows to the chest, and by falls. Increased intraluminal pressure with a closed glottis may be a factor. Tremendous cervical and facial emphysema ("the puffball man") may be rapidly fatal. Tension pneumothorax (Topic 31–5) may require treatment. In some cases, immediate tracheotomy (Topic 17–11) followed by thoracotomy may have a successful outcome; in all cases, immediate hospitalization is indicated.

55–37. **Whiplash injuries.** See Topic 45–11,B, and Topic 47–4,K.

55–38. **Wringer injuries.** See Topic 48–61.

55–39. **Zipper injuries.** See Topic 48–62.

56. *STINGS*

See also Topic 27 (*Bites*); and Topic 62 (*Venoms*). About 50% of deaths from venomous stings are due to hymenoptera (ants, bees and wasps); 80% of these deaths occur within 2 hours of the sting.

56–1. **Bee stings**

These are common and may be dangerous. Symptomatic local treatment consisting of cold compresses, application of ammonia or baking soda, or magnesium sulfate (Epsom salts) soaks will usually give relief. The "stinger" should be identified and removed if present.

Extremely great sensitivity (natural or acquired) to hymenoptera venom may be encountered and constitutes an acute emergency. These patients present the clinical picture of severe anaphylactic shock and require immediate energetic handling as a lifesaving measure (Topic 24). Epinephrine hydrochloride (Adrenalin), 0.5 to 1 ml. 1:1000 solution, should be given subcutaneously at once, followed by shock therapy (Topic 15–7) and hospitalization.

56–2. **Fire ant stings.** (See also Topic 27–2 and 10.)

Although these ants bite, toxic effects are caused by venom injected through a spine on the ant's abdomen. Since the ants move and sting quickly (each ant 3 or 4 times) 3000 to 5000 stings have been reported on one person following disturbance of an ant mound.

A. Signs and Symptoms

1. Immediate development of an umbilicated pustule surrounded by a reddened acutely painful halo.
2. Severe, burning, stinging pain at, and for some distance around, the site of the sting.
3. Temperature elevation.
4. Dyspnea and cyanosis; occasionally, acute respiratory depression.

B. Treatment

1. Artificial respiration in severe cases.
2. Treatment of allergic reactions (Topic 24–1).
3. Protective sterile dressing over pustular areas.
4. Control of pain. Narcotics may be necessary for 12 to 24 hours.

C. Prognosis. Although fatalities from respiratory collapse have been reported from multiple stings, complete recovery in 3 to 5 days usually occurs.

56–3. **Portuguese Man-of-War stings**

Stings from these marine creatures are relatively common in sports divers. Severe pain, local swelling and severe anaphylactic shock (Topic 24) may occur.

Treatment

1. Remove any adherent tentacles at once, with the hands wrapped in cloth or protected by gloves.
2. Treat shock (Topic 15–7).
3. Wash with water followed by dilute ammonia; coat with sodium bicarbonate paste.
4. Give tripelennamine hydrochloride (Pyribenzamine), 50 mg., orally every 4 hours.
5. Inject 10 ml. of 10% calcium gluconate intravenously.

56–4. **Scorpion stings**

Usually these cause only severe discomfort in adults, but in children they may be dangerous.

Treatment

1. Iced compresses.
2. Control of pain by intravenous calcium gluconate (10 ml. of 10% solution) and rapid-acting barbiturates. Small doses of narcotics may be necessary.
3. Dextrose, 5% in saline, intravenously.
4. Hospitalization for supportive therapy and possible use of antiserum.

56–5. **Sea nettle stings**

Signs and symptoms of toxicity and treatment are the same as outlined for Portuguese Man-of-War stings (56–3, above).

56–6. **Sting ray** (Stingaree).

Wounds caused by the sting ray are common in the South Pacific and have been reported from Gulf of Mexico and California resorts where sport diving is popular. They are characterized by:

1. Large, jagged, irregular wounds which may in themselves be fatal.
2. Severe localized pain or, in some instances, numbness of the whole affected extremity, caused by venom carried in the integumentary sheath of the ray's serrated stinger.
3. Nausea and vomiting.
4. Headache and dizziness.
5. Painful, shallow respiration, with pallor and cyanosis.
6. After 1 or 2 hours, development of severe intractable generalized myalgia, often associated with muscle spasm.

7. Severe shock which may be irreversible and terminal if the chest or abdomen has been penetrated.

Treatment

1. Thorough irrigation of the wound (provided the pleura or peritoneum has not been perforated).
2. Sedation by intramuscular or intravenous barbiturates.
3. Control of severe pain by local heat and morphine sulfate subcutaneously or intravenously.
4. Surgical removal of the serrated stinger or sheath as soon as possible.
5. Hospitalization for care in all cases after treatment of shock (Topic 15–7). Unless extensive debridement is done, large, slow-healing ulcers may develop at the site of the sting.

56–7. **Tropical catfish whiskers**

These can cause severe local reactions. For treatment see 56–3, above.

56–8. **Tropical jellyfish stings**

These cause local pain and generalized myalgia. Severe systemic reactions are rare. This muscle pain usually yields readily to intravenous administration of 5 to 10 ml. of 10% calcium gluconate solution, but in some cases codeine or morphine sulfate may be necessary. Local treatment as given under Portuguese Man-of-War stings (56–3, above) should be used.

56–9. **Wasp (hornet) stings**

Wasp stings may cause reactions similar to, but more severe than, bee stings (56–1, above). Acute anaphylactic reactions (Topic 24) may be terminal. The treatment is the same as for bee stings except that there is no buried stinger to be removed.

56–10. **Wooly worm stings**

Contact with the hollow spines on the dorsal surface of these worms releases a rapidly acting toxin which causes toxic effects.

A. Signs and Symptoms

1. Intense local burning and swelling.
2. Lymphadenopathy.
3. Convulsions.
4. Shock.

B. Treatment

1. Control of severe pain by narcotics.
2. Treatment of shock (Topic 15–7).

     3. Epinephrine hydrochloride (Adrenalin) hypodermically, dosage according to age (Topic 5).

     4. Calcium gluconate, 10 ml. of 10% solution, intravenously.

56–11. Stings of unidentified etiology

Any stings suspected of being dangerously toxic should be treated as follows:

     1. Application of a tourniquet if on an extremity.

     2. Chilling of the site of the sting by ice packs.

     3. Intravenous injection of 10 ml. of 10% calcium gluconate for acute myalgia. If relief is obtained, this injection can be repeated as needed; if not, the tourniquet and ice packs with symptomatic measures should be continued until the patient can be hospitalized for observation.

57. TEMPERATURE VARIATION EMERGENCIES

57–1. Cold injuries (*Cold Allergy or Sensitivity, Chilblain, Foxhole Foot, Frostbite, Immersion Foot, Trench Foot*)

The exact mechanism of injury from exposure to low temperatures is unknown, but vascular changes with sludging of the blood are undoubtedly important factors. There is a wide variation in the ability of different individuals to tolerate cold. The chances of injury by exposure to low temperature are increased by:

     1. A darkly pigmented skin.

     2. Advanced age or poor general physical condition.

     3. Anoxia, as in high altitude climbing or flying.

     4. Previous trauma, especially cold injury.

Accurate determination of the extent of tissue damage at the time of the original examination is impossible.

A. Treatment

     1. Rest in a recumbent position.

     2. Rapid rewarming by moist heat. The solution should be kept between 31° C. (87.9° F.) and 38° C. (100.4° F.).

     3. After rewarming, exposure to air at room tempera-

ture. [Between 21° C. (69.4° F.) and 24.4° C. (76° F.) is most satisfactory.]

4. Administration of analgesics for severe pain. Morphine sulfate, 8 to 15 mg., subcutaneously or intravenously, or dihydromorphinone hydrochloride (Dilaudid), 2 to 4 mg., subcutaneously may be necessary in severe cases; codeine sulfate, 0.06 gm., or meperidine hydrochloride (Demerol), 50 to 100 mg., may give relief if the pain is moderate.

5. Administration of tetanus antitoxin or toxoid (Topic 19).

6. Adequate prophylactic antibiotic therapy.

7. Observation until the extent of damage can be determined.

B. Do Not

1. Rub or compress the affected part with ice, snow or cold water. Massage or friction of any type is harmful.

2. Allow use, especially weight bearing, unless absolutely necessary (evacuation from disaster areas, etc.).

3. Allow excessive use of tobacco or snuff.

4. Apply pressure dressings or ointments of any type.

5. Administer anticoagulants, corticosteroids or vasodilators; they are of no value and may do harm.

6. Debride sloughing areas or perform any type of amputation except in the presence of a spreading virulent infection; unnecessary loss of tissue may result.

57–2. Heat cramps

A. Signs and Symptoms

1. Pale skin; excessive perspiration.

2. Nausea and dizziness.

3. Rapid but strong pulse.

4. Normal or slightly elevated temperature.

5. Extreme thirst.

6. Muscular twitching, sometimes generalized as in epilepsy.

7. Severe abdominal cramps.

B. Treatment

1. Complete rest in a cool place.

   2. Normal salt solution, 1000 ml., intravenously to combat dehydration.
   3. Complete rapid recovery practically always occurs. Hospitalization is generally not required.
57–3. Heat exhaustion (Sunstroke). See 57–8, below.
57–4. Heat stroke (Heat Retention)
   A. Signs and Symptoms
   1. Dry, hot skin; high temperature; fast, full pulse.
   2. Early loss of consciousness.
   3. Dilated pupils.
   4. Deep breathing at first, later becoming shallow and Cheyne-Stokes type.
   5. Offensive body odor.
   6. Muscular twitching.
   7. Epileptiform convulsions.
   B. Treatment
   1. Reduction of body temperature by alcohol sponges, ice compresses, chilled water enemas, evaporation of water sprayed on the body, and application of hypothermia blankets. THE RECTAL TEMPERATURE MUST BE REDUCED TO 39° C. (102.2° F.) OR BELOW.
   2. Administration of cardiac and respiratory stimulants —in severe cases, intravenously.
   3. Control of convulsions by heavy sedation with rapidly acting barbiturates, chloral hydrate or paraldehyde. During convulsions protection from injury, especially tongue biting, and insurance of an adequate airway are essential.
   4. Hospitalization as soon as possible.
57–5. Hypothermia. (For localized effects, see 57–1, above.) Chilling of the whole body from exposure to natural elements or during therapeutic procedures (cardiac and vascular surgery, treatment of certain poisonings, etc.) results in progressive decrease of physiologic processes which eventually becomes irreversible. The ability to survive hypothermia depends on:
   1. Length of exposure.
   2. Inherent constitutional factors; some persons tolerate low temperatures better than others.
   3. Environmental factors (altitude, barometric pressure, humidity).

    4. Physical condition (age, nutritional status, pre-existent disease).

Survival from rectal temperatures as low as 23.3° C. (74° F.) has occurred.

Treatment

A. Slow Rewarming.

    1. Application of blankets.

    2. Determination of urinary output by retention catheter. Intravenous fluids must be limited until kidney function is re-established, usually 12 to 18 hours after treatment is begun.

    3. Careful search for, and treatment of, underlying disease processes. Hypothermia may completely mask the usual signs and symptoms of infection and other diseases and make the effects of commonly used drugs such as digitalis, steroids, insulin and anticoagulants completely unpredictable until the body temperature approaches normal.

B. Rapid Rewarming is necessary if the rectal temperature is close to the lethal limit.

    1. Application of heat under close supervision by any and all means available, including hot fluids by mouth, electric blankets, electric heaters, hot water bottles, gastric lavage with warm solutions, and warm water enemas. The rate of body temperature increase is not related to the methods used and rarely exceeds 0.6° C. (1.2° F.) per hour.

    2. Insertion of a retention catheter for observation of kidney function.

    3. Recognition and symptomatic treatment of the two frequent complications of rapid rewarming:

        a. Cardiac arrythmias which may progress to cardiac arrest (Topic 29–2).

        b. Hypertension.

    4. Recognition and treatment of underlying pathologic conditions (see 57–5,A,3, above).

    5. Avoidance of measures outlined in 57–1,B, above.

57–6.   **Iatrogenic heat stroke.** (Also see 57–4, above.)

During periods of excessively hot weather with high humidity, hospitalized persons with impaired sweat secretion are especially susceptible to heat stroke. The significance of the clinical picture of impending heat stroke may be overlooked or misinterpreted in the following patients:

1. Patients under anesthesia, if drapes and coverings prevent adequate heat loss.
2. Quadriplegics, hemiplegics and paraplegics in whom the perspiration-control mechanism has been short-circuited.
3. Persons on medications which inhibit sweating, especially atropine and its derivatives and phenothiazines.
4. Psychiatric patients whose mental symptoms are dramatic enough to divert attention from signs of impending heat stroke (57-4,A, above).

Treatment. See 57-4,B, above.

57-7. Low salt syndrome

Hot, humid temperatures increase the body's need for salt; hence, the widespread use of salt tablets in industries where high temperatures are the usual environment (steel and aluminum furnaces, engine rooms of ships, etc.).

Infants and small children are peculiarly susceptible to the effects of hot weather salt depletion, which may be confused with other serious conditions such as brain concussion or contusion.

A. Signs and Symptoms

1. Lethargy.
2. Loss of appetite.
3. Nausea and vomiting.
4. Opisthotonus.
5. Convulsive seizures.
6. Stupor deepening into coma.

B. Treatment

1. Oxygen by face mask or tent as required.
2. Intravenous administration of normal saline solution for correction of salt deficiency and fluid imbalance (Topic 7).
3. Control of convulsions by sedative suppositories [dosage according to age (Topic 5)].
4. Prophylactic measures for hospitalized children:
   a. Infants: Daily oral administration of Darrow's solution and glucose water.

b. Older children: Add 0.5 to 1.5 gm. of salt to daily
diet.

57–8. **Sunstroke** (Heat Exhaustion)

A. Signs and Symptoms
1. Pale, clammy skin; normal or subnormal temperature.
2. Generalized weakness.
3. Nausea; occasionally vomiting.
4. Fast and weak pulse; hypotension.
5. Dilated pupils.
6. Stupor deepening into coma.

B. Treatment
1. Loosen clothing.
2. Allow fluids as desired if able to swallow; if not, give
normal saline intravenously.
3. Give stimulants if the pulse is weak or hypotension
is severe.
   a. Strong black coffee by mouth, or caffeine sodiobenzoate, 0.5 gm., intramuscularly.
   b. Amphetamine sulfate, 15 mg., slowly intravenously.
   c. Atropine sulfate, 1.0 to 1.5 mg., subcutaneously
or slowly intravenously.

58. TOOTHACHE

58–1. **Pain** from injuries, disease or extraction of the teeth
may be very severe. Temporary relief of acute discomfort can
often be given.

Treatment
1. Codeine sulfate, 0.03 to 0.06 gm., and acetylsalicylic
acid (aspirin), 0.6 gm., by mouth every 2 to 4
hours.
2. Application of oil of cloves. A local anesthetic ointment such as 4% butacaine (Butyn) with 1:1500
nitromersol (Metaphen) rubbed into the painful
area and surrounding gum tissues will usually
give relief for 4 to 6 hours.

    3. Packing of cavities with a thick paste prepared by mixing oil of cloves and powdered zinc oxide. A few cotton fibers may be added for body.

    4. The need for dental care at the earliest possible opportunity should be stressed.

58–2. Aerodontalgia

A minute pocket of air beneath a filling or cap may cause excruciating pain in divers on ascent to the surface. Treatment consists of replacement of the dental repair even if ordinary methods of detection fail to show any defect.

58–3. Alveolar abscesses. See Topic 23–4.

58–4. Postextraction bleeding. See Topic 8–4,J,3.

59. TOXIC REACTIONS TO AVERAGE DOSES OF COMMONLY USED DRUGS

(For acute poisoning from excessive amounts, see under Topic 49.)

Many individuals are acutely sensitive to therapeutic doses of drugs. The commonly administered or prescribed substances listed in the following paragraphs are some of those which in THERAPEUTIC DOSES may cause symptoms and signs acute enough to require emergency care.

59–1. Acetylsalicylic acid (Aspirin)

Aspirin can cause gastric bleeding in certain individuals.

59–2. ACTH (Adrenocorticotropic Hormone)

This very potent anterior pituitary hormone has many adverse physiologic side effects, any combination of which may bring the patient for emergency care.

    A. Signs and Symptoms

      1. Headaches, dizziness and transient blurring of vision.

      2. Bizarre paresthesias.

      3. Nervousness and insomnia; fatigue and exhaustion.

      4. Psychoneurosis.

      5. Signs of fluid balance disturbance (edema, anasarca, polydipsia, etc.).

      6. Alkalosis with lowered potassium levels.

    B. Treatment. Development of any of the symptoms listed

above calls for immediate discontinuance of therapy and hospitalization for thorough investigation, evaluation and restoration of normal fluid balance (Topic 7).

59–3.　Aminophylline (Theophylline ethylenediamine)

In adult patients this very dangerous drug is often injected intravenously in the treatment of asthma and coronary disease by physicians who are not cognizant of its toxicity or of the marked variation in reactions of different individuals (or of the same individual at different times). The smallest size suppositories commercially available (0.25 gm.) can cause acute toxic symptoms (irritability, restlessness, vomiting, convulsions and respiratory depression) in children under 3 years of age.

A. Signs and Symptoms following TOO RAPID Injection
1. Cardiac palpitation.
2. Mydriasis.
3. Syncope.
4. Death from respiratory and circulatory collapse.

B. Treatment
1. Prophylactic—slow injection.
2. Oxygen inhalations by face mask and rebreathing bag.
3. Caffeine sodiobenzoate, 0.5 gm., subcutaneously in mild cases. Severe cases may go into severe shock and require use of vasoconstrictor drugs (Topic 15–7) for a lengthy period as a lifesaving measure.
4. Immediate hospitalization for observation and symptomatic treatment. Although usually rapidly absorbed, in some individuals aminophylline has a prolonged and cumulative effect.

59–4.　Aminopyrine and antipyrine

(Also known as amidopyrine, aminophenazone, dimethyl-aminoantipyrine, dimethylaminophenazone and pyramidon.) Common commercial preparations are:

Aminophen Pulvules　　　　Felsol Powder and Tablets
Amytal and Aminopyrine　　Optalidon
　　Pulvules　　　　　　　　Ray-Pyrine
Cibalgine

These very toxic preparations are sold without prescription except in Denmark, Sweden and the United States. Therapeutic doses recommended by the manufacturer may cause hypersensitivity reactions—especially agranulocytosis.

For acute toxicity signs and symptoms see *Acetanilid* (Topic 49–11).

59–5. Ammonium chloride

In the presence of even slightly impaired liver or kidney function the usual dose of ammonium chloride continued for a few days may cause accumulation of toxic amounts of ammonia [Topic 3–10 (*Hepatic Coma*)]. Acidosis and coma may develop if long continued use of ammonium chloride has embarrassed ammonia synthesis in the body. Hypoproteinemia also may develop.

If given with sulfonamides the danger of deposit of sulfa crystals in the kidneys is markedly increased.

Treatment is primarily preventive:
1. Limitation of therapeutic use of ammonium chloride to not more than 4 days in persons with normal renal function.
2. Avoidance of administration to persons with impaired liver or kidney function.
3. Avoidance of administration at the same time as sulfonamide therapy.

59–6. Amphetamine (Benzedrine, Dexedrine, D-Desoxyephedrine)

A. Signs and Symptoms
1. Severe headache, irritability and insomnia.
2. Anorexia and diarrhea.
3. Cardiovascular reactions—palpitation, arrhythmias.
4. Acute psychoses.

B. Treatment
1. Stop the medication at once.
2. Start oxygen therapy if necessary.
3. Sedate by rapid-acting barbiturates.

59–7. Anabolic-androgenic steroids

A. Preparations
Methandriol (Neostene, Stenediol)
Methandrostenolone (Dianabol)
Nandrolone phenpropionate (Durabolin)
Norethandrolone (Nilevar)
Oxymetholone (Adroyd, Anadrol)
Testosterone

Indiscriminate use of the basic steroid, testosterone, and its analogues, is common and may result in toxic effects.

B. Signs and Symptoms
1. Liver damage with BSP retention.
2. Sodium retention and edema.
3. Increase in serum cholesterol level.
4. Retarded growth in children due to premature epiphysial closure.
5. Masculinizing effects (acne, hypertrophy of clitoris, penis and prostate, menstrual abnormalities or suppression, abnormal hair growth, voice changes).
6. Acceleration of growth of prostatic carcinoma.

C. Treatment
1. Immediate discontinuance of the steroid preparation.
2. Fluid replacement and balance as required (Topic 7).
3. Symptomatic treatment. Unfortunately, many of the changes outlined above are irreversible.

59–8. Anesthetics, inhalation. [See also *Chloroform* (Topic 49–137) and *Trichlorethylene*, (Topic 49–620).]

The gases most commonly used for inhalation anesthesia are ether, chloroform, nitrous oxide, ethyl chloride and ethylene. Although there is a marked difference in the margin of safety for each gas, the symptoms of toxicity and treatment are approximately the same for all.

A. Signs and Symptoms
1. Deepened unconsciousness.
2. Rapid heart beat.
3. Loss of reflexes.
4. Respiratory and/or cardiac failure.

B. Treatment
1. Stop administration of the anesthetic as soon as any of the signs of incipient cardiac arrest (Topic 29–2,B) develop.
2. Start oxygen inhalations under positive pressure at once, preferably by means of an endotracheal catheter and rebreathing bag.
3. Inject caffeine sodiobenzoate, 0.5 gm., intramuscularly or intravenously.
4. Give pentylenetetrazol (Metrazol), 0.2 gm., intramuscularly.
5. If cardiac arrest occurs, the circulation of the blood must be re-established within 5 minutes if irversible degenerative changes caused by anoxia are to be avoided (Topic 29–2).

59–9. **Anesthetics, intravenous.** See *Pentothal Sodium* (Topic 49–444).

59–10. **Anesthetics, local.** (See also Topic 49–52.)

The widespread use of local anesthesia in present-day medicine and dentistry has resulted in the recognition of three important types of toxic reactions.

A. Allergic Reactions. (See also Topic 24.) This type of toxic reaction occurs in persons who are allergic by heredity (atopic) and fortunately is relatively rare. It may be so overwhelming that death occurs in a few minutes.

Characteristics

1. Skin wheals (Topic 54–16).
2. Angioedema; swelling of the soft tissues of the throat may be severe enough to require tracheotomy (Topic 17–11).
3. Bronchospasm (Topic 53–1).

Treatment

1. The best treatment is prevention. Patients should be questioned regarding any family or personal history of allergy before the local anesthetic is used. In these cases, intracutaneous tests for sensitivity are of absolutely no value. Instead, a small amount of the solution to be used should be applied intranasally by means of an applicator. In an atopic patient, itching, burning and congestion will develop within 10 minutes. If the test is negative, injection of the local anesthetic can be considered as relatively safe; if positive, injection of even a minute amount may be fatal.
2. Maintenance of a clear airway and prevention of anoxia by whatever means are necessary.
3. Epinephrine hydrochloride (Adrenalin), 0.5 to 1.0 ml. of 1:1000 solution, subcutaneously.
4. Tripelennamine hydrochloride (Pyribenzamine), 50 to 100 mg. orally, or 25 to 50 mg. intramuscularly.
5. Hydrocortisone sodium succinate (Solu-Cortef), 100 mg., intravenously.

Prognosis. Complete recovery unless the onset has been overwhelming and fatal. The need for avoidance of the offending drug, or of others of similar chemical structure, should be stressed to the patient. Constant wearing of a "dog tag" specifying the offending substance should be recommended.

B. Immediate Toxic Blood Level Reactions
Causes
1. Accidental injection into a blood vessel.
2. Use of too concentrated a solution.
3. Extremely rapid absorption through an unusually vascular area.

Onset. Acute toxic symptoms develop WITHIN A FEW SECONDS after injection or topical application. If death occurs, it is usually due to complete circulatory and respiratory collapse within 1 or 2 minutes of the onset of the toxic picture.

Treatment. Although in many cases the onset is too overwhelming and death too rapid for any emergency measures to have any effect, the treatment given under Delayed Toxic Blood Level Reactions (next section, below) should be attempted.

C. Delayed Toxic Blood Level Reactions
Cause. A relatively slow development of toxicity due to the gradual building up of a toxic blood level following injection or topical use.

Onset. Never less than 5 or more than 30 minutes after injection or local application. The average time of onset is 15 to 20 minutes.

Signs and Symptoms
1. Gradual development of somnolence which may progress to coma. This sleepy stage in certain persons may be replaced by marked euphoria, excitement and elation. Generally, the patient feels that there is something wrong and will tell the physician so.
2. Progressive decrease in rate and quality of pulse.
3. Development of facial pallor and of a cold and clammy skin.
4. Twitching of the face, hands and feet.
5. Hypotension and syncope.
6. Convulsions.
7. Respiratory and circulatory failure, sometimes irreversible and terminal.

Treatment
1. MENTAL CHANGES require no specific treatment. However, these patients should be watched carefully for at least 30 minutes for evidence of more severe reactions.
2. HYPOTENSION with slow weak pulse, cold clammy skin, intermittent apnea and dyspnea should be treated as primary shock (Topic 15–7).
3. CONVULSIONS must be controlled as quickly as possible by rapid-acting barbiturates. Pentothal Sodium is the drug of choice. Six ml. of a 2½% solution should be injected intravenously, followed by 2 to 3 ml. every 2 minutes until the convulsions have ceased. If Pentothal Sodium is not available, sodium pentobarbital (Nembutal), 0.12 to 0.25 gm., can be given intramuscularly as an initial dose; after 3 minutes 60 mg. more can be given.

Prognosis. Good, if the early symptoms are recognized and proper treatment given; very poor, if extreme hypotension and convulsions are allowed to develop or persist.

59–11. **Antabuse** (Disulfiram). [See also *Thiram* (Topic 49–602) and *Zerlate* (Topic 49–664).]

Two types of reactions to this drug used in the treatment of chronic alcoholism may occur.

A. Side Effects from Administration of Excessive Doses. Although there is marked individual variation in tolerance, one 0.5 gm. tablet daily usually is adequate for the desired therapeutic effect; larger doses increase the incidence of side effects very markedly.

Signs and Symptoms
1. Drowsiness, especially in the morning.
2. Headache.
3. Loss of appetite, with a constant feeling of fatigue.
4. Psychosis. Activation of a previously latent psychosis may occur, but in most cases the drug seems to be the direct cause. This is the only absolute contraindication to the use of disulfiram.

Treatment. Unless a psychosis has developed, nothing is required except reduction of the size of the dose. If psychotic symptoms are present, disulfiram should be discontinued at once and symptomatic treatment begun. Complete recovery within 1 to 2 weeks almost invariably occurs if the drug is the causative factor.

B. Antabuse—Alcohol Reactions may be brought on by ingestion of ALCOHOL IN ANY FORM—drinks, foods cooked in wine, wine vinegar, salad dressing or medications in alcoholic vehicles. Generally, the amount of alcohol ingested determines the severity of the reaction, but in some individuals even small amounts may cause very severe, even dangerous, toxic changes.

Signs and Symptoms

1. Flushed skin, severe headache, burning of the eyes, salivation and dyspnea, coming on within ½ hour after ingestion of the alcohol-containing substances.
2. Nausea and vomiting.
3. Feeling of tightness in the chest. This may be severe enough to be mistaken for a cardiac condition.
4. Hypotension.
5. Cyanosis.
6. Severe shock (Topic 15).

Treatment

1. Mild cases will respond immediately to oxygen inhalations and oral administration of an antihistaminic drug.
2. Severe cases require intravenous administration of diphenhydramine hydrochloride (Benadryl) and immediate shock therapy (Topic 15–7). Chlorpromazine hydrochloride (Thorazine), 50 mg., intramuscularly will usually control severe vomiting.

Prognosis. Complete recovery within a short time. Even if untreated, all except the most severe cases in profound shock will make a complete recovery in 8 to 12 hours.

59–12. **Antibiotics**

A. Achromycin (Tetracycline, Polycycline, Steclin, Tetracyn). See *Tetracyclines* (59–12,I, below).

B. Aureomycin (Chlortetracycline). See *Tetracyclines* (59–12,I, below).

C. **Bacitracin** (Parentracin). Acute hypersensitivity reactions (Topic 24) requiring epinephrine hydrochloride (Adrenalin), oxygen and supportive therapy may result from topical use. In addition, acute renal failure may occur.

Treatment
1. Discontinue use of the antibiotic.
2. Symptomatic supportive therapy.

D. **Chloromycetin** (Chloramphenicol). In addition to all types of allergic reactions (Topic 24), this very valuable antibiotic in therapeutic doses may cause toxic side effects.

Signs and Symptoms
1. Nausea and vomiting.
2. Diarrhea.
3. Mucous membrane lesions.
4. Aplastic anemia and agranulocytosis.

Treatment
1. Discontinue administration at once.
2. Treat acute symptoms due to hypersensitivity (Topic 24).
3. Prescribe bismuth subcarbonate, 5 gm., by mouth every 2 to 4 hours.
4. If possible, stop all antibiotics since cross-sensitization may occur.

E. **Neomycin** (Mycifradin). Hypersensitivity reactions (Topic 24) are rare but do occur; they are relatively mild as compared with the other commonly used antibiotics.

Treatment
1. Discontinue use.
2. Symptomatic and supportive therapy as required.

F. **Penicillin**. This may cause severe anaphylactic reactions (Topic 24). Characterized by rapid onset of muscular twitching and convulsions followed by respiratory and cardiac collapse, this type of overwhelming reaction with a high mortality rate may occur with either oral or parenteral use. More common but less serious allergic reactions usually do not appear until from 4 to 7 days after the first injection or oral dose.

Signs and Symptoms

1. Generalized skin rash often associated with severe persistent itching.
2. Angioedema.
3. Severe myalgia and arthralgia.
4. Occasional convulsions.
5. Blood dyscrasias.

Treatment

1. As a preventive measure, prescribe or administer penicillin in any form ONLY IF THERE IS A DEFINITE INDICATION FOR ITS USE.
2. Stop administration of the antibiotic.
3. Start antihistaminic agents:
   a. In severe cases give diphenhydramine hydrochloride (Benadryl), 5 to 10 mg. in 20 ml. of saline, intravenously, or epinephrine hydrochloride (Adrenalin), 0.5 to 1.0 ml. 1:1000 solution, subcutaneously.
   b. In milder cases prescribe tripelennamine hydrochloride (Pyribenzamine), 50 to 100 mg., orally 3 times a day.
   c. Apply calamine lotion with phenol 1% locally for itching. (Do not compress.)
   d. Hospitalize severe cases, especially those with respiratory embarrassment from edema. Marked skin involvement may require referral to a dermatologist for treatment.

Prognosis. Mild cases usually clear within 12 hours; severe cases may require 5 to 7 days. If administration of penicillin is imperative and the patient gives a history of sensitivity, antihistaminics should be given before, with and after the antibiotic.

G. Streptomycin (Dihydrostreptomycin). In certain individuals therapeutic doses may cause toxic effects.

Signs and Symptoms

1. Urticaria and angioedema; sometimes shock.
2. Varied types of acute skin reactions.
3. Acute conjunctival irritation.
4. Labyrinthitis and deafness, especially in persons with renal impairment.
5. Acute gastrointestinal symptoms.
6. Liver and kidney damage.

7. Cardiac arrhythmias; sometimes cardiovascular collapse.

8. Progressive anemias; agranulocytosis.

Treatment

1. Stop administration of the drug at once.

2. Treat allergic manifestations (Topic 24).

3. Treat shock (Topic 15–7) if present.

4. Hospitalize severe cases.

H. Terramycin (Oxytetracycline). See *Tetracyclines* (59–12,I, below).

I. Tetracyclines (Achromycin, Aureomycin, Polycycline, Steclin, Terramycin, Tetracyn). Overenthusiastic employment of these very useful antibiotics, especially in futile prophylaxis and treatment of minor ailments, has resulted in increasing numbers of:

1. Allergic reactions of all types (Topic 24).

2. Gastrointestinal disturbances, especially persistent diarrhea.

3. Vaginal and anal urticaria from monilial infections.

4. Staphylococcal enteritis.

Treatment

1. Stop use of drug and of all other antibiotics if possible. Cross-sensitization may occur.

2. Give symptomatic and supportive therapy.

59–13. Anticoagulants

Of the commonly used oral anticoagulant drugs, coumarin derivatives have less side effects than those of the indandione group (Danilone, Hedulin).

A. Signs and Symptoms

1. Conjunctivitis; paralysis of ocular accommodation.

2. Nausea and vomiting; bloody diarrhea.

3. Hematuria.

4. Steatorrhea.

5. Jaundice and liver damage.

6. Agranulocytosis.

B. Treatment

1. Discontinue drug.

2. Control of hemorrhage as outlined in Topic 8–4,C.

59–14. Antihistaminics

Signs and Symptoms

1. Drowsiness, dizziness and headaches; sometimes intractable insomnia.

2. Flushing of the skin.
3. Dryness of the mouth.
4. Dilation of the pupils.
5. Nausea and vomiting, diarrhea or constipation.
6. Mental confusion—occasionally visual and olfactory aberrations.
7. Hypotension followed by collapse and unconsciousness.
8. Agranulocytosis.

Treatment
1. Stop administration of the drug at once.
2. Give amphetamine sulfate (Benzedrine), 5 to 10 mg., by mouth or intravenously.
3. Arrange for adequate follow-up medical supervision.

Prognosis. Complete recovery usually occurs within a few hours unless agranulocytosis has developed.

59–15. Belladonna alkaloids. (See also Topic 49–78.)

Especially in children, toxic symptoms from atropine and scopalamine in therapeutic doses are fairly common.

Signs and Symptoms
1. Dry, hot skin with increased temperature.
2. Dryness of the mouth with difficulty in swallowing.
3. Weak and rapid pulse with increased blood pressure.
4. Dilated pupils.
5. Restlessness, confusion and incoordination; sometimes speech disturbances, delirium and convulsions. In elderly arteriosclerotic patients, transient hallucinations are common.
6. Urinary retention, especially if prostatic hypertrophy is present.
7. Respiratory and circulatory depression in severe cases.

Treatment
1. Gastric lavage with 1:5000 potassium permanganate solution if the drug has been taken by mouth.
2. Pilocarpine hydrochloride, 5 mg., subcutaneously; repeat at 20-minute intervals until the dryness of the mouth and the difficulty in swallowing have been controlled.
3. Sodium pentobarbital (Nembutal), 0.1 to 0.2 gm., orally. Chloral hydrate, 1 to 2 gm., by mouth; or paraldehyde, 4 to 6 ml., by mouth or intramus-

cularly, may be given during the acute excitement stage.

4. During the severe depressant stage amphetamine sulfate (Benzedrine), 10 to 20 mg., intravenously, may be of value.

Prognosis. Complete recovery without sequelae unless very severe depressant symptoms are terminal.

59–16. **Chenopodium** (Wormseed). See Topic 49–126.

59–17. **Chlordiazepoxide** (Librium)

This sedative-tranquilizer in commonly used dosages may cause toxic side effects.

1. Hypotension.
2. Mental confusion.
3. Extra-pyramidal disturbances.
4. Edema, especially pretibial.
5. Decreased libido.

Treatment

1. Stop the drug.
2. Give symptomatic treatment for the uncomfortable but not dangerous withdrawal symptoms.

59–18. **Chlorpromazine hydrochloride** (Thorazine). [See also 59–53, below (*Phenothiazines*).]

This valuable drug has multiple actions and may give a wide variety of toxic side effects. Primarily it is a central nervous system depressant but it has also a mild antispasmodic and antihistaminic action. The amount required to cause undesirable side effects varies markedly in different individuals but, in general, these side effects are more uncomfortable than dangerous.

A. Signs and Symptoms

1. HYPOTENSION. Although this is usually mild and transient, it may be very severe and require shock therapy (Topic 15–7). With even small doses the patient should be lying down when the drug is given and kept under observation for at least 20 minutes. Intravenous administration should not be used. Arteriosclerosis and heart disease are definite contraindications to Thorazine therapy.

2. DROWSINESS AND DIZZINESS. These symptoms are transient but may occur after small oral doses. All patients receiving chlorpromazine hydrochloride (Thorazine) should be warned against driv-

ing a motor vehicle for 30 to 40 minutes after taking the drug.

3. TRANSIENT SYNCOPE.

4. TACHYCARDIA.

5. ALLERGIC REACTIONS. Generally a mild urticaria (Topic 24).

6. PARKINSONIAN SYNDROME SYMPTOMS. These may follow very large doses but will disappear rapidly on cessation of therapy.

7. AUTONOMIC NERVOUS SYSTEM SYMPTOMS (nasal congestion, dryness of the mucous membranes, constipation, etc.). These are mild and require no treatment.

8. SECONDARY SYMPTOMS. These may be caused by the tendency of chlorpromazine to accentuate and prolong the effects of sedatives, narcotics, analgesics and anesthetics.

9. JAUNDICE. This is usually transient and benign.

B. Contraindications to Chlorpromazine Therapy

1. Arteriosclerotic or cardiovascular disease.

2. Coma due to alcohol, barbiturates or opiates (Topic 3).

3. Recent administration of large doses of sedatives, analgesics, narcotics or anesthetics, because of the prolongation and accentuation of the effect caused by chlorpromazine.

C. Prognosis. Good for rapid, complete recovery. The drug has a wide margin of safety.

59–19.   **Colchicine.** See Topic 49–154.

59–20.   **Cortisone.** See Topic 49–160, and 59–2, above (*ACTH*).

59–21.   **Dicodid** (Eucodal). See Topic 49–186.

59–22.   **Dicumarol.** See Topic 49–187.

59–23.   **Diethylstilbestrol.** See Topic 49–190.

59–24.   **Digitalis.** See Topic 49–191.

59–25.   **Dilantin** (Sodium Diphenylhydantoinate). See Topic 49–193.

59–26.   **Ephedrine**

Overdosage usually occurs as a result of too frequent use of ephedrine-containing nose drops or sprays.

A. Signs and Symptoms

1. Nervousness, tremor and insomnia.

   2. Headaches and dizziness.

   3. Dyspnea and weak pulse.

   4. Excessive perspiration.

   5. Dilation of the pupils.

   6. Precordial pain and palpitation.

B. Treatment

   1. Stop administration of the drug at once.

   2. Give sodium pentobarbital (Nembutal), 0.1 to 0.2 gm., by mouth, or sodium phenobarbital, 0.1 to 0.2 gm., intramuscularly for sedation.

C. Prognosis. Complete recovery in from 4 to 6 hours.

59–27. Epinephrine (Adrenalin)

In certain hypersensitive persons even minimal therapeutic doses may produce uncomfortable but rarely dangerous symptoms. For clinical picture and treatment, see Topic 49–214.

59–28. Ergotamine (Gynergen)

Therapeutic doses may cause acute ergot poisoning. See Topic 49–218.

59–29. Eserine. See under *Physostigmine* (Topic 49–463).

59–30. Estrogens

These may cause true drug addiction with increased tolerance and withdrawal symptoms.

Treatment

   1. Controlled withdrawal.

   2. Sedation as required.

   3. Psychotherapy if indicated.

59–31. Fowler's solution. See Topic 49–63 (*Arsenic*).

59–32. Glucagon

Used in the treatment of insulin shock (Topic 3–3,D) this substance increases the blood sugar at the expense of liver glycogen. Too rapid intravenous injection of the usual dose (0.5 to 1.0 mg.) may cause transient nausea, vomiting and hypotension. No treatment is required.

59–33. Gold salts. See Topic 49–257.

59–34. Heparin. See Topic 49–266. For treatment of hemorrhage see Topic 8–4,C.

59–35. Homatropine. See Topic 49–274.

59–36. Hyoscine. See Topic 49–71 (*Atropine Sulfate*).

59–37. Imipramine (Tofranil)

Used in the treatment of severe mental depression, this drug has many side effects.

Signs and Symptoms
1. Disturbance of motor function; tremor.
2. Hypotension; syncope.
3. Increased intra-ocular tension.
4. Jaundice.
5. Parkinsonian-like symptoms.
6. Cardiac arrhythmias; sometimes congestive failure.

These manifestations of toxicity usually clear slowly when the drug is discontinued.

59–38. Insulin. For differential diagnosis and treatment of insulin shock, see Topic 3–3.

59–39. Lithium chloride. See Topic 49–320.

59–40. Mecholyl (Acetyl-beta-methylcholine). See Topic 49–334.

59–41. Meprobamate (Equanil, Miltown). (See also Topic 49–336.)

Usual doses may cause toxic side effects.

A. Signs and Symptoms
1. Drowsiness or excitement; generalized muscle weakness.
2. Acute hypersensitivity reactions (Topic 24).
3. Gastric distress with abdominal cramping, flatulence and diarrhea.
4. Diplopia.

B. Treatment
1. Withdrawal or reduction of dosage of the drug.
2. Treatment of hypersensitivity reactions (Topic 24).

59–42. Mercury diuretics. See Topic 49–345.

59–43. Methenamine (Urotropin). See Topic 49–354.

59–44. Methyl salicylate (Oil of Wintergreen). See Topic 49–363.

59–45. Methysergide maleate (Sansert)

This congener of ergonovine is used for prevention of migraine attacks. Its toxic effects are similar to those caused by ergot (Topic 49–218), plus the following:
1. Acute apprehension and excitement.
2. Nightmares.
3. Hallucinations.
4. Precipitation of psychotic states.

Treatment
1. Discontinuance of the drug.
2. Sedation as required.
3. Therapy as given under ergot (Topic 49–218).

59–46. Metrazol (Pentylenetetrazol). See Topic 49–364.

59–47. Mineral oil

Habitual use may cause fibrosis of the lung or even pneumonia. The section of the lung involved depends on the user's position in bed after his nightly dose.

59–48. Muscle relaxant drugs

The toxic effects of average doses of drugs commonly used for muscle relaxation are uncomfortable but rarely serious. Among these drugs are:

Carisoprodol (Soma, Rela)   Orphenadrine citrate (Norflex)
Chlormethazanone (Trancopal) Phenyramidol hydrochloride
Chlorzoxazone (Paraflex)   (Analexin)
Methocarbamol (Robaxin)   Styramate (Sinaxar)

Signs and Symptoms

1. Drowsiness and apathy.
2. Anorexia; nausea (rarely vomiting).
3. Headache.
4. Dizziness.
5. Dryness of the mouth and throat.

All disappear slowly when the drug is discontinued.

59–49. Myochrysine. See Topic 49–257 (Gold Salts).

59–50. Oxyquinoline derivatives. See Topic 49–428.

59–51. Paraldehyde. See Topic 49–437.

59–52. Phenacemide (Phenurone)

This anticonvulsant drug may cause severe, even terminal, liver damage. Early signs of toxicity resemble infectious hepatitis (Topic 63–8,A). The hepatic damage is reversible if detected early.

59–53. Phenothiazines

Used widely in the treatment of gastrointestinal and psychiatric complaints, phenothiazines may cause characteristic side effects following average as well as excessive doses.

A. Common Preparations

Chlorpromazine (Thorazine)   Thiopropazate (Dartal)
Methoxypromazine (Tentone)   Trifluoperazine (Stelazine)
Perphenazine (Trilafon)   Triflupromazine (Vesprin)
Prochlorperazine (Compazine)   Trimeprazine (Temaril)

B. Extrapyramidal Reactions

1. Dyskinesia and dystonia.
   a. Opisthotonus with intense cervical muscle spasm.
   b. Facial muscle spasm (trismus, sardonic grin, etc.).

    c. Protrusion and lack of control of the tongue.

    d. Bizarre involuntary movements of the extremities.

    e. Embarrassment of respiration.

  2. Parkinsonian symptoms.

    a. Drooling.

    b. Tremor.

    c. Rigidity; abnormal posture and gait.

  3. Restlessness and turbulence.

    a. Inability to relax or sit quietly (akathisia).

    b. Profuse speech.

Treatment

1. Discontinue or decrease the dose of the medication.
2. Give diphenhydramine (Benadryl), 25 mg. intravenously, or 50 mg. intramuscularly; in milder cases, oral administration may be substituted.
3. Administer barbiturates for sedation.
4. Support respiration as needed.
5. If continuation of phenothiazine therapy is necessary, decrease the dosage and give antiparkinsonian agents.

C. Hypotension and Shock. For treatment see Topic 15–7.

D. Jaundice, Dermatitis and Agranulocytosis. These may persist for lengthy periods after the drug has been stopped.

E. Somnolence. This usually clears rapidly when the phenothiazine is discontinued.

59–54. Phenylbutazone (Butazolidin) and **Oxyphenbutazone** (Tandearil)

Both of these drugs have very important toxic side effects.

A. Signs and Symptoms

1. Acute gastrointestinal symptoms including activation of healed ulcers.
2. Fluid retention.
3. Acute skin changes; sometimes very severe exfoliative dermatitis.
4. Stomatitis.
5. Sore throat.
6. Serious progressive blood changes which may develop rapidly, even with small doses, and which may be irreversible.

B. Prevention and Early Recognition of Toxic Reaction

1. Limitation of dosage to 300 mg. daily. A base-line complete blood count should be established.

    2. Discontinuance at the end of one week if no clinical improvement.

    3. Hematologic examinations every week for the first 6 weeks of treatment; then every 4 to 6 weeks for as long as therapy is continued.

C. Treatment

    1. Stop administration at once.

    2. Symptomatic care, local or general. Mild cases, as a rule, do well under home care; severe cases require hospitalization for control of edema and fluid imbalance, transfusion, etc.

59–55. **Phenylhydrazine.** See Topic 49–454.

59–56. **Picrotoxin.** See Topic 49–465.

59–57. **Posterior pituitary extracts.** Apparently, considerable variation in the tolerance of the human organism for these substances exists. The most commonly used extracts are posterior pituitary (Pituitrin), oxytocin (Pitocin) and vasopressin (Pitressin). All are oxytocic agents and all may cause toxic effects.

A. Signs and Symptoms

    1. Nausea, vomiting and intestinal cramping.

    2. Extreme facial pallor.

    3. Cramping similar to menstruation in women.

B. Treatment. No physiologic antagonist to posterior pituitary extracts is known; therefore, symptomatic treatment consisting of oxygen inhalations, sedation by barbiturates and moderate doses of vasopressor drugs is all that is indicated.

C. Prognosis. Complete and rapid disappearance of symptoms, provided the offending extract has been discontinued.

59–58. **Privine** (Naphazoline Hydrochloride). See Topic 49–477.

59–59. **Pyrogallol.** See Topic 49–486.

59–60. **Quinicrine** (Atabrine). See Topic 49–492.

59–61. **Quinidine**

A. Indications of Cardiotoxicity

    1. Ventricular premature beats—1 or more every 6 normal beats.

    2. ECG changes (increase of QRS width).

    3. Fibrillation (ventricular).

    4. Circulatory collapse.

    B. Treatment. Intravenous administration of 100 to 125 ml. of molar sodium lactate solution.

59–62.   Rauwolfia serpentina (Reserpine, Raunorine)

Rauwolfia in therapeutic doses may cause toxic side effects.

    A. Signs and Symptoms
1. Epistaxis secondary to nasal congestion.
2. Acute gastrointestinal symptoms; occasionally, flare-ups of healed ulcers.
3. Acute colitis simulating an acute surgical abdomen.
4. Acute mental depression.
5. Parkinsonism.

    B. Treatment. Decrease in dosage or stopping the administration of the drug usually results in spontaneous and complete clearing of symptoms.

59–63.   Saccharin. See Topic 49–507.

59–64.   Salicylates. See Topic 49–511.

59–65.   Salyrgan (Mersalyl and Theophylline). See Topic 49–345 (*Mercury Diuretics*).

59–66.   Serum reactions

    A. Serum Disease
1. ONSET. Seven to 12 days after injection of antiserum. Horse serum is the most common offender.
2. SIGNS AND SYMPTOMS
    a. Severe headache accompanied by a high temperature.
    b. Diffuse erythema usually followed by urticarial wheals with severe itching and marked edema.
    c. Nausea, vomiting and abdominal cramping.
    d. Generalized adenopathy.
    e. Severe joint and muscle pain.
3. TREATMENT
    a. *Mild Cases*
      (1) Control of itching by sodium bicarbonate paste or calamine lotion.
      (2) Tripelennamine hydrochloride (Pyribenzamine), 50 to 100 mg., orally every 4 hours.
    b. *Severe Cases*
      (1) Epinephrine hydrochloride (Adrenalin), 0.5 to 1.0 ml. 1:1000 solution, subcutaneously.
      (2) Procaine (0.1% solution) injected SLOWLY intravenously. The usual dose is 4 mg. per kilogram of body weight administered over

a 20 to 30 minute period. The development of any of the symptoms of an atopic or toxic blood level procaine reaction (59–10, B, above) calls for immediate discontinuance of the injection.

4. PROGNOSIS. Complete recovery, although uncomfortable and sometimes disabling symptoms may persist for 10 to 14 days.

B. Serum Shock

1. ONSET. Immediately following injection. Death may occur in a few minutes from respiratory and circulatory collapse. Horse serum is the most frequent offender.

2. TREATMENT

a. Prevention is the only sure treatment. INTRA-CUTANEOUS (INTRADERMAL) TESTS FOR SENSITIVITY SHOULD ALWAYS BE DONE BEFORE ANTISERUM OF ANY TYPE IS GIVEN, although the absence of dermal hypersensitivity does not always indicate that there will be no general hypersensitivity reaction. If the intracutaneous test is positive, the method outlined in Topic 14 for desensitization should be used if administration of antitoxin is essential, and no other animal or human antiserum is available. Daily intake of a sustained release capsule of an antihistaminic may prevent, or decrease the severity of, the hypersensitivity reaction.

b. Epinephrine hydrochloride (Adrenalin), 1 ml. of 1:1000 solution intramuscularly if the patient shows any signs of serum shock.

c. Oxygen inhalations under positive pressure by face mask or catheter and rebreathing bag.

d. Caffeine sodiobenzoate, 0.5 gm., subcutaneously or intramuscularly. Support of the blood pressure by controlled intravenous infusion of 4 ml. of a 0.2% solution of arterenol bitartrate (Levophed) in 1000 ml. of 5% dextrose in saline may be necessary.

e. Hospitalization for observation and treatment if the patient survives the initial shock. This applies even if complete recovery apparently has taken place.

3. PROGNOSIS. Full-fledged serum shock may be overwhelming and rapidly fatal, but if the patient survives for 5 minutes or more there is a good chance that he will make a complete recovery. If proper intracutaneous (intradermal) skin tests (Topic 14) are done and interpreted accurately, serum shock will rarely occur.

59–67. **Sodium thiocyanate.** See Topic 49–600 (*Thiocyanates*).

59–68. **Sulfonamides.** (See also Topic 49–569.) Toxic manifestations of greater or lesser degree occur in about 50% of adults and 20% of children. Although the symptoms may be very alarming, few fatalities have been reported.

A. Minor Toxic Effects

1. Fever, usually accompanied by skin rashes suggestive of measles.
2. Cyanosis.
3. Gastrointestinal irritation.
4. Precordial and abdominal pain.
5. Acidosis.
6. Central nervous system disturbances: confusion, restlessness, headache, vertigo, nausea and vomiting, depression or elation, and lassitude.

Treatment

1. Temporary decrease or discontinuance of the drug.
2. Administration of oxygen by face mask and rebreathing bag.
3. Referral of the patient if possible back to the physician who prescribed the medication. A brief summary of the symptoms, signs and treatment should be sent with the patient.

B. Dangerous Toxic Effects

1. SKIN RASHES. Generalized, very serious, exfoliative dermatitis may occur, sometimes associated with hepatitis.
2. JAUNDICE. The causative acute hemolysis apparently has no relationship to the level of sulfonamides in the blood. There is usually an associated hemoglobinuria.
3. ACUTE HEMOLYTIC ANEMIA with hemoglobinuria, severe leukopenia and agranulocytosis.
4. RENAL CALCULI with resultant suppression of kidney function.

Treatment
1. Discontinue all sulfonamides at once.
2. Transfer to a hospital equipped for the complete laboratory studies essential for accurate evaluation and proper therapy.

59–69. Thiazide diuretics

This group of drugs has practically replaced mercurial diuretics for oral use. Among the preparations available are:

Benzydroflumethiazide (Naturetin)
Benzthiazide (NaClex)
Chlorothiazide (Diuril)
Flumethiazide (Ademol)
Hydrochlorothiazide (Esidrex, Hydro-Diuril, Oretic)
Hydroflumethiazide (Saluron)
Methyclothiazide (Enduron)
Polythiazide (Renese)
Quinethazone (Hydromox)
Spironolactone (Aldactone)—a thiazide plus a mercurial diuretic
Trichlormethiazide (Metahydrin, Naqua)

Usual therapeutic doses of any of these may cause many side effects, including aggravation of pre-existent systemic conditions such as diabetes and gout and accentuation of the effects of drugs such as digitalis. Potassium depletion often requires replacement therapy (Topic 7).

Other Side Effects Are
1. Muscular weakness.
2. Gastroenteritis.
3. Pancreatitis.
4. Jaundice; hepatic cirrhosis.
5. Glomerulonephritis.
6. Photosensitization.
7. Blood dyscrasias (rare).

Treatment
1. Discontinuance of offending thiazide.
2. Symptomatic therapy is all that is required except in extreme cases requiring correction of potassium depletion (Topic 7).

59–70. d-Tubocurarine chloride (Tubadil). See Topic 49–168 (*Curare*).

59–71. Vitamin K₁

Therapeutic doses may cause flushing, sweating and a sense

of constriction of the chest. Acute allergic reactions (Topic 24) are fairly common. In certain susceptible persons usual doses may cause hypotension, rapid irregular pulse, severe chest pain, cyanosis and coma.

Recovery occurs rapidly under symptomatic supportive therapy after the drug has been discontinued.

59–72. Viosterol. See Topic 49–644.

60. VASCULAR DISORDERS

Various types of severe catastrophes can occur from acute pathology involving the vascular system (arteries, veins and lymphatics).

60–1. Arterial injuries

Immediate recognition of severe injuries to major arteries, followed by prompt and proper surgical treatment, may be life-saving or may eliminate the necessity for amputation. Modern surgical techniques allow repair of the aorta, axillary, brachial, iliac, femoral and popliteal arteries. Even small arteries sometimes may be repaired successfully under a microscope.

A. Types of Arterial Injury

1. CONTUSIONS. Vasospasm resulting from damage to the intima may give the same clinical picture and results as complete transection.

2. COMPRESSION against a bony prominence, usually near the elbow or knee.

3. LACERATIONS may result in fatal hemorrhage or in superficial or deep hematomas. Bleeding may be more pronounced than with complete severance because the injured vessel cannot retract into the surrounding soft tissues.

4. SEVERANCE—complete.

B. Signs and Symptoms of Severe Arterial Damage

1. HEMORRHAGE of spurting bright red blood if open; rapid development of a tense hematoma if closed. Exsanguination may occur unless immediate control is accomplished (Topic 8–1).

2. DECREASED OR ABSENT PULSATIONS in the arteries distal to the injury.
3. SHOCK (Topic 15).
4. INTENSE PAIN from ischemia.
5. INCREASED, DISTURBED OR DECREASED SENSATION; tingling, numbness.

C. Treatment
1. CONTROL OF HEMORRHAGE (Topic 8–1). This may be a lifesaving measure.

METHODS
a. Application of a pressure bandage.
b. Clamping with a hemostat just proximal to the injury. To prevent additional damage to the artery the hemostat should be placed as close as possible to the site of injury.
c. Packing with sterile gauze.
d. Application of a tourniquet to an extremity proximal to the injury. The pressure of the tourniquet must be above arterial systolic pressure. Every effort should be made to preserve collateral circulation.

2. TREATMENT OF SHOCK (Topic 15–7).
3. RELEASE OF COMPRESSION by reduction of displaced fractures or dislocations. This should be done as soon as evidence of arterial compression is recognized, or whenever the possibility of compression of a major artery is suspected from the position of the bone fragments or joint surfaces.
4. HOSPITALIZATION for definitive surgical care AS SOON AS POSSIBLE in all cases of known or suspected major arterial damage. The time lag between injury and repair must be kept to a minimum for a successful result.

60–2. **Intracranial bleeding.** See also Topic 43–18.
A. Epidural Hemorrhage. See Topic 43–20; and Topic 48–22 (*Extradural Hemorrhage in Children*).
B. Intracerebral Hemorrhage
1. ETIOLOGY
a. Degeneration of cerebral arteries and arterioles secondary to arteriosclerosis and atherosclerosis.
b. Hypertension.

c. Blood dyscrasias, either primary or secondary to medications such as anticoagulants (Topic 8–4).

d. Trauma.

e. Damage of arterial walls secondary to arteritis, infection and toxins.

2. SIGNS AND SYMPTOMS

a. Sudden onset, usually with activity.

b. Intense headache.

c. Nausea and vomiting.

d. Coma (frequently).

e. Neurologic signs of paralysis and paresis depending upon location and extent of hemorrhage.

f. Blood in the spinal fluid. Secondary meningeal irritation may be present.

3. TREATMENT

GENERAL SUPPORTIVE MEASURES

a. Clear airway and maintain patency.

b. Treat shock (see Topic 15–7); use caution in increasing blood pressure above adequate perfusion level as further hemorrhage may occur.

c. Institute preventative skin and joint care at once; turn every 2 hours, pad pressure areas and properly position joints.

d. Maintain hydration and electrolyte balance (Topic 7) intravenously if the patient is unconscious or stuporous.

e. Give sedatives as necessary for pain and restlessness. Avoid narcotics.

SPECIFIC MEASURES

a. Treat any contributing blood-clotting disorders [as from heparin or warfarin-like drugs (Topic 8–4)].

b. Reduce moderate to severe hypertension cautiously. Rapid reduction with inadequate perfusion levels (although "normal") may cause the clinical condition to deteriorate.

C. **Subarachnoid Hemorrhage** of severe degree occurs most frequently from a ruptured saccular aneurysm. Signs, symptoms and precipitating causes are similar to those outlined under intracerebral hemorrhage (60–2,B, above); however, in general, the onset is more catastrophic, the coma is more severe, and the cerebrospinal fluid shows more red blood cells.

TREATMENT AND PROGNOSIS. Treatment is similar to that outlined for intracerebral hemorrhage (60–2,B,3, above) except that surgery may provide definitive therapy. If the only neurologic signs are meningeal irritation from blood, IMMEDIATE angiograms, followed by surgery if indicated, give the best statistical chance of survival. Hypothermia may be of value in some cases.

D. Dissecting Aneurysm. The defect which leads to weakening of the aortic wall is usually cystic central necrosis. Increased stress on the aortic wall from hypertension, trauma and extreme exertion may precipitate acute changes.

1. SIGNS AND SYMPTOMS
   a. Abdominal or thoracic pain which may be excruciating or minimal, sudden or progressive.
   b. Evidence of widening of aorta by palpation or aortography.
   c. Pallor, sweating and shock (Topic 15).
   d. Discrepancy in the blood pressure and pulses between the two arms or between the arms and the legs.
   e. Signs of ischemia or infarction of the brain, spinal cord, myocardium or kidney.

2. TREATMENT
   a. Immediate hospitalization.
   b. Absolute rest.
   c. Barbiturates and opiates as necessary for control of restlessness, pain and apprehension.
   d. Treatment of shock (Topic 15–7). The blood pressure should be kept at a level just high enough to maintain perfusion of vital organs. Cautious reduction of moderate or severe hypertension is indicated.
   e. Evaluation for possible surgical treatment.

3. PROGNOSIS. The mortality is in the 75 to 80% range.

60–3. Embolism

An embolus of either cardiac or noncardiac origin may cause infarction of any organ of the body. The diagnosis is usually made by evidence of sudden infarction and/or malfunction of the involved organ plus determination of the presence of a probable source of the embolus. In general, emergency therapy is designed to be supportive, to reduce the source or likelihood of other emboli and to allow performance of a surgical embolectomy if indicated and possible.

A. Cerebral Embolism usually is caused by a cardiac source such as myocardial infarction, chronic atrial fibrillation or endocarditis. The onset of symptoms and signs, which correspond to the cerebral artery occluded, is sudden.

Treatment
1. Supportive.
2. Variable results have been reported following surgical removal of emboli lodged in the carotids; even in the middle cerebral artery.
3. Anticoagulation may be considered for reduction of thrombotic emboli if evidences of infection and secondary hemorrhage are *not* present.

B. Pulmonary Artery Embolism
1. MASSIVE EMBOLISM, large enough to plug one of the main branches of the pulmonary artery itself.

TREATMENT. Since sudden collapse and death within 5 minutes usually occurs, little can be done except gentle restraint and oxygen inhalations while awaiting the extent of the involvement.

2. EMBOLISM OF A MEDIUM-SIZED BRANCH OF THE PULMONARY ARTERY
a. *Signs and Symptoms* vary with the size and location of the occluded artery but, in general, are characterized by SUDDEN ONSET of:
(1) Severe agonizing pain in the chest.
(2) Pallor or cyanosis.
(3) Extreme anxiety and apprehension. Unless in collapse, the patient is generally sitting up, panting for air, with a look of terror on his face. Hemoptysis, sometimes severe, may occur.
(4) Although large infarcts sometimes can be located by careful percussion and auscultation or a pleural friction rub may be present, physical examination is often within normal limits.

(5) Shock (Topic 15).

(6) Sudden rise in temperature or pulse rate.

(7) X-rays may show the area of infarction or some pleural effusion but often are within normal limits.

(8) Electrocardiograms are of little value for early diagnosis although an incomplete right bundle branch block or right axis deviation may be present.

b. *Prophylactic Treatment.* Persons who have had previous emboli, cardiac patients, those suffering from phlebothrombosis, thrombophlebitis and varicose veins, and victims of accidents seem to be especially prone to develop pulmonary emboli. Although prophylactic treatment is not properly a part of emergency care, the essential features are outlined here because their importance is so often overlooked. The measures given below should be carried out, if possible, with the patient under absolute control in a hospital.

(1) Maintenance of proper fluid balance and prevention of dehydration (Topic 7).

(2) In postoperative patients, insistence on early activity and frequent changes in position. Active and passive leg exercises should be encouraged.

(3) Application of heat to the legs but not above body temperature.

(4) Application of compression bandages or elastic stockings from toes to midthigh.

(5) Administration of anticoagulant therapy under careful control and observation. Heparin is the drug of choice.

3. EMBOLUS OF PERIPHERAL ARTERIES. Whether the blocking of a peripheral artery is due to embolism, thrombus or arteriosclerosis, the emergency treatment is the same. Recognition of the condition and proper handling may be the deciding factors in saving a limb or life.

a. *Signs and Symptoms*

(1) Acute pain, usually very severe.

  (2) Pallor, coldness and numbness of the affected extremity. Elevation causes increased pallor.

  (3) Lack of pulsation in the arteries distal to the lesion.

  (4) Puffiness and pitting edema if there is venous involvement.

 b. *Treatment*

  (1) Lower the extremity.

  (2) Relieve pain and vasospasm by:

   (a) Morphine sulfate, 15 to 30 mg., subcutaneously or intravenously.

   (b) Papaverine hydrochloride, 0.2 gm., by mouth.

   (c) Codeine sulfate, 60 mg., subcutaneously.

   (d) Atropine sulfate, 0.6 mg., subcutaneously or intravenously.

  (3) Apply local heat, but not above body temperature.

  (4) Transfer to a hospital as soon as possible since immediate embolectomy or nerve blocks may be indicated. Transportation should be by ambulance with the leg DOWN.

  (5) After obtaining control specimens, anticoagulation therapy, preferably with heparin, may be begun if indicated.

4. AIR EMBOLISM (Arterial Embolism). [See also Topic 26–5 (*Diving Hazards*).] In an adult of average weight, 100 to 150 ml. of air in the vascular tree is usually considered to be a lethal amount, although the speed of entry, pressure and position of the patient may cause marked variations in the amount which can be tolerated.

 a. *Etiology*

  (1) Intrinsic air in the alveoli, pulmonary cavity, or pleural cavity (pneumothorax).

  (2) Extrinsic air injected during diagnostic procedures, open operations and traumatic incidents, or aspirated from the fallopian tubes. Arteriovenous fistulas are rare causes.

 b. *Signs and Symptoms*

  (1) Dizziness.

   (2) Cold and clammy skin; thready pulse; extreme hypotension.
   (3) Dyspnea and cyanosis often followed by Cheyne-Stokes respiration.
   (4) Convulsions and coma.
   (5) Localized neurologic signs (hemiplegia, blindness, etc.).

c. *Confirmatory Findings*
   (1) Detection of air in the retinal vessels by ophthalmoscopic examination.
   (2) Appearance of sharply defined areas of pallor in the tongue (Liebermeister's sign) and of "marbling" of the skin.
   (3) Bubbling of air mixed with blood from a skin incision.
   (4) X-ray demonstration of air in the cerebral vessels.
   (5) Coronary involvement with characteristic electrocardiographic changes.

d. *Treatment*
   (1) Keep the patient's head down.
   (2) Give symptomatic supportive therapy (artificial respiration, oxygen under positive pressure, support of circulation, etc.).
   (3) Hospitalize immediately for further treatment.

60–4. Syncope (Fainting, Vasodepressor Syncope)

Transient loss of consciousness is not a serious condition unless the patient injures himself in falling. Various mechanisms may lead to collapse of arterial vasomotor tone and temporary insufficiency of cerebral circulation; thorough investigation should be made to determine the underlying cause. See Topic 51–9,C, for differential diagnosis.

Treatment
   1. Recumbent position until recovered.
   2. Prevention of repeated falling; instructions for gradual arising in orthostatic hypotension.
   3. Treatment of any injuries sustained in falling.
   4. Inhalations of aromatic spirits of ammonia.
   5. Ephedrine, 25 mg. to 50 mg., orally.

60–5. Thromboangiitis obliterans (Buerger's Disease)

The extremely severe pain caused by this progressive condition may bring the patient for emergency relief.

Treatment of Acute Episodes

1. Bed rest with the involved extremity in such a position that it does not blanch.
2. Papaverine hydrochloride, 30 to 60 mg., intravenously. Larger doses, up to 100 mg. intravenously, may be given with safety in severe cases.
3. Tetraethylammonium chloride (Etamon), 200 mg. dissolved in 4 ml. of physiologic salt solution, intravenously. This solution should be given very slowly with close observation for the onset of hypotension, nausea and abdominal distention.
4. For severe pain, codeine sulfate, morphine sulfate or dihydromorphinone hydrochloride (Dilaudid) can be given, AFTER THE PHYSICIAN HAS MADE SURE BY THOROUGH EXAMINATION AND A CAREFUL HISTORY THAT THE PATIENT IS NOT ADDICTED TO THESE DRUGS.
5. Hospitalization may be indicated if the acute pain cannot be controlled by the measures given above, or if the patient is addicted to narcotics.

60–6. Thrombosis

A. Cerebral and Major Arteries of Neck. Signs, symptoms and treatment are similar to emboli (60–3, above) occurring in the same arteries, except that the onset is frequently slower. Thrombolysins have not proved their value in emergency treatment. Use of anticoagulation in the emergency situation is equivocal, and statistics favor nonuse except in vertebral-basilar artery thrombosis. Surgery for thrombectomy is usually too late for preservation or restoration of cerebral function.

B. Peripheral Artery Thrombosis. See 60–3, above.

60–7. Transient focal cerebral ischemia ("Paradoxical Stroke")

Recurrent episodes of cerebral ischemia lasting from seconds to a few minutes may give any of the signs and symptoms of a "stroke," but the patient reverts to his prior normal state.

Treatment

1. Obtain and record an accurate history of events.
2. Refer the patient to a vascular surgeon for diagnostic work-up. Surgical removal of large atherosclerotic lesions in major branches of the aortic arch and arteries of neck may prevent recurrences.

3. Anticoagulation is effective in reducing the number of recurrences.

60–8. Venous air embolism

A. Etiology

1. Associated with pregnancy and its complications (curettage, Rubin test).
2. Following diagnostic injections of air (peritoneum, pleura, subarachnoid space).
3. Retroperitoneal trauma.
4. Operations on the head and neck and on the genito-urinary tract.
5. Accompanying administration of fluids into, or removal of blood from, any vein.
6. Changes in atmospheric pressure [Topic 26 (*Barotrauma*)].

B. Signs and Symptoms

1. Deep inspiration followed by coughing exhalation; then a few attempts at breathing followed by apnea.
2. Hypotension; pulse very weak or imperceptible.

C. Treatment

1. Immediate left lateral position.
2. Artificial respiration followed by administration of oxygen under positive pressure by endotracheal catheter and rebreathing bag.
3. Aspiration of air from the right atrium by open operation or through the chest wall in urgent cases. Open operation is preferable.
4. Hospitalization as soon as the patient's condition will allow.

60–9. Phlebothrombosis

Few clinical signs may be produced even by the sudden development of large intravenous clots, usually in the deep veins of the lower extremities. These thrombi may become dislodged because of their strong retractile power. Phlebothrombosis is the most common cause of pulmonary embolism (60–3,B, above).

A. Signs and Symptoms

1. Moderate elevation of temperature.
2. Unilateral leg edema with enlargement of thigh and calf.

  3. Positive Homans' sign (pain in the calf of the involved leg on forced dorsiflexion of the foot).

B. Treatment
  1. Absolute rest. Physiologic quiet for the involved extremity is essential.
  2. Application of moist heat.
  3. Application of a snug elastic bandage.
  4. Elevation of the limb.
  5. Referral to a hospital for observation and care. Transfer should be by ambulance with minimal handling of the patient.
  6. Anticoagulation, initially with heparin.

60–10. Thrombophlebitis

  A. Etiology. The cause of thrombophlebitis is probably a diseased vein, with infection and varicosities contributing factors. The commonest sites are the veins of the lower extremities, especially the femorals and iliacs, although veins in any portion of the body may be involved.

B. Signs and Symptoms
  1. Severe pain with redness and induration over the course of the vein.
  2. Fever, sometimes chills.
  3. Swelling of the extremity.
  4. Emboli may become detached and cause pulmonary occlusion of varying degrees of severity (60–3,B, above). This is much less common with thrombophlebitis than with phlebothrombosis.

C. Treatment
  1. Rest, preferably in bed.
  2. Heat (hot, moist compresses are best) at about body temperature.
  3. Elevation of the extremity about 6 inches above the heart level to allow lymphatic venous drainage.
  4. Avoidance of dehydration by oral and intravenous administration of fluids (Topic 7).
  5. Antibiotics may be of benefit.
  6. Hospitalization if the condition persists, if massive deep involvement is present, or if any signs of breaking loose of emboli are present. Thrombectomy followed by anticoagulant therapy is the treatment of choice in many instances.

     7. Evaluation for paravertebral block if severe pain and reflex arterial vasoconstriction are present.

60–11. **Varicose veins**

  A. Esophageal Varices. See Topic 39–4,A and B.

  B. Hemorrhoids. See Topic 39–6,C.

  C. Postinjection Thrombophlebitis. Inflammation of a vein wall of varying degrees of severity may follow local injection of varicose veins with sclerosing solutions. For treatment see 60–10,C, above.

  D. Postligation Hemorrhage. Bleeding may occur several days after surgical procedures for ligation of veins, especially of the lower extremities.

Treatment

    1. Sedation by barbiturates subcutaneously or intravenously.

    2. Application of local pressure.

    3. Hospitalization if bleeding is persistent or if blood loss has been extreme.

  E. Pruritus Due to Varicose Eczema. The itching caused by chronic eczema, especially that secondary to degenerative changes in the vessels of the lower legs, may be severe enough to bring the patient for emergency care.

Treatment

    1. Sedation by barbiturates.

    2. Application of local anesthetic preparations such as calamine lotion with 1% phenol (DO NOT BANDAGE OR COMPRESS) or dibucaine (Nupercaine) ointment.

    3. Referral to a dermatologist for definitive care.

  F. Rupture of a Varicose Vein of an Extremity. Rupture of a varicosity may be spontaneous or traumatic and may cause stubborn and persistent bleeding severe enough to result in secondary anemia. The bleeding is rarely sufficiently severe to cause symptoms of shock.

Treatment

    1. Elevate the extremity; restrict activity.

    2. Apply direct pressure by an elastic bandage or gauze fluffs held in place by roller elastic bandage.

    3. Administer sedation as needed, preferably by rapid-acting barbiturates.

4. Place mattress sutures of No. 40 or 50 cotton, under local anesthesia if necessary.
5. Refer for further surgical care, preferably within 24 hours.

G. Varicose Ulcers with Secondary Infection and Cellulitis
Treatment
1. Limit activity.
2. Elevate the extremity.
3. Give penicillin, 600,000 units, intramuscularly, supplemented by tetracyclines orally.
4. Apply petrolatum or bacitracin (Parentracin) gauze dressings covered with fluffs and an elastic bandage for gentle pressure.
5. Hospitalize if the cellulitis is extensive or spreading in spite of conservative treatment or if the cooperation of the patient in regard to limitation of activity cannot be obtained.

60–12. **Subdural hemorrhage.** [See also Topic 43–21; and Topic 48–8 and 28 (*Head Injuries in Children*).]

This condition usually arises from a tear in one of the cerebral veins entering the dural sinuses, caused by direct trauma to the frontal or occipital region. Since the hemorrhage is venous and its pressure less than in extradural hemorrhage, signs are slower in developing, sometimes requiring weeks. However, acute subdural hematoma, suspected on the basis of alteration of conscious state, unilateral pupillary dilation, focal sensory and motor changes will require emergency care.

    Treatment: Hospitalization for diagnostic localizing examinations and for burr hole procedures.

60–13. **Lymphatic system emergencies**
    A. Lymphangitis. Uncontrolled infection in an extremity, frequently of streptococcal origin, will cause involvement of the lymphatics and adjacent blood vessels. The condition is identified by pain, tenderness, swelling and characteristic red streaks in the involved extremity.

    Treatment
1. Antibiotics, broad spectrum or penicillin.
2. Moist heat and hypertonic solutions such as magnesium sulfate locally.
3. Rest and elevation of the extremity.
    B. Obstruction. Enlargement of lymph nodes secondary to

various types of pathology (infection, neoplasm) may cause acute obstruction of the superior vena cava or extrahepatic bile ducts.

Treatment is primarily referral of the patient to a surgeon for definitive procedures.

61. VENEREAL DISEASES

61–1. Chancre (Hard Chancre)

[See 61–6 (*Primary Lesions*).] No medication or treatment which might block the diagnosis should be prescribed, or be allowed to be applied, until a darkfield examination has been done.

61–2. Chancroid (Soft Chancre)

No emergency treatment is indicated. The patient should be referred to a physician or to a venereal disease clinic for care and should be warned against the application of medications of any type, since this may block diagnosis by darkfield examination.

61–3. Gonorrhea

No matter what history is given by the patient, if a urethral discharge is present in a male, a smear should be taken by the attending physician and, if facilities are available, stained and examined. Additional smears and cultures should be sent to a laboratory for examination. The same applies to females with profuse whitish vaginal discharge. If the clinical picture is that of gonorrhea, the treatment should be started without waiting for the laboratory findings.

Treatment

1. Penicillin, 600,000 units, intramuscularly daily for 3 days.
2. Sulfadiazine, 2 gm. at once, followed by 1 gm. three times a day for 3 days.
3. General measures:
    a. Support of the scrotum and contents by a suspensory or athletic supporter.
    b. Limitation of activity.
    c. Intake of large amounts of fluids, avoiding alcoholic drinks of all types.

   4. Instruction to male patients to obtain further medical
      attention within 3 days even if the discharge
      clears. Female patients should be impressed with
      the need for gynecologic care as soon as possible.

For prophylactic measures see 61–9 (below).

Gonorrhea is a reportable disease (Topic 12).

61–4. Lymphopathia venereum (Venereal Lymphogranuloma,
Lymphogranuloma Inguinale)

This is caused by a virus which is transmitted by sexual
contact.

A. Signs and Symptoms

   1. Minute, often undemonstrable, lesions at site of
      entry.
   2. Development of enlarged lymphatic nodes ("buboes")
      which may suppurate and become fistulous.
   3. Scarring and stricture of the rectum.

B. Treatment

   1. Instruction regarding sterilization of dressings, cloth-
      ing, towels, etc.
   2. Penicillin, 600,000 units, intramuscularly.
   3. Sulfadiazine, 1 gm., orally every 4 hours.
   4. Arrangement for further medical care or reference
      to a public health clinic.

61–5. Syphilis

61–6. Primary lesions (Chancres)

These should not receive emergency treatment. The patient
should be told not to apply any medication of any type but to
report to his physician or to a venereal disease clinic as soon
as possible for diagnosis and treatment.

61–7. Secondary lesions require no emergency treatment.

61–8. Tertiary (late) syphilis

A. Gastric Crisis in Tabes

This condition may simulate an acute surgical abdomen.
Since the vomiting is of central origin, the usual antispasmodics
are of little value.

Treatment

   1. Put the patient to bed and give a retention enema
      prepared as follows:

> Chloral hydrate, 2–4 gm.
> Sodium bromide, 2–4 gm.
> Water to make 15 ml.

2. If 1, above, does not give complete relief after 2 or 3 hours of observation, the patient should be hospitalized.

3. The use of morphine sulfate and other opiates or synthetic narcotics should be avoided in gastric crises because of the strong possibility of addiction. Codeine sulfate in effective doses may be given orally, subcutaneously or intramuscularly.

B. Lightning Pain in Tabes

Treatment. Any and all types of therapy are symptomatic, empirical and usually unsuccessful.

1. Penicillin, 600,000 units, intramuscularly.
2. Thiamine hydrochloride, 20 mg., intravenously.
3. Narcotics may be necessary but should be used with caution because of possible addiction. Codeine sulfate is the narcotic of choice.

C. Paretic Mental Disturbances

These conditions all require hospitalization after temporary control of the patient by large doses of barbiturates and/or chloral hydrate. Physical restraint is often necessary until adequate sedation can be accomplished. Chlorpromazine hydrochloride (Thorazine), 50 to 100 mg., intramuscularly may assist markedly in sedation.

61–9. Prophylaxis

A. **If Facilities Are Available,** the following venereal prophylactic routine may be used for male patients at the discretion of the physician:

1. Have the patient urinate.
2. Instruct the patient to wash the external genitalia thoroughly with soap and water.
3. Irrigate the anterior urethra with either
   a. Potassium permanganate solution 1:8000, or
   b. Mild protein silver solution, 10%.
      The patient should be shown how to prevent extension into the posterior urethra by pressure at the base of the penis.
4. Rub 2 to 4 gm. of mild mercurous (calomel) ointment, preferably containing 10% sulfathiazole, into the genitals and surrounding area.
5. Give penicillin, 600,000 units, intramuscularly.
6. Instruct the patient to report to his physician or to a public venereal disease clinic for further care.

B. If Facilities and Time Are Not Available for the procedure outlined above, the patient should be:

1. Referred to his physician for care.
2. Given the address of the closest public health prophylactic station.
3. Given 600,000 units of penicillin intramuscularly.
4. Instructed in the procedures above and given prescriptions for the necessary medications for home use.

C. Female Patients should be instructed to obtain medical care at once. Penicillin, 600,000 units, should be given intramuscularly, together with instructions for cleansing and douching.

61–10. **Reporting of syphilis**

The reverse side of the standard Confidential Morbidity Report (Topic 12) must be completed.

SYPHILIS Diagnostic Information·

INFECTIOUS
- ☐ PRIMARY
- ☐ SECONDARY
- ☐ EARLY LATENT

EPIDEMIOLOGIC NOTE: TO MINIMIZE SPREAD, PROMPT CONTROL MEASURES ARE ESSENTIAL. PLEASE PHONE REPORTS FOR INFECTIOUS CASES.

NON-INFECTIOUS
- ☐ LATE LATENT
- ☐ NEUROSYPHILIS, ASYMPTOMATIC
- ☐ NEUROSYPHILIS, CLINICAL
- ☐ CARDIOVASCULAR
- ☐ OTHER LATE_____
- ☐ CONGENITAL   SPECIFY

REMARKS

REQUEST MORBIDITY BOOKS	NUMBER	NAME AND ADDRESS

DEPARTMENT OF PUBLIC HEALTH

Reverse side of Confidential Morbidity Report. (See page 47.)

62. VENOMS

SOURCE	LOCAL REACTION	TYPE OF TOXIC REACTION	SEVERITY	DANGEROUS TO LIFE?
Ants (except fire ants) (Topic 27–2)	Severe	Endothelial	++	Only to hypersensitive persons
Bee (Topic 56–1)	Moderate	Endothelial	++ (Acute sensitivity common)	No, except in cases of extreme sensitivity
Black widow spider (Topic 27–5)	Severe pain for 10–15 minutes, recurrence later	Neurotoxic	++ to ++++	Rarely fatal in adults unless an especially vascular part of body has been bitten; high mortality in children
Brown spider (Topic 27–6)	Blebs followed by sloughing	Necrotizing	++	No
Bushmaster (Topic 27–17)	Marked swelling	Hemolytic and neurotoxic	++++	Yes
Cantril (Topic 27–17)	Swelling and discoloration	Hemolytic, neurotoxic and hemotonic	++++	Yes
Centipede	Moderate pain, swelling	Local irritant only	+	No
Cobra (Topic 27–17)	Minimal	Hemolytic and neurotoxic	++++	Yes
Copperhead (highland moccasin) (Topic 27–17)	Severe pain and swelling	Mixed hematoxic and neurotoxic	++++	Yes; death is caused by a curare-like paralysis (see Topic 49–168)

Coral snake (harlequin snake) (Topic 27–17)	Minimal	Neurotoxic	+++	Yes
Fer-de-lance (Topic 27–17)	Severe local pain	Neurotoxic	++++	Yes
Fire ants (Topic 56–2)				
Flea (Topic 27–11)	Varies in individuals	Allergic reactions common	+	No
Gila monster (Topic 27–12)	Severe	Hematoxic	+++	Yes; mortality rate is 1% an adults, 5% in small children
Insects (hymenoptera, Topic 56)	Moderate; allergic reactions common	No systemic reaction unless transmitters of disease or acute allergic reaction	+	Fatalities may occur from anaphylactic reactions (Topic 24)
Mosquito (Topic 27–15)	Varies, may be severe	Allergic	+ to ++	No
Rattlesnake (Topic 27–17)	Marked swelling and discoloration	Mixed hematoxic, neurotoxic and histaminic	++++	Yes, about 11% of reported rattlesnake bites are fatal
Sandflies (Topic 27–16)	Very slight	Febrile, acute arthralgic	++	No
Scorpion (Topic 56–4)	Usually numbness, rarely severe pain	Hemolytic and neurotoxic	+++	Yes, 100% fatal in children under 1 year; adults generally survive
Tarantula (Topic 27–19)	Moderate to very severe, especially in children	None	++	No

SOURCE	LOCAL REACTION	TYPE OF TOXIC REACTION	SEVERITY	DANGEROUS TO LIFE?
Wasp (hornet, yellow jacket) (Topic 56–9)	Moderate	None	++ (Acute sensitivity common)	Only in hypersensitive persons
Water moccasin (cottonmouth, gapper, trapjaw) (Topic 27–17)	Moderate pain and swelling	Mostly neurotoxic, but some hematoxic	+++	Yes
Water snakes (common type) (Topic 27–17)	Moderate due to tooth marks	None	+	No
Wood ticks (certain varieties) (Topic 27–20)	None	Neurotoxic	++	Yes, progressive paralysis may cause death if tick is not completely removed (Topic 27–20,C)

63. VIRUS INFECTIONS

63–1. **Arbovirus infections** (Arthropod-borne Viruses)
    A. Syndromes
        1. Encephalitis or meningoencephalitis caused by numerous viral strains:
          a. Eastern equine.
          b. Western equine.
          c. St. Louis.
          d. California.
          e. Japanese B.
          f. Russian spring-summer and diphasic meningo.
          g. Murray Valley (Australia).
        2. DENGUE-LIKE FEVERS (63–4, below). 3 to 7 days days duration.
          a. Colorado tick fever.
          b. Sandfly fever (Topic 27–16).
          c. Chikungunya and o'nyong nyong fevers (Africa).
        3. HEMORRHAGIC FEVERS
          a. Yellow fever (63–24, below; and Topic 32–38).
          b. Hemorrhagic fevers of South Asia, Crimea and Argentina.
          c. Kyasanur Forest disease (India).
            All tend to occur in epidemics and all except the dengue-like fevers result in considerable mortality.
    B. Treatment. No specific therapy is available. Antibiotics are of no value and should be used only in the presence of bacteriologic complications. Efficient symptomatic and supportive care are very effective.

63–2. **Chickenpox** (Varicella). See Topic 32–3.

63–3. **Common cold.** [See also Topic 53–3 (*Coryza*).]
    A. Signs and Symptoms
        1. General malaise.
        2. Coryza, sore throat, cough.
    B. Treatment. Symptomatic only. The following measures may be advised although the most effective measures (1 and 2, below) will rarely be carried out by the patient.

1. Bed rest.
2. Large amounts of fluids by mouth.
3. Acetylsalicylic acid (aspirin), 0.6 gm., orally every 4 hours.
4. Mild sedation by small doses of barbiturates by mouth.
5. Phenylephrine hydrochloride (Neo-Synephrine) nose drops (0.25% buffered solution). Amphetamine (Benzedrine) inhalers may give temporary relief; however, excessive or prolonged use will result in rebound edema of the mucous membranes.
6. Any thick, syrupy cough mixture to allay throat tickling. Brown mixture and elixir terpin hydrate, with or without codeine sulfate or dihydrocodeinone bitartrate (Hycodan), are satisfactory. Vaporizers or aerosols may give subjective relief.

63–4. **Dengue** (Dandy Fever, Breakbone Fever)

This acute but rarely fatal virus infection is transmitted by the *Aedes* mosquito. Although it is more common in tropical climates, it has been reported in more temperate zones. The incubation period is 5 to 10 days.

A. Signs and Symptoms

1. Sudden rise in temperature—39.4 to 40.6° C. (103 to 105° F.).
2. Slow pulse.
3. Intense headache with general malaise and prostration, often associated with severe myalgia and arthralgia, especially of the muscles of the back.
4. Cyanotic, blotchy appearance of the face.
5. Soreness behind the eyeballs with severe pain on eye movements.
6. Generalized adenopathy with splenic enlargement.
7. Deferred appearance of a generalized morbilliform rash, usually starting on the back of the hands and feet.
8. Leukopenia.

B. Treatment

1. Bed rest, preferably in a darkened room to minimize movements of the eyes.
2. Large doses of salicylates, with or without codeine, by mouth for headache and hyperpyrexia.

3. Calcium gluconate, 10 ml. 10% solution, intravenously for acute muscle and joint pain.

C. Prognosis. Complete recovery in from 10 to 14 days. Hospital care is necessary.

63–5. **Encephalitis, acute**

Many conditions which have been reported as being due to infectious organisms are grouped together under this general heading. (See 63–1,A,1, above.) In addition, the following clinical entities are among those which may manifest themselves as encephalitis:

1. Chickenpox (Topic 32–3).
2. Measles (Topic 32–15).
3. Mumps (Topic 32–17).
4. Herpes simplex (63–9, below; and Topic 37–14).
5. Lymphopathia venereum (Topic 61–4).
6. Poliomyelitis (Topic 32–21).

A. Laboratory investigation is necessary to determine the etiology since, in general, all are characterized by the following signs and symptoms:

1. High fever, often to 41.1° C. (106° F.).
2. General malaise; acute restlessness.
3. Severe headache.
4. Severe, generalized myalgia; sometimes palsies.
5. Delirium, convulsions (especially in children) and coma. Blood specimens for identification of viral strains must be refrigerated, packed in special containers, and sent at once to a properly qualified laboratory.

B. Treatment

1. SYMPTOMATIC
   a. Tepid sponges to reduce fever.
   b. Codeine sulfate, 0.03 gm., and acetylsalicylic acid (aspirin), 0.6 gm., by mouth for headaches.
   c. Chloral hydrate, 0.5 to 1.0 gm., by mouth; repeated as necessary for adequate sedation.
   d. Barbiturates, preferably sodium pentobarbital (Nembutal), 120 to 200 mg., intravenously for extreme restlessness or convulsions.
2. Immediate transfer to a hospital equipped for isolation and treatment.

63–6. **Foot and mouth disease** (Aphthous Fever)

This is characterized by a moderate temperature elevation

and the formation of vesicles on the buccal membrane of the mouth and between the fingers and toes. The acutely contagious virus may be transmitted from infected animals by milk and butter.

> *Treatment.* Symptomatic only. Mouthwashes may be prescribed. Complete recovery within 2 weeks is to be expected.

63–7.   **German measles** (Rubella). See Topic 32–24.

63–8.   **Hepatitis**

Two types are recognized:

> **A. Infectious Hepatitis.** IH is characterized by an abrupt acute onset, usually with a high fever. It is transmitted by oral secretions and has an incubation period of 15 to 60 days.
>
> *Treatment.* Immediate hospitalization. Hemorrhagic complications may be serious.
>
> **B. Homologous Serum Hepatitis.** SH is transmitted by administration of infected blood or plasma or by the use of inadequately sterilized instruments. This type is rarely encountered as an emergency because its onset is usually insidious, with an incubation period of 2 to 5 months.
>
> *Treatment.* Hospitalization on a nonemergency basis for study, determination of the amount of liver damage, and supportive therapy.

63–9.   **Herpes simplex.** (See also Topic 37–14.)

All adults probably have latent infection. Vesicles may form when the body resistance is low for any reason, or after direct stimuli such as bright sunlight. Encephalitis may be a serious complication, especially in children.

> *Treatment.* Local application of zinc oxide ointment to prevent cracking and secondary infection, followed by referral to an internist or dermatologist for further care, is all that is required in most cases, unless the eyes are involved (Topic 37–14). In some cases injection of proteolytic enzymes (Protamide) will give subjective relief and prevent the development of acutely painful postherpetic neuralgia. Acute encephalitis requires immediate hospitalization (see 63–5, above).

63–10.   **Influenza.** (See also Topic 32–11.)

> **A. Incubation Period.** 1 to 5 days.

B. Signs and Symptoms
1. Sudden onset, usually with acute catarrhal symptoms and fever of 38.9 to 40.6° C. (102 to 105° F.).
2. Severe, generalized myalgia; chest pain.
3. Marked pharyngitis and purulent bronchitis, often associated with sinusitis. In children, otitis media (Topic 34–12,B) may develop. Pneumonia, usually involving both lower lobes, may occur.
4. Acute gastrointestinal symptoms.
5. Leukopenia.

C. Treatment
1. Home care is usually possible except when a severe pneumonic process is indicated by clinical or x-ray examination.
   a. Bed rest.
   b. Large amounts of fluids, especially fruit juices, by mouth.
   c. Soft diet.
   d. Magnesium sulfate (Epsom salts), 30 gm., or citrate of magnesia, 240 ml., by mouth.
   e. Phenylephrine hydrochloride (Neo-Synephrine) nose drops (0.25% buffered solution).
   f. Control of high fever by repeated sponging or application of cold compresses. These measures, with sedation by sodium pentobarbital (Nembutal) suppositories, are essential to prevent the development of convulsions or coma in children.
2. Antibiotics and sulfonamides have no effect on influenzal conditions and should be used only for associated bacterial infections.

63–11. **Interstitial pneumonia** (Virus Pneumonia)
[See also Topic 48–41 (*Pneumonia in Children*).] The etiology of acute interstitial pneumonia may be a filterable virus or a specific rickettsial organism.

A. Incubation Period. 10 to 14 days.

B. Signs and Symptoms
1. Insidious onset with constitutional symptoms more marked than respiratory symptoms.
2. Severe headaches and general malaise.
3. Slight intermittent temperature rise, usually not over 38.8° C. (102° F.). Pulse relatively slow.

4. Minimal physical signs in the lungs.
5. Striking x-ray changes: .
   a. Increase in size of hilar shadow.
   b. Soft, patchy infiltration, most marked near the hilum. Parts of more than one lobe may show changes.
6. Normal or decreased white blood count.

C. Treatment

1. Acetylsalicylic acid (aspirin), 0.6 gm., with or without codeine sulfate; or sodium salicylate, 1 gm., with sodium bicarbonate, orally every 4 hours for joint and muscle pain. If the myalgia is very severe, 10 ml. of 10% calcium gluconate intravenously may give relief.
2. Large amounts of fluids by mouth or intravenously if the patient shows evidence of dehydration (Topic 7).
3. Oxygen therapy if dyspnea or cyanosis is present.
4. Ammonium chloride or dihydrocodeinone bitartrate (Hycodan) cough mixtures.
5. Bed rest at home is generally adequate. Hospitalization is rarely necessary.

D. Prognosis. Complete recovery almost invariably occurs. Complications are rare although extreme weakness and lassitude may persist for several weeks.

63–12. **Lymphopathia venereum.** See Topic 61–4.
63–13. **Measles** (Rubeola). See Topic 32–15.
63–14. **Mumps** (Epidemic Parotitis). See Topic 32–17.
63–15. **Myositis** (Myofibrositis). See Topic 45–10.
63–16. **Pleurodynia**

Supposedly caused by a virus, pleurodynia may be encountered as an emergency because of the sudden onset of high fever associated with rapid breathing and acute chest pain. In children, acute abdominal pain may simulate a surgical emergency.

Treatment

1. Bed rest.
2. Codeine sulfate, 0.06 gm., and acetylsalicylic acid (aspirin), 0.6 gm., by mouth. Morphine sulfate in small doses subcutaneously may be necessary for relief of acute pain in older children and adults.

3. Because acute symptoms usually subside in 24 hours
    with recurrence within a few days, medical
    check-up during the quiescent period should be
    recommended.

63–17. Poliomyelitis (Infantile Paralysis, Heine-Medin Disease). See Topic 32–21; and Topic 47–5.

63–18. Psittacosis (Ornithosis, Parrot Fever)

A history of contact with parrots, parakeets, lovebirds, or laboratory birds or animals infected with the disease is essential for a provisional diagnosis of psittacosis. The disease has also been reported in pheasants and barnyard fowl.

A. Incubation Period. 5 to 21 days.

B. Signs and Symptoms
1. Acute onset with chills, general malaise and fever to
    40.6° C. (105° F.). The pulse remains relatively
    slow.
2. Splitting headache.
3. Photophobia.
4. Nausea and vomiting.
5. Herpetic skin lesions.
6. Acute sore throat. Pulmonary involvement with persistent cough and signs of patchy consolidation
    may develop in a few hours.
7. Severe cases may show pinkish oval papular lesions
    on the trunk, and develop diplopia, hallucinations
    and stupor.

C. Treatment
1. Control of headaches by oral administration of codeine sulfate, 0.06 gm., and acetylsalicylic acid
    (aspirin), 0.6 gm., every 4 hours.
2. Morphine sulfate, meperidine hydrochloride (Demerol), or dihydromorphinone hydrochloride (Dilaudid) may be given IN SMALL DOSES subcutaneously for very severe pain but if possible
    should be avoided.
3. Chloramphenicol (Chloromycetin), 250 mg., orally
    every 4 hours if hospitalization is delayed.
4. Transfer as soon as possible to a hospital equipped
    to handle acute infectious diseases.

63–19. Rabies (Hydrophobia)

This acute infectious disease has been reported in badgers, bats (insectivorous and vampire types), cats, coons, coyotes, dogs, foxes, jackals, mongooses, skunks, squirrels, wildcats and wolves. It may be transmitted to human beings by:

1. A bite of a rabid animal.
2. Licking of any superficial abrasion of the skin by a rabid animal.
3. Contact of oral secretion from a patient suffering from rabies with any break in the attendant's skin.
4. Exposure to (possibly inhalation of) dust in caves infested with rabid bats.

A. Incubation Period. Two weeks to 12 months, usually 15 days to 5 months.

B. Signs and Symptoms

1. Redness, swelling and pain around the healed scar at the point of entry.
2. Severe encephalitic symptoms—headache, insomnia, restlessness, irritability and increased sensitivity to stimuli.
3. Development in 2 or 3 days after the initial symptoms of an acute excitement stage characterized by:
   a. Extreme restlessness with intermittent maniacal outbursts.
   b. Spasm of the muscles of deglutition and respiration.
   c. Frothing at the mouth, bloody saliva and vomitus.
   d. Slow rise in temperature to 41.7° C. (107° F.).
4. Terminal paralytic stage characterized by complete total exhaustion, coma and death from complete cardiac collapse.

C. Treatment

1. IF THERE IS NO SUSPICION OR PROOF THAT THE ANIMAL IS RABID, the treatment should consist of
   a. Local cleansing. Lacerations should be thoroughly washed with green soap and water, debrided, irrigated and sutured.
   b. Administration of tetanus antitoxin (3000 to 5000 units) intramuscularly after testing for sensitivity and densensitization if necessary (Topics 14 and 19). A booster injection of tetanus toxoid may be substituted or added if the patient gives a history of adequate active immunization.

   c. Penicillin, 300,000 to 600,000 units, intramuscularly followed by chlortetracycline (Aureomycin) or oxytetracycline (Terramycin), 250 mg., every 4 hours by mouth.

   d. Immediate reporting of the incident to the proper local authorities for impounding, observation and possible postmortem examination of the animal. As a rule, impounded animals are kept under observation for 10 days; if they show no evidence of illness during this period, the danger of rabies is negligible. THE ANIMAL SHOULD NEVER BE DESTROYED by the victim, his family or friends; if it has been killed, the body must be saved and turned over as soon as possible to the proper public health authorities.

  2. IF THE ANIMAL IS KNOWN TO HAVE, OR SUSPECTED OF HAVING, RABIES, treatment should consist of:

   a. Thorough local cleansing of the wound with green soap and water. Lacerations should be spread and the depths of the wound washed thoroughly. Puncture wounds should NOT be probed or extended surgically because of the danger of spreading the virus.

   b. Administration of tetanus antitoxin (3000 to 5000 units) after testing for sensitivity to horse serum and desensitization if necessary (Topic 14). If the patient has been actively immunized at any time in the past, a booster of tetanus toxoid should be given in addition to the antitoxin.

   c. Administration of hyperimmune serum (HIS), 55 units per kilogram (2.2 lb.) of body weight, and/or rabies vaccine (RV) as outlined in 63–19,E, below. Hyperimmune serum must be given as soon as possible; it has no effect after 72 hours.

D. Treatment of Established Rabies

  1. Transfer to a properly equipped hospital as soon as possible.

  2. Give morphine sulfate, 15 to 30 mg., subcutaneously or intravenously AS OFTEN AS NECESSARY TO CONTROL PAIN.

3. Control convulsions and spasm by:
    a. Ether, chloroform or ethyl chloride inhalations—
       to the point of coma if necessary.
    b. Chloral hydrate, 1 to 3 gm., rectally.
    c. Tribromoethanol (Avertin), 60 to 100 mg., rectally.
4. ALL PERSONS WHO COME IN CONTACT WITH THE PA-
   TIENT MUST WEAR RUBBER GLOVES AND OBSERVE
   EXTREME PRECAUTIONS. The saliva, even if dry,
   is very infectious for 12 to 18 hours.

E. Treatment Outline

TYPE OF EXPOSURE	CONDITION OF ANIMAL At Time of Exposure	After 10 Days' Observation	TREATMENT HIS = Hyperimmune Serum. RV = Rabies Vaccine (Duck Embryo)
Licking—skin intact	Rabid	Dead	RV daily × 14
Licking—abrasions present	Rabid	Dead	HIS daily × 2; RV daily × 14
	Healthy	Signs of rabies	Start RV at first sign
Bites other than of face and head	Healthy	Healthy	None
	Healthy	Signs or proof of rabies	Start RV at first signs
	Signs suggestive of rabies	Healthy	Start daily RV at once; discontinue on 5th day if animal is healthy
	Rabid, escaped, not identified, any wild animal	—	HIS daily × 2; RV daily × 14
Bites of face or head	Healthy	Healthy	HIS daily × 2
	Signs suggestive of rabies	Healthy	HIS daily × 2; RV daily—discontinue on 5th day
	Rabid, escaped, not identified; any wild animal		HIS daily × 2; RV daily × 14

F. Prognosis. Rabies has a very high mortality rate if the disease has become established. Fortunately, the lag in the development of symptoms after exposure allows time for observation of the animal and laboratory proof of rabies by examination of the brain for Negri bodies. Recent development of a fluorescent-dye method by which rabies can be detected in animals in 15 minutes may allow more prompt and efficient management of suspected cases of rabies in the near future.

63–20. **Sandfly fever**

This fever is caused by a virus transmitted to humans by sandfly bites. Its course is brief and never fatal.

A. Signs and Symptoms
1. Fever—usually not over 39.4° C. (103° F.)—lasting 3 to 4 days.
2. Painful joints and muscles.
3. Slow recovery of normal strength; weakness and lassitude often persist for several weeks.

B. Treatment
1. Limited activity, preferably bed rest.
2. Copious fluids.
3. Local heat and codeine sulfate, 0.03 gm., and acetylsalicylic acid (aspirin), 0.6 gm., for myalgia. Severe cases may require intravenous injection of 10 ml. of 10% calcium gluconate solution.

63–21. **Smallpox** (Variola). See Topic 32–30.

63–22. **Trachoma**

This infectious conjunctivitis is due to a virus which is spread by personal contact. It may cause severe scarring; occasionally, blindness.

Treatment
1. Instruction regarding disposition of infected handkerchiefs, towels, etc.
2. Sulfadiazine, 0.5 to 1 gm., by mouth 3 times a day.
3. Penicillin, 600,000 units, intramuscularly.
4. Sulfathiazole ophthalmic ointment.
5. Reference to an ophthalmologist.

63–23. **Whooping cough** (Pertussis)

This is probably caused by the Borget-Gengou bacillus in symbiosis with the virus.

Treatment. See Topic 32–37.

63–24. **Yellow fever.** (See also Topic 32–38.) In this age of rapid transportation when intercontinental travel within the 3- to 6-day incubation period is not only possible but common, the physician must be aware of this very serious virus infection transmitted by the *Aedes aegypti* mosquito. Yellow fever is still endemic in parts of South America and West Africa.

A. Incubation Period. 3 to 6 days.

B. Signs and Symptoms
  1. INITIAL STAGE
      a. Sudden onset of chills and fever, associated with severe headache, particularly in the frontal area.
      b. Temperature to 40° C. (104° F.). THE PULSE GOES DOWN WHILE THE FEVER GOES UP.
      c. Generalized acute myalgia.
      d. Red eyes, bloated face.
      e. Anorexia, nausea; occasionally, vomiting.
      f. Apparent remission after 2 to 3 days.
  2. MIDDLE STAGE
      a. Severe vomiting with coffee-ground appearance of the vomitus.
      b. Extreme thirst, acute dehydration.
      c. Gastrointestinal hemorrhage.
      d. Extreme generalized jaundice.
      e. Anuria, or scanty urine with marked albuminuria.
  3. FINAL STAGE. A crisis usually occurs on the sixth or seventh day; either the patient dies or the beginning of recovery is indicated by rapid fall of body temperature and increased secretion of urine.

C. Treatment. No specific therapy is known. Immediate hospitalization is indicated since the outcome will depend to a considerable extent upon adequate nursing care. Symptomatic treatment, especially for dehydration, should be given before and during transfer for hospitalization.

64. WARTIME EMERGENCIES

Injuries and illnesses of every conceivable type and severity may result among the civilian population during wartime as a result of bombing of various types. Explosions, bullet and shrapnel wounds, poison gases, and bacterial and viral infections, burns, concussions, contusions, dislocations, fractures, infections and contagious diseases, lacerations, perforating wounds, the effects of "nerve gases" and radioactivity, and aggravation of pre-existent conditions may all require the best possible treatment in the shortest possible time. When tremendous numbers of casualties occur, as in area saturation bombing or nuclear blasts, on-site treatment must of necessity be restricted to the simplest possible effective procedures, with removal at the earliest opportunity to a safer area for definitive care.

In wartime, the emergency treatment of many conditions will vary in important details from that outlined in previous sections in this book. The most important points are summarized in the following paragraphs.

64–1. **Bacterial or virus infections** (Biological Warfare)

Inoculation of the population in a given area through bombing or sabotage is always a possibility during wartime, in spite of highly publicized and supposedly sacred covenants between nations. It is impossible to outline in advance any emergency procedures to cope with such a situation. However, the well-known public health principles applicable to any epidemic should be put into effect as soon as possible. These principles are:

A. Segregation of cases.

B. Decontamination.

C. Symptomatic treatment, followed by specific treatment and preventive inoculations as soon as the causative organisms have been identified and their sensitivities determined.

Decrease in resistance of the body to infection may also be expected to occur following mass or nuclear bombing or other wartime emergencies. Interference with normal sleep, poor

food, extreme fatigue and mental strain may also contribute
to this morbid picture.

64–2. **Blast injuries**

A. *Direct Blast Effects* usually consist of multiple massive
contusions of the lungs and are characterized by
dyspnea, cyanosis and unconsciousness. External
signs of trauma may be completely absent. Cardiac
contusion cases may be in shock or show marked
bradycardia and irregularities.

Treatment

1. Insurance of an adequate airway.
2. Administration of oxygen under positive pressure by
   face mask or endotracheal catheter and rebreathing bag. Mouth-to-mouth methods of artificial
   respiration (Topic 17–1) may be necessary while
   awaiting mechanical facilities or if such facilities are not available in sufficient quantity.
3. Strong coffee or tea by mouth or injection of caffeine
   sodiobenzoate, 0.5 gm., intramuscularly.
4. Treatment of shock (Topic 15–7). Administration of
   excessive amounts of fluids should be avoided
   because of the danger of development of pulmonary edema (Topic 52).
5. Transfer from the disaster site for definitive care as
   soon as possible.

B. *Indirect Blast Effects* are caused by striking, or being
struck by, objects and are similar to those encountered in industry, automobile accidents, explosions or in the home. Although therapy may of
necessity have to be modified by lack of supplies
and properly trained personnel, the best emergency
treatment possible under the circumstances should
be administered, with arrangements for evacuation
as soon as possible to an area where more thorough care can be given.

64–3. **Explosive and fire bombs**

These may cause many casualties if employed in saturation
or area bombing. The types of injuries to be expected are the
same as given under blast injuries (64–2, above) and nuclear
bombs (64–4, below), except that the effects of radioactivity
(64–4,B, below) would not be present.

64–4. Nuclear (atomic, hydrogen) bombs

Although nuclear bombs have been characterized as "just bigger and better bombs," certain effects resulting from ionizing radiation are peculiar to them. If an atomic or hydrogen bomb is exploded at a considerable distance above the earth's surface, gamma rays and, under certain circumstances (see B,4, below), neutrons may cause serious and fatal injury. Extreme thermal radiation also may cause flash burns (Topic 28–15) as well as secondary burns. If the fireball comes in contact with the earth's surface, the blast and thermal effects are decreased, but the ground or water is contaminated with fission products. Radioactive fallout, although it may have serious delayed effects, is not an urgent emergency problem in the ordinary sense; however, determination of the intensity of radioactive contamination is essential for estimating prognosis.

A. *Blast Injuries,* if direct (64–2, above) need no practical consideration following nuclear bombing since any person close enough to be injured by blast pressure would undoubtedly be killed by other effects. For indirect blast injuries, see B, above.

B. *Ionizing Radiation Effects* may be caused by:

1. ALPHA RAYS, emitted by unfissioned bomb residue containing plutonium or uranium. If even small amounts of an alpha-emitting substances are deposited in the bones, under certain circumstances serious damage may occur from long-term bombardment of tissues.

2. BETA RAYS, emitted from fission products. Although they are relatively nonpenetrating as compared with gamma rays, the products by which they are emitted may enter the body through inhalation, ingestion or through a break in the skin. Many of these products have the same tendency as alpha rays to localize in the bones and cause severe signs and symptoms, often delayed, through constant bombardment.

3. GAMMA RAYS, liberated for only a few seconds after a high air burst and similar in effect to a high energy x-ray machine. Their range in air varies directly with the size of the bomb, and they may be lethal for several miles from the point of explosion. These rays have a tremendous penetrat-

ing power and are the most important causative
factor in radiation injuries.

4. NEUTRONS, formed by the combination of a positively
charged proton and an electron. These particles
have a relatively short range as compared with
gamma rays; their chief importance is that, on
striking the surface of the earth, they may cause
fission products which emit beta or gamma rays.
Since their penetrating power is very great, persons relatively close to a nuclear blast may be
shielded by a barrier from gamma rays but may
develop acute toxic pictures from neutron exposure.

64–5. **Evaluation and treatment of radiation injuries**

The distance from the exploding bomb and the measurement
of the amount of radiation exposure have been considered as
possible criteria for determining the need for, and extent of,
treatment. Too many variables are involved to make either
method alone practical, but a combination of this information
with the tempo of the effects and the clinical picture is a
feasible method by which radiation injuries can be divided into
three groups:

A. Supralethal Doses of Radiation. In these cases survival
is improbable.

Signs and Symptoms
1. Development of vomiting not more than 2 hours after
exposure, rapidly becoming persistent and severe,
and followed by high fever, diarrhea, tenesmus
and dehydration.
2. Rapid development of extreme prostration, with death
in a few hours or days.

Treatment of this group of cases based on the hope that
prolongation of life might conceivably result in re-
generation of damaged tissues would be prolonged
and expensive and consume large amounts of supplies and drugs which could be better utilized in
caring for persons with a greater chance of survival (see B and C, below). Therefore, it is probable
that refusal of all treatment to persons receiving
supralethal doses of radiation would be necessary.

If treatment of this category of patients were
decided upon, transfer from the disaster site to an

adequately equipped hospital would be necessary. If, by use of sedatives and antispasmodics and by maintenance of fluid balance (Topic 7), the patient could be kept alive for 10 to 12 days, it would be possible (although not probable) that recovery might take place. A relatively small percentage of cases would fall into this group because of the more rapid lethal blast and thermal effects.

1. FOR SEDATION. Any available barbiturates can be used, preferably those such as phenobarbital with a relatively prolonged effect. Paraldehyde, chloral hydrate and bromides also may be of value, as may any of the numerous tranquilizer drugs.

2. FOR CONTROL OF NAUSEA AND VOMITING
   a. Amphetamine sulfate (Benzedrine) or dextroamphetamine sulfate (Dexedrine), 10 mg., three to four times daily by mouth.
   b. Meclizine hydrochloride (Bonamine or Bonine), 25 mg., in tablets or chewing gum.
   c. Atropine sulfate, 0.5 to 1.0 mg., subcutaneously or intravenously three times a day.
   d. Adiphenine hydrochloride (Trasentine), 30 mg. with, or without phenobarbital, 20 mg., by mouth three or four times a day.
   e. Chlorpromazine hydrochloride (Thorazine), 25 to 50 mg., by mouth or intramuscularly.
   f. Prochlorperazine dimaleate (Compazine), 5 to 10 mg., by mouth.
   g. Pyridoxine hydrochloride (Vitamin B_6), 50 to 100 mg., orally three or four times daily, or 25 to 50 mg., intravenously.

3. FOR CARDIOVASCULAR SUPPORT
   a. Ephedrine sulfate, 50 mg., by mouth three times a day, or 25 to 30 mg. in 500 to 1000 ml. of 5% dextrose in saline, intravenously.
   b. Arterenol bitartrate (Levophed) intravenously, or metaraminol bitartrate (Aramine) intramuscularly or intravenously.

4. FOR FLUID AND ELECTROLYTE REPLACEMENT (Topic 7)
   a. Saline and other fluids—by mouth if possible. One level teaspoonful of table salt and ½ teaspoon-

ful of baking soda dissolved in 1000 ml. of
water makes a satisfactory hypotonic solution.

b. Sodium bicarbonate, 1000 ml. of 2% solution, by
rectum per day.

c. Saline or Ringer's solution intravenously if supplies and equipment are available.

B. Potentially Lethal Doses of Radiation. Survival of members of this group of patients will depend to a great
extent upon adequate medical care. The clinical
picture of potentially lethal dosage is as follows:

1. Nausea and vomiting coming on within a short time
after exposure, not more than 1 to 2 hours.

2. Spontaneous cessation of vomiting within 24 hours.

3. An asymptomatic period of 1 to 3 weeks.

4. Late (after 1 to 3 weeks) development of:
   a. Marked infections.
   b. Purpura and epilation.
   c. Oral and cutaneous lesions.
   d. Bloody diarrhea.

Treatment. The only emergency treatment indicated is that
aimed at the acute symptoms of the first few hours;
that is, sedation, administration of antispasmodics
and fluid replacement (Topic 7).

C. Sublethal Doses of Radiation. Symptoms and signs in
this group will, in general, be the same as for
potentially lethal doses of radiation (64–5,B,
above) except that:

1. There will usually be no vomiting on the day of the
bombing.

2. Late symptoms will be much milder or may not appear at all.

3. The late development of a leukopenia may be the
only clinical evidence of radiation damage.

Treatment. At the present time no emergency treatment
of any kind is known which will influence the development or severity of late symptoms in any way.

Do Not

1. Waste whole blood, plasma, plasma volume expanders or intravenous fluids as emergency supportive measures in this group of patients unless
other associated conditions make their use imperative. Replacement fluids (Topic 7) should

not be given intravenously if oral or rectal administration is practical. Increased bleeding tendencies and decreased resistance to infection may make any type of hypodermic administration hazardous.

2. Administer antibiotics. They will be far more useful in treatment of other conditions.

3. Prescribe corticosteroids; they do no good and possibly may do harm.

64–6. Thermal effects

Burns of all degrees and extent, often associated with other severe injuries, may follow a nuclear blast. These burns differ in no way from those encountered in civilian emergency practice (Topic 28 and Topic 48–10).

Treatment. Through instruction of Civilian Defense units and stockpiling of supplies, the following method of management would seem to be practical:

1. Treat shock (Topic 15–7). Whenever possible, hypotonic solution should be given by mouth, supplemented if necessary by plasma volume expanders (Topic 7). As much as 10 liters (quarts) of hypotonic solution, prepared by dissolving one level teaspoonful of table salt (sodium chloride) and ½ teaspoonful of baking soda (sodium bicarbonate) in 1000 ml. (1 quart) of water, can be given orally to severe burn cases during a 24-hour period.

2. Cut off or remove soiled or charred clothing.

3. Cleanse gently with soap and water and a weak detergent solution after administration of anodynes or narcotics if pain is severe. No debridement should be attempted and no antiseptic or disinfectant solutions should be used.

4. Apply a securely anchored sterile dressing. This may consist of petrolatum gauze or a similar material if available, or of a simple type of dry dressing stockpiled in many localities. This dressing consists of a large cellulose pad faced with fine mesh gauze which is applied directly to the burned surface and held in place with bandage or adhesive. With this method elastic pressure bandages are not necessary.

5. Fasten burn dressings so that slipping will not take place. Although the original dressing may become discolored from serous drainage, it should not be disturbed for at least a week unless evidence of gross infection is present.

6. DO NOT apply any of the following substances to burns of any degree or extent:

    a. Alcoholic preparations of any type.

    b. Aluminum powder.

    c. Antibiotic solutions, salves, ointments or creams.

    d. Boric, picric or tannic acid.

    e. Butter, grease, lard, paraffin or wax.

    f. Gentian violet or other dyes.

    g. Proprietary burn salves, creams or lotions.

    h. Silver nitrate solutions.

7. Splint to prevent motion of the burned areas.

8. Arrange for disposition of cases:

    a. Hospitalize if:

        (1) More than 25% of the body surface of an adult is involved. (For children, see Topic 48–10.)

        (2) Less than 25% of the body area is involved, but the eyes, eyelids, nose, mouth, trachea, genitalia or feet are severely damaged.

        (3) Other severe injuries are present.

        (4) Severe electrical or chemical burns are present.

    b. Arrange for ambulatory care for all other burn cases.

64–7. Bullet wounds

On-site treatment should be limited to control of hemorrhage (Topic 8–1) and shock (Topic 15–7), with transfer as soon as possible to a hospital equipped for definitive care.

64–8. Burns

No matter what the causative agent, the treatment of burns in wartime is as given in detail under thermal effects (64–6, above).

64–9. Fractures and dislocations

Reduction of fractures or dislocations of any type under wartime conditions should not be attempted unless there is evidence of acute circulatory embarrassment or nerve pressure. The injured part should be immobilized in a position of minimal discomfort, pain controlled by necessary measures, and evacuation arranged. Compound (open) fractures should be covered with a protective dressing, sterile if possible, and given tetanus antitoxin or toxoid (Topic 19). No sulfonamide powder, antibiotic powder or ointment of any kind should be applied to any compound (open) fracture. Antibiotics should be given only if a long delay before definitive treatment is anticipated.

64–10. **Medical emergencies.** (Also see 64–1, above.)

In wartime many chronic medical conditions undoubtedly would be aggravated sufficiently to require emergency care. Poor food, nervous strain, exposure, prolonged excitement and overexertion might well trigger disabling increases in symptoms primarily caused by pre-existent metabolic disorders, infections and other chronic conditions. Even small doses of ionizing radiation will cause decreased general body resistance with the usual complications.

It has been estimated that about 2% of all casualties following a major wartime catastrophe would involve known or latent diabetics. Persons requiring insulin would be given just enough insulin to control their condition so that they could be evacuated from the disaster area. Using the Benedict urine test, dosage of insulin can be calculated accurately enough for this purpose according to the following schedule:

BENEDICT TEST	UNITS OF REGULAR INSULIN
Blue, negative	None
Green, 1 plus	5
Yellow, 2 plus	10
Orange, 3 plus	15
Red, 4 plus	20

The Clinitest and Acetest methods are also of value in determination of the severity of diabetes.

For differential diagnosis and treatment of diabetic coma and insulin shock, see Topic 3–3.

64–11. **Poison gases** (Chemical Warfare)

If chemical warfare is ever used again, it is probable that the "nerve gases" will almost completely replace lacrimators, pulmonary irritants, irritant smokes and vesicants [Topic 49–648 (*War Gases*)]. All "nerve gases" are strongly cholinesterase-inhibiting and result in profound stimulation of the parasympathetic nervous system. For treatment see Topic 49–421 (*Organic Phosphates*).

ADMINISTRATIVE, CLERICAL and
MEDICOLEGAL PRINCIPLES and
PROCEDURES

65. ABANDONMENT

65–1. Acceptance of patients

No physician is compelled legally to respond to any emergency call or undertake emergency examination or treatment in any situation whatever, just as he is not compelled legally to respond to any other request for his services. He need give no explanation for his refusal to render aid or accept responsibility for the case. Once he has advised or given treatment, however, the physician-patient relationship has been established. From then on the attending physician is responsible for the patient's care until this responsibility has been shifted to another physician either by the original attendant or by the patient or his agents.

65–2. Grounds for possible legal action

Failure of the attending physician to take reasonable steps to complete specific arrangements for follow-up care after emergency treatment and to stress the possible ill-effects of lack of such care may constitute a basis for legal action by the patient (or his natural or legal guardians) on the grounds of abandonment.

65–3. Prevention

A practical method of prevention of such legal action consists of sending the patient (or his legal guardian) a brief letter explaining the need for further medical care and outlining the possible consequences of lack of care. This letter should be sent by registered mail, with return receipt requested. A copy of the letter and the return receipt (or the undelivered original letter) should be made a part of the patient's record.

As an added protection the form on page 604 has been found to be of value, especially in clinics, offices and stations where large numbers of emergency cases are treated. This form should be completed in duplicate. The original should be given to the patient when emergency care is completed and the copy placed in the patient's record.

INSTRUCTIONS FOR FOLLOW-UP CARE

The examination and treatment which you have received has been on an emergency basis only and has not been intended to be a substitute or replacement for complete medical care. For your protection, I hereby suggest that in order to prevent possible complications you follow the recommendations checked below:

☐ Telephone your private physician for an appointment

on_____
                                (Date)

☐ Report at once to your private physician.

☐ Report at once to_____Hospital.

☐ Telephone for an appointment in the_____

   Clinic at_____on_____
                    (location)   (date)

☐ Report back to this Emergency Department on_____

   _____at   A.M.
          (date)   P.M.

☐ Other (specify)_____

   Date_____ Signed_____M.D.

66. CERTIFICATES

66–1. Birth certificates

The signature of the attending physician (or licensed midwife in some localities) in black permanent ink is required on all certificates covering live births and stillbirths.

For uniformity in reporting to public agencies the following criteria are in general use:

66–2. Live birth

Any infant born at any age which after birth shows any sign of life, even momentarily (heart beat, impulse in cord or respiratory activity).

66–3. Premature birth

Any infant under 2500 gm. (5½ lbs.) in weight, regardless of length or age.

66–4. Stillbirth

Any infant born dead (no heart beat, impulse in cord or respiratory activity) and weighing 1000 gm. (2 lbs. 3 oz.) or more, regardless of length or age.

66–5. Abortion

Any infant born dead and weighing under 1000 gm. (2 lbs. 3 oz.), regardless of length or age.

66–6. Death certificates

A. Whenever an infant weighing 2500 gm. or more shows any signs of life (66–2, above), even momentarily, both a birth certificate (66–1, above) and a death certificate must be completed and signed by the attending physician or coroner. Abortions (66–5, above) do not require completion of any certificate; however, a notation must be made in the emergency record and signed by the attending physician.

B. A death certificate must be completed within a given time (usually 15 to 24 hours) on every death case, no matter what the cause. For detailed information regarding coroner's (medical examiner's) responsibility see Topic 4–5.

67. EMERGENCY CASE RECORDS

In many instances, legal actions against physicians and hospitals are based upon incidents alleged to have occurred at the time of initial emergency treatment (Topic 69). Therefore, to protect the physician and hospital as well as the patient, meticulous care should be used in completion, filing and safekeeping of detailed, accurate, legible records in all emergency cases.

67–1. Emergency charts, cards or sheets

A detailed record of each emergency case interviewed, examined and/or treated should be written and signed by the attending physician as soon as possible after the patient is seen.

The record on each case should be written legibly in ink and should contain the following information:

A. Chief Complaints. What brings the patient in?

B. History of Onset
    1. Illnesses—duration, type of onset, symptoms, previous attacks.
    2. Injuries—When? Where? How? Previous injuries?

C. Physical Findings. Temperature, respiration, pulse and blood pressure should be recorded in severe cases or when shock or evidence of infection is present. Neurologic examination should be done whenever the history or findings suggest possible head, spinal cord or peripheral nerve injury. Negative as well as positive findings should be recorded.

D. X-Rays. The attending physician's interpretation of any films should be recorded (Topic 21). Careful examination of the wet films generally will disclose any pathology present. A confirmatory reading by a roentgenologist should be obtained as soon as possible.

E. Laboratory Results. The results of any laboratory tests performed by, under the direction of, or by order of the attending physician should be recorded.

F. Diagnosis or Impression. Whenever possible, a specific diagnosis should be given. If this is not possible, the impression or working diagnosis can be used. "DEFERRED" SHOULD NEVER BE USED.

G. Treatment
    1. Medications administered or prescribed.
    2. Acute shock therapy—time and amount.
    3. Splints—type, time applied.
    4. Supportive measures—artificial respiration, analeptics, oxygen, etc.
    5. Gastric lavage—with what? Results?
    6. Tourniquet—time applied and removed.
    7. Surgical repair—anesthesia, number and type of sutures.
    8. Immunizing or prophylactic procedures—tetanus antitoxin or toxoid, gas bacillus antitoxin, etc.
    9. Antibiotics.
    10. Instructions regarding home treatment, with number of doses of medication prescribed.

H. Disposition
    1. Sent home? How? With whom? At what time?

    2. Referred? To whom? (Specify name and address of physician.) A follow-up care form (Topic 65–4) should be completed in duplicate and the original given to the patient. The duplicate copy should be made a part of the patient's record.

    3. Hospitalized? Where? At what time? By private car or ambulance?

Note: If the patient and/or his family or legal guardian refuse to follow the advice of the attending physician regarding disposition or treatment, it should be explained in the presence of witnesses that the attending physician will not be responsible for further developments. The patient (or the parents or guardian) should be given a "Release from Responsibility" form to sign (67–3, below). This should be witnessed by two persons over 21 years of age (NOT by the attending physician) and should be made a part of the patient's record. Refusal to sign the "Release from Responsibility" form should be indicated by a witnessed note to that effect in the record.

As further protection for the physician whose advice has been refused, a letter specifying that the patient-physician relationship has been severed and that further medical care should be obtained elsewhere should be sent as soon as possible to the last known address of the patient (or his guardian). This letter should be sent by registered mail, with return receipt requested. A copy, together with the returned receipt (or the undelivered original letter), should be incorporated in the patient's record.

I. Estimated Temporary Disability. This information is often necessary for completion of insurance forms. Whenever the patient is told by the physician to discontinue work (housework or in industry), it should be indicated as:

    Estimated Temporary Disability (ETD) . . . .
    (days, weeks, months).

J. All emergency records MUST be signed by the attending physician with his full name. INITIALS ONLY SHOULD NEVER BE USED.

67–2. **Emergency case log**

In those offices, admitting departments, stations or wards which handle emergency cases, a current and chronologic emergency log should be kept by clerical or nursing personnel in addition to the records or charts completed by the attending physician. This log should be a permanent record, typed or written in ink, and should contain the following information:

A. Classification code (private, industrial, insurance coverage, etc.).

B. Date and time registered.

C. Name in full, including middle name (no middle name, indicate as N.M.I.). If the patient is a minor, the legal guardian's name, address and telephone number should be given.

D. Address and telephone number.

E. Date of birth (if not known, indicate apparent age).

F. Sex, race or color.

G. Brought for emergency care by (self, family, guardian, friends, police, ambulance, etc.).

H. Brought from (home address, site of accident, name of hospital, etc.).

I. Type of case (pediatric, surgical, medical, obstetric, undetermined).

J. Diagnosis. If a specific diagnosis has not been given on the medical record by the examining physician, the working or symptom diagnosis should be entered. "DEFERRED" SHOULD NEVER BE USED.

K. Treatment, in brief.

L. Disposition—home, to work, hospitalized, referred (to whom?), etc.

M. Condition—good, fair, poor, critical, deceased.

N. Time discharged from emergency care.

O. Out by (self, friends, ambulance).

P. Name (not initials), address, and telephone number of the attending physician.

67–3. **Release from responsibility**

Occasionally a patient, or his guardian, will refuse to follow the recommendations for treatment or disposition made by the examining physician. In cases of this type a "Release from Responsibility" form (page 609) should be signed by the patient (or his natural or legal guardian) in the presence of two witnesses. This signed and witnessed release should be made a permanent part of the emergency record.

RELEASE FROM RESPONSIBILITY
(*Cross out portions which do not apply*)

Date_____Time_____m.

I hereby certify that of my own free will I am removing my

_____from the
(self, son, daughter, husband, wife, ward)

_____
(Office, Clinic, Hospital)

against the recommendation and advice of_____M.D.,
and that I am hereby refusing further examination, tests, and
treatment. I hereby acknowledge that I have been informed of, and
understand, the possible consequences of such removal and/or refusal. Having full knowledge of the risks involved, and realization of
the dangers that may result from removal of the patient and/or refusal of recommended examination, tests, and treatment, I hereby

agree to hold the_____
(Office, Clinic, Hospital)

and_____, M.D.

and all others concerned blameless and free from any and all liability
for any direct or indirect injuries or ill-effects which may result by
reason of removal of the patient, and/or refusal of examination,
tests, and treatment.

Witness_____Signed_____

Witness_____   Relationship to Patient_____
                               (self, mother, father, husband,
                               wife, guardian)

67–4. Unusual occurrence reports

Emergency practice is prone to unusual occurrences because
of the types of cases which are handled. Any incidents which
fall into any of the following categories should be covered by
a detailed note made in the patient's record and by an entry
in the emergency log (67–2, above).

A. Omission, incorrect administration or improper dosage
of any drug or medication ordered by the attending
physician.

B. Incidents which cause, or which might be construed as
causing, bodily injury to a patient or other persons.

C. Serious reactions caused by drugs or other substances administered in the treatment of emergency conditions.

D. Incidents, accidents or breaks in technique during examination and/or treatment.

E. Incidents occurring in the entrance to, or on the property or grounds of, the Emergency Station, office, clinic, ward, or hospital, which might be construed as causing or contributing to, mental or physical suffering or injury to a patient or visitor. (Injuries to emergency personnel, police officers, etc., are covered under the compensation acts and require the usual industrial form.)

F. Loss, or alleged loss, of money, jewelry or other personal effects.

G. Complaints of any nature made by a patient or visitor —no matter if trivial or apparently unsubstantiated.

67–5. **Permits, consents and authorizations.** See Topic 70.
67–6. **Death cases.** See Topic 4.
67–7. **Subrogation (liability) cases.** See Topic 68.
67–8. **Workmen's compensation (industrial) cases.** See Topic 76.

68.   LIABILITY AND SUBROGATION CASES

A. Many of the cases treated as emergencies result from direct or indirect trauma (assault, auto accidents, railroad wrecks, industrial accidents, etc.) which may be the basis for future litigation of considerable complexity; therefore, it is the responsibility of the attending physician to see that ON FIRST EXAMINATION all evidences of injury are noted in detail on the patient's chart. These include superficial contusions, abrasions and lacerations, as well as more serious injuries. The exact location and severity (slight, moderate, severe) should be noted in detail on the emergency record.

B. X-rays should be taken whenever necessary to establish, confirm or rule out traumatic, pre-existent or other relevant conditions (Topic 21–1).

C. Any evidence of, or tests for, any degree of intoxication from alcohol, narcotics or other drugs should be entered on the clinical record with enough detail to refresh the physician's memory in case he should be required to testify in court at a later date.

69. MALPRACTICE

69–1. Negligence

Malpractice actions against physicians are usually based on allegations of negligence. In order to prove negligence, the complainant must, as a rule, present evidence concerning the following points (sometimes referred to as the "FOUR D's"):

A. Duty. The existence of a physician-patient relationship (Topic 65–1) assumes a duty of the physician toward the patient.

B. Dereliction of Duty. See 69–3, below.

C. Direct Causation. An unbroken chain of causation from the derelict act, or acts, to the condition of which the patient complains must be proved.

D. Damages. Proof of general damages (pain, suffering, physical dysfunction or disfigurement, etc.) and/or special damages (loss of earnings, medical and hospital expenses, necessary travel and other indirect costs) must be presented.

Negligence may consist of:

A. Omission of proper and recognized methods of examination and treatment.

B. Commission of improper, experimental or nonrecognized methods of examination or treatment.

The criteria by which proper and recognized methods of examination and treatment are determined vary in different localities and circumstances. A general practitioner in a small country town, for example, would not be expected to possess the same skill and knowledge as a specialist in a large urban medical center.

69–2. Statutes of limitation

This rule varies in different jurisdictions, but generally statutes of limitation run from the time that the patient becomes aware of the damaging incident, not from the date of the procedure which resulted in the injury.

69–3. Standards of care in emergency cases

It is sometimes assumed that a lower standard of care is required in the management and treatment of emergency cases than in nonurgent situations and that the ordinary criteria for determining negligence do not apply in these circumstances. No reliable legal support can be found for these assumptions. The standard of care in emergencies can be more easily understood if it is remembered that a general legal rule applies as a guide in all types of cases, regardless of their urgency. This general rule is usually stated as follows:

> "A physician is required to exercise or use such reasonable and ordinary care, skill, and diligence as a physician in good standing in the same area in the same general line of practice, ordinarily uses in like cases."

The available time or degree of urgency (Topic 20) does not in any way modify a physician's duty to use reasonable care; this duty remains the same at all times. However, the degree of skill required of the physician may vary according to the skill that good physicians exercise in like cases and circumstances. A correct test is whether or not the physician took such action as a skillful and experienced physician might have taken UNDER SIMILAR CIRCUMSTANCES.

69–4. Malpractice insurance

All physicians, especially those who handle a large volume of emergency cases, should be covered adequately by malpractice insurance with a reliable company.

69–5. Routine safeguards against malpractice actions

    A. Completion and careful preservation of accurate, detailed and legible records on every patient. The length of time that these records are required by law to be preserved varies in different localities, but records on children must be kept until they reach their majority.

    B. Utilization of maximum skill, knowledge and judgement in examination, treatment and disposition.

    C. Insistence on competent consultation in problem cases.

    D. Avoidance of quasi-experimental, controversial, or non-accepted procedures.

    E. Explanation to the patient (or his legal guardian) IN ADVANCE of the purpose, extent, expected results, possible complications and estimated expense of any procedure. Under no circumstances should any express, specific, or implied guarantee or warranty be given.

F. Notation in the patient's record, in detail and in a noncritical fashion, of any complications or unusual situations related directly or indirectly to the management of the case.

G. Avoidance of direct, indirect or implied criticism of the work of, or the results obtained by, other physicians, even under extreme provocation.

H. Use of courtesy, kindness, sympathy and tact in all relationships with the patient, family, relatives, friends or other interested parties.

70. *PERMITS, CONSENTS AND AUTHORIZATIONS IN RELATION TO EMERGENCY CASES*

(Some of the forms in this section are modified from "Medicolegal Forms with Legal Analysis" published by the Law Department of the American Medical Association and from "Reference Manual of Permits, Consents and/or Releases; Hospital Administrative Procedure No. 1–10" prepared by the office of the Area Administrator, Kaiser Foundation Hospitals, Oakland, California.)

Some of the following forms have been referred to in the preceding text. All have been found useful in the management of emergency cases.

70–1.   **Access to emergency records** (Also see 70–8, below)

To_____, Administrator, _____Hospital.
I hereby authorize you to furnish a copy of the hospital records of

_____, covering the period from
(Name of patient or "myself")

_____19_____to_____19_____to, or to allow

those records to be inspected or copied by,_____

I hereby release_____Hospital, all members of its
staff, and you personally from all legal responsibility or liability that
may arise from the act I have authorized above.

                        Signed_____

                        Date_____

Witness_____

Approved_____M.D., Attending Physician.

70–2.   **Admission of observers**

                        Date_____19_____

Patient_____ Age_____

Room or Ward_____

    I hereby authorize my attending physician_____M.D.

and the_____Hospital
to permit the presence of such observers as they may deem fit to
admit, in addition to physicians and hospital personnel, while I
am undergoing operative surgery, childbirth, examination, treatment.

(Cross out portions   Signed_____
  which do not apply)
                        Spouse_____

                    Witness_____

70–3. **Autopsy permit.** (See Topic 4–6.)

NAME OF DECEASED_____AGE_____SEX_____

RACE_____MARITAL STATUS_____DATE OF BIRTH_____

1. I hereby authorize_____M.D., and such persons as he may designate, to perform and attend a complete autopsy, including brain and spinal cord, on the remains of my

_____for the purpose of determining the cause of death. Authority is also granted for the preservation and study of any and all tissues or parts which may be removed. This authority shall be limited only by the following express conditions:

_____

2. It is understood that due care will be taken to avoid mutilation or disfigurement of the body.

Signature of spouse,
legal guardian or
next of kin*_____

Address_____

Relationship to
the deceased_____

Signature of Witness_____

Address_____

City and State_____ Date_____

* For explanation of "Next of Kin," see Topic 4–6,B,1.

70–4. Blood alcohol test. (See Topic 18–1,B.)

Witnesses should be disinterested adults, NOT the attending physician, his nurse or a law enforcement officer.

Date_____Time_____

I, the undersigned, hereby authorize withdrawal of blood for the purpose of determination of the alcohol content.

Witness_____　　Signed_____

Witness_____

— — — — — — — — — — — — —

We request a blood specimen for alcohol content from_____

(Patient's name)

_____

(Address)

by authorization of my supervisor, _____

(Capt., Sgt., or Chief)

Witness_____ Signed_____

Witness_____

Badge No._____

Police Dept._____

Date_____Time_____.

70–5. **Blood transfusion.** [See also 70–31, below (*Refusal of Blood or Blood Derivatives*).]

To:_____M.D.
(Attending physician)

and_____Hospital. Date_____19___

    1. I hereby request and authorize administration of a blood

transfusion to_____and
(Insert "myself" or name of patient)
such additional transfusions as may be deemed necessary and advis-

able by_____M.D. or physicians specifically
designated by him.

    2. It is understood and agreed that_____M.D., or the physicians designated by him, will be responsible only for the performance of their own individual professional acts, and that blood typing and selection of compatible blood are the responsibilities of those who actually perform the necessary laboratory tests.

    3. It has been fully explained, and it is understood, that blood transfusions do not always produce a desirable result and that there is a possibility of ill-effects, including hepatitis and/or other diseases, from such transfusion or transfusions.

    4. It has been clearly explained, and it is understood, that circumstances may make detailed cross-matching tests impractical or impossible and that immediate need may make necessary the use of existing stocks of blood which may not include the most compatible blood types.

    5. It is understood, and hereby expressly agreed, that blood supplied in accordance with this agreement is incidental to the rendition of services and that no requirement, guarantee or warranty of fitness or quality shall apply.

                         Signature of patient_____

        When patient is a minor or incompetent to give consent:

            Signature of person authorized to sign consent for

            patient_____

            Address_____

            Relationship to
            patient_____

Witness_____

Address_____

70–6. **Blood plasma transfusion.** [See also 70–31, below (*Refusal of Blood or Blood Derivatives*).]

To_____M.D. and
                    (Attending physician)

_____Hospital. Date_____19___

   1. I hereby request and authorize administration of blood plasma

to_____in such amounts and at such
  (Insert "myself" or name of patient)

times as may be deemed necessary and advisable by_____M.D.
or physicians specifically designated by him.

   2. It has been fully explained, and it is understood, that blood
plasma does not always produce a desirable result and that it is a
product made from mixed blood obtained from many persons and
that sometimes it may cause hepatitis and/or other diseases.

   3. It is understood, and hereby expressly agreed, that the blood
plasma supplied in accordance with this agreement is incidental to
the rendition of services and that no requirement, guarantee or
warranty of fitness or quality shall apply.

                  Signature of patient_____

       When patient is a minor or
       incompetent to give consent:

       Signature of person authorized to sign consent for patient

       _____

       Address_____

       Relationship to patient_____
Witness:

  Signature_____

  Address_____

70–7. **Diagnostic procedures** (spinal puncture, myelograms,
sternal punctures, abdominal paracentesis, etc.).

PATIENT_____AGE_____

DATE_____TIME_____A.M.

   I hereby request and authorize_____M.D.

to perform upon_____the following
              ("myself" or name of patient)

diagnostic procedure:_____.

I have been fully informed of the risks and possible consequences
involved and understand that unforeseen results may occur.

          Signed_____

          Relationship to patient_____

The foregoing consent was read, discussed and signed in my presence,
and in my opinion the person so signing did so freely and with full
knowledge and understanding.

          Witness_____

70–8. Disclosure of information by patient's physician

   1. I hereby authorize_____M.D.

to disclose complete information to_____

concerning medical findings and treatment of_____
                          (name or "myself")

from about_____19_____until the date of conclusion
of such treatment.

   2. Furthermore, I authorize the physician specified above to testify
without limitation as to all medical findings and to all treatment
administered to the undersigned, in any legal action, suit or pro-
ceedings to which I am, or may become, a party, and I hereby waive
on behalf of myself and any persons who may have an interest in
the matter, all provisions of law relating to the disclosure of confidential medical information.

          Signed_____

          Place_____

          Date_____

Witness_____

70–9. **Disposal of body** (Antemortem bequest)

I hereby instruct that my body be delivered immediately after death

to the_____Hospital, _____,

(address)

through the local coroner, to be preserved and used in such manner
as may seem desirable for purposes of medical teaching and research.

Signature_____

Address_____

Date_____

Witnesses: Addresses:

_____   _____

_____   _____

70–10. **Disposal of dead fetus***

Date_____

We hereby authorize and request that_____
Hospital preserve for scientific purposes, or dispose of, the dead fetus

or body of the baby born to_____on_____, 19___
in accordance with customary medical practice. All claims to the
body are hereby relinquished.

Signed_____(mother)

Signed_____(father)

Witness_____

* This consent should be executed by both parents if possible. An unmarried mother's consent is sufficient.

70–11. Disposal of a severed or amputated part or organ

Date_____

  I hereby authorize the_____Hospital
to preserve for scientific purposes, or for use in grafts upon living
persons, or to otherwise dispose of in a proper and suitable manner,

the tissues, parts, or organs of_____
                             (Name of patient or "myself")
specified below.

_____
               (Parts or organs)

               Signed_____

               Relationship to patient
               (Self, parent, legal guardian)_____

Witness_____

Witness_____

70–12. Emergency care without a surgery permit
The degree of emergency as evaluated by the examining
physician is the deciding factor in the handling of patients who
are unable to sign their own operative permits because of
minority or mental condition, and whose natural or legal guardians are not available. These cases can be divided into three
main groups by means of the time element:

    A. Immediate Treatment Required. [Gross hemorrhage,
        acute poisoning, cardiac emergencies, respiratory
        embarrassment, etc. (Topic 20).] In these cases
        there is a definite POSITIVE obligation for treat-
        ment without delay. While the patient is being pre-
        pared for, and undergoing, treatment, every effort
        should be made to locate the natural or legal guard-
        ian by telephone, telegraph or other means. The
        cooperation of law enforcement and social service
        agencies of the community can often be obtained.

        Before emergency surgery or procedures of any
        type are undertaken, the Immediate Treatment

Form (D, below) must be signed by TWO licensed physicians and made a part of the patient's permanent record.

In addition, a standard treatment permit (17–14,B, below) signed by the natural or legal guardian, or telegraphic (70–30,B, below) or telephonic permission (70–30,C, below), should be obtained at the earliest opportunity.

B. Treatment within 6 to 12 Hours Required (lacerations, compound fractures, etc.). In these cases, further attempts should be made by the means previously outlined to obtain permission from the natural or legal guardian. If the SAFE PERIOD OF DELAY has passed without obtaining permission, an Immediate Treatment Permit form (D, below) should be completed and treatment given.

C. Treatment Postponable for Over 12 Hours without Danger to the Life or Health of the Patient (simple fractures, dislocations without nerve or vascular pressure symptoms, etc.). In these cases, every attempt should be made within the set time limit to obtain proper authorization before proceeding with surgical or other care. Copies of telegrams, letters, etc., should be attached to the patient's record. In order to retain control of the patient, hospitalization while attempting to locate the natural or legal guardian may be indicated. If proper written, telephonic or telegraphic authority has not been obtained at the end of the SAFE WAITING PERIOD, the treatment necessary to prevent injury to health or serious permanent disability may be performed, provided full information regarding the need for the procedure has been made a part of the record, and an Immediate Treatment Permit (D, below) has been signed by TWO licensed physicians in the presence of two witnesses.

D. Immediate Treatment Permit

Date_____Time_____m.

(Patient a minor or unable to sign because of condition; natural or legal guardian not available.)

We, the undersigned physicians, licensed to practice in the State

of_____, hereby certify that it is our considered

opinion that_____, _____, is in
(Name of patient)   (Age)

need of immediate treatment to save life and/or to prevent serious disability and/or deformity. We further certify that unsuccessful attempts have been made for a reasonable time to communicate with the parents, spouse, or legal guardian of the patient named above, and that in our professional judgement further delay in rendering treatment will seriously increase the danger to the patient's life and health.

Witness_____ Signed_____, M.D.

Witness_____ Signed_____, M.D.

E. Miscellaneous Provisions Concerning Emergency Permits

1. The signer must be clearly aware of the nature of his consent.

2. Persons witnessing signatures must be 21 years of age or older.

3. When emergency procedures are performed without the signature of the patient or his natural or legal guardian, A PROPERLY SIGNED PERMIT SHOULD BE OBTAINED AT THE EARLIEST POSSIBLE OPPORTUNITY.

4. Permits signed with an "X" should be witnessed by TWO adult persons able to write their names.

5. Surgery or other treatment necessary to prevent only a cosmetic or functional defect requires a validly signed operative or treatment permit (70–14,B, below). This requirement also applies to elective surgery of any type. These procedures cannot be performed under an Immediate Treatment Permit.

6. No person who has temporary custody only of a minor

has any legal right to authorize treatment of any kind.

7. The authority of a duly appointed legal guardian supersedes that of a parent or spouse.

8. Grandparents, adult brothers, sisters, close relatives, etc., CANNOT SIGN A PERMIT FOR A MINOR [except *IN LOCO PARENTIS* (70–20,D, below)].

9. Permits should be signed BEFORE ANY PREOPERATIVE MEDICATION IS GIVEN TO THE PATIENT.

10. If a patient qualified to sign his own permit specifically prohibits any procedure before becoming incompetent or irresponsible, the procedure cannot be performed under any circumstances, even as a lifesaving measure, in many localities (see 70–31, below).

11. Because the father and mother are charged equally with the control and custody of a child, express prohibition by one parent prevents any treatment even though the other has given permission. This applies even if the parents are separated and can be overruled only if the laws in the particular locality provide for the issuance of treatment orders by juvenile or other courts.

12. When marriage of a minor, divorce, annulment, legal guardianship, or IN LOCO PARENTIS relationship is claimed as a basis for exceptions to the usual rules regarding treatment permits, adequate proof to substantiate the claim should be required.

70–13.　Entrustment of care of minors

Parents or legal guardians who wish to leave their children or wards under the care of another adult during working hours, overnight, while on vacation trips, etc., can ensure prompt emergency care by completing and signing a document of the type shown on page 625. The signed and witnessed document should be kept in the possession of the adult responsible for care during the parents' or guardian's absence, to be presented to the attending physician in the case of an emergency involving the persons specified thereon.

TO WHOM IT MAY CONCERN:

(Cross out words which do not apply)

This is to certify that I/we,_____

_____the_____
      (names in full)   (mother, father, legal guardian)

of the persons listed below, do hereby constitute and appoint

_____
      (name in full)   (address)

my/our true and lawful attorney, solely, and with the power, to authorize and consent to the administration of any anesthetic or medical treatment to, and the performance of whatever operations or removal of tissue decided to be necessary by the attending physician,

on the below named minor(s) for the period from_____to
                                        (date)

_____, inclusive.
   (date)

NAME	AGE OR DATE OF BIRTH
_____	_____
_____	_____
_____	_____
_____	_____

WITNESSED BY:

_____	_____
Name	Name Relationship
_____	_____
Address	Name Relationship
_____	_____
Name	Address
_____	
Address	

      Date of signing_____

70–14. **Informed consent**

A. No longer is a blanket authorization covering all conceivable medical, surgical and laboratory procedures considered to be adequate permission for emergency or other medical care. In some areas it is becoming generally accepted that the patient has the right to accurate detailed information regarding not only the projected operation but also the possible complications and risks entailed before he signs the authorization. Another viewpoint is well summarized in this quotation from a recent Wyoming Supreme Court decision: "Whether or not a surgeon is under a duty to warn of the possibility of adverse results depends upon the circumstances of a particular case and upon the general practice followed by the medical profession in the locality."

B. The following authorizations reconcile both viewpoints and have been found satisfactory for emergency use.

OPERATIVE PERMIT (Adults) Date_____Time_____M.

I hereby authorize_____M.D., to perform the

operation specified below upon_____
(name of patient or "myself")

and to proceed with any other operation which he may consider necessary without further authorization. I hereby consent to the administration of any anesthetic(s) which he, or an anesthetist or anesthesiologist designated by him, may consider advisable.

Name or Description of Operation

_____Signed_____

_____Witness_____

OPERATIVE PERMIT
(Patient a Minor or Mentally Incompetent)
(Cross out portions which do not apply)

Date_____Time_____M.

I (we), the parent(s), legal guardian of a minor, mentally incom-

petent person, hereby authorize_____M.D.,

to perform the operation specified below upon_____

_____, my (our) son, daughter, ward, and
to proceed without further authorization with any other operation
deemed necessary by him.

I (we) hereby consent to the administration of any anesthetic(s)
deemed necessary by the physician specified above or by the anesthetist or anesthesiologist designated by him.

Name or Description of Operation   Signed_____

                                       Relation to Patient_____

_____   Signed_____

_____   Relation to Patient_____

_____   Witness_____

70–15. **In loco parentis.** See 70–20,D, below.

70–16. **Mature minors.** See 70–19,C, below.

70–17. **Nalorphine hydrochloride.** (Nalline) Test authorization.
See Topic 18–3,C.

70–18. **Operative and treatment permits.** [See also 70–14,
above (*Informed Consent*).]

    A. General Considerations. Whenever possible, a treatment
permit including permission for operative procedures (70–14,B, above) should be signed by the
patient (or his natural or legal guardian), properly
witnessed, and made a permanent part of the medical record BEFORE ANY TREATMENT IS GIVEN.
Legally, treatment against the explicit or implied
wish of the patient or of his natural or legal guardian may constitute actionable assault. Practically,
it is generally considered that the following types
of treatment can be given without authorization and

that omission may be considered as evidence of improper care and negligence (Topic 69–1 and 3).

1. Cleansing and irrigation of a wound (*not* debridement) with coaptation of the edges by adhesive straps or "butterflies" and application of protective sterile bandages.

2. Application of temporary splints (*not* casts) to prevent aggravation of an injury by motion.

3. Oral or rectal administration of medications.

4. Artificial respiration, or assistance to respiration, by any expired air, manual or mechanical means, including inhalation by tent, catheter or mask of oxygen or other nonanesthetic gases.

B. In contrast, the following procedures should NOT be done without a properly signed permit unless an *immediate* threat to life or health is present:

1. Surgical procedures, major or minor, emergency or elective.

2. Administration of local or general anesthesia.

3. Insertion of a needle for any reason whatsoever. This includes intracutaneous, subcutaneous, intramuscular, intravenous or intraspinal injections of all types, as well as the withdrawal of blood, spinal fluid, etc., for diagnosis or treatment.

4. Gastric lavage or gavage.

5. Catheterization.

6. Application or changing of corrective splints or casts.

C. The best definition of a danger or threat to life or health which would warrant proceeding without proper authorization is as follows:

"It must involve a threat which carries danger of major incapacities, permanent or irreversible, through impairment or loss of a function, organ, or structural unit of the body."

70–19. **Persons who may sign their own emergency treatment permits**

A. Any mentally competent person over 21 years of age. The decision regarding mental competency must be made by the attending physician, provided it has not been established by court action.

B. Any mentally competent male over 18, or female over

16, who is married or divorced, or whose marriage has been annulled. Such persons are considered as being emancipated from parental control; hence, they can sign their own permits in many states.

C. "Mature" minors. In some states, unmarried minors between 16 and 21 may, under certain circumstances, sign emergency permits. These circumstances are as follows:

1. When the consent of the natural or legal guardian cannot be obtained within the time limit available to save life or prevent suffering or permanent disability.

2. When the natural or legal guardians are not available, but the minor has presented himself for treatment accompanied by older relatives and with a parent's knowledge, provided there is no reason to suspect that one or both of the parents' consent would not have been given had they been available.

70–20. **Persons who may sign permits for minors**

A. *A Natural Parent.* If the parents have been legally divorced, the parent to whom the court has awarded custody of the child must sign the permit. The signatures of both parents are desirable, although not essential, in cases of this type.

In the rare instances where there is a difference of opinion between undivorced parents, emergency treatment of any type CANNOT BE GIVEN if specifically prohibited by one of the parents, unless there is a provision in the law of the specific locality for the issuance of a treatment order by juvenile or other courts.

B. *A Legal Guardian,* duly appointed by court order.

C. *The Husband of a Married Female over 16, or the Wife of a Married Male over 18,* if the patient is mentally incompetent, and provided the patient has not expressly prohibited the procedure before the onset of mental incompetence.

D. *In Loco Parentis.* Any person who, in the *permanent* absence of the parents, has assumed parental obligations without the formalities of legal adoption is IN LOCO PARENTIS. For example, if an uncle or grandparent receives a niece, nephew or grandchild into his household as a member of his family, he assumes the rights and duties of the lawful parent. Since *permanent*, not temporary, custody is required, the important factor to determine in each case is whether the child has actually been deserted or abandoned by the parents. To constitute abandonment there must be actual desertion, accompanied by the intention to sever completely, or as completely as possible, the parental relationship.

70–21. Persons who may sign permits for legally adjudged mentally incompetent adults

A legally appointed guardian, usually a parent, spouse or close relative, but in some instances a nonrelated person. In this case, the legal guardian alone can sign permits, and his decision takes precedence over that of a parent or spouse.

70–22. Persons who may sign permits for adults who are temporarily mentally incompetent from serious disease or injury

A. A Spouse, provided that the patient has not expressly prohibited the procedure before becoming mentally irresponsible.

B. A Legal Guardian. If a mentally irresponsible patient is brought for emergency care without accompanying identification (transients, auto accident cases, alcoholics, attempted suicides, etc.), handling must be in accordance with the rules outlined under 70–12, above (*Emergency Care without a Surgery Permit*).

70–23. Photographing of patients

A. By News Cameramen, etc. Photographing by newspaper cameramen of injured or ill persons who are undergoing emergency care should never be allowed without the written permission of the patient or, if a minor, of a parent or legal guardian. Under no circumstances should photographs of unconscious, dazed or mentally irresponsible adult patients be allowed, even if a permit has been signed by the spouse, unless such photographs are required by law enforcement agencies for possible identification.

B. For Medical Articles, Teaching, etc. The following permit is acceptable:

CONSENT TO TAKING AND PUBLICATION OF PHOTOGRAPHS

Patient_____

Place_____

Date_____

   In connection with the medical services which I am receiving from my physician, _____M.D., I consent that photographs may be taken of me, or of parts of my body, under the following conditions:

   1. The photographs may be taken only with the consent of the physician designated above and under such conditions and at such times as he may approve.

   2. The photographs shall be taken by my physician or by a photographer approved and designated by him.

   3. Any and all photographs taken as specified above shall be used for medical purposes only.

   4. If, in the judgment of my physician, medical research, education, or science will be benefited by their use, such photographs, and information relating to my case, may be published and republished, either separately or in connection with each other, in professional journals or medical books, or used for any other purpose which my physician may deem proper in the interest of medical education, knowledge, or research; provided, however, that it is specifically understood that in any such publication or use I shall not be identified by name.

   5. The aforementioned photographs may be modified or retouched in any way that my physician, in his discretion, may consider desirable.

                    Signed_____
                                  (patient)

                    Witness_____

70–24. Sterilization permit

   If a surgical procedure which might cause sterility must be performed on an emergency—not elective—basis, the following authorization MUST be signed by both husband and wife and properly witnessed BEFORE THE OPERATION IS BEGUN.

I hereby authorize and direct_____M.D.,

or the attending physicians of the_____Hospital, to

perform the following operation upon_____,

(name of patient or "myself")

and to perform any other procedures which they may, in their absolute discretion, deem advisable or desirable during this operation.

_____

(name or description of operation)

_____

It has been explained to me, and I understand, that as a result of the operation or operations specified above I may (or will probably) be sterile. I understand that the word "sterility" means that I will be unable to reproduce, and, in giving my consent to the operation specified above and/or other procedures deemed desirable, I have in mind the possibility or probability of such a result. I hereby release

_____M.D., the attending physicians of the

_____Hospital, and the hospital, its agents and employees from any liability or responsibility for my present condition or for any condition that may result from said operation or procedures.

Date_____Hour_____Signed_____

(Patient)

Witness_____

Witness_____

I join in authorizing the performance upon my wife (husband) of the operation and procedures specified and consented to above. It has been explained to me, and I understand, that as a result of the operation, and/or procedures, my wife (husband) may be sterile.

Date_____Hour_____Signed_____

(Husband) (Wife)

Witness_____

70–25. **Tacit consent.** See Topic 18–1,B,1 (Blood Analysis).
70–26. **Telegraphic consent.** See 70–30,B, below.
70–27. **Telephonic consent.** See 70–30,C, below.
70–28. **Televising of operation**

PATIENT_____PLACE_____DATE_____

In the interest of medical education and knowledge, I hereby consent to the televising of the operation which is scheduled to be

performed upon me on or about_____19_____

I hereby authorize_____M.D. and the_____
Hospital to admit to the operating room the cameramen and technicians and other persons who are to participate in the televising of this operation.

Witness_____   Signed_____

70–29. **Termination of pregnancy permit.** (Not to be used for therapeutic abortion—this is not an emergency procedure.)

TERMINATION OF PREGNANCY RELEASE: (Other than therapeutic abortion)

I, the undersigned, am advised by the attending physicians of the

_____Hospital that I may be in a condition of abortion. I hereby declare that neither the physicians nor any persons employed by or connected with said hospital have performed any act which may have contributed directly or indirectly to the interruption of my pregnancy and do hereby release said hospital and the attending physicians from any liability or responsibility for my condition. I hereby consent and direct the attending physicians to terminate my pregnancy as an urgent medical necessity and for my physical welfare. I further release the attending physicians and the hospital and its employees from all liability for any results and consequences that may occur from the termination of my pregnancy.

Date_____Hour_____Signed_____
(Patient)

Witness_____Approved_____
(Husband)

Witness_____Approved_____

_____
(Parents, if a Minor)

70–30. **Types of valid emergency treatment permits**
    A. ***Written.*** Authorizations should always be signed if possible. If the patient is illiterate or physically unable to write, but is mentally competent, he should make

an X, with assistance if necessary. The certification by two witnesses should be as follows:

"John Doe (his mark)"　　Witness_____

　　　　　　　　　　　　Witness_____

B. Telegraphic. A copy of the telegraphic authorization must be made a permanent part of the record.

C. Telephonic. This is valid provided two persons listen in on the line and both record the time and circumstances in the patient's record. A substantiating written authorization should be obtained as soon as possible.

D. Verbal. Verbal permission or silent (tacit) acquiescence of a mentally competent adult is a valid consent, but often difficult or impossible to prove at a later date. Therefore, a properly witnessed written consent (70–14,B, above) should be obtained at the earliest possible opportunity.

70–31. **Refusal of Blood or Blood Derivatives**

At least one religious group (Jehovah's Witnesses) will not allow administration of blood or blood derivatives, even as a lifesaving measure. In circumstances of this type, to protect the attending physician and the hospital, the following form should be signed by the patient and spouse, by parents of a minor, or by the legal guardian of a mentally incompetent person.

I request that no blood or blood derivatives be administered to

_____during this hospitalization. I hereby release the hospital, its personnel and my attending physician from any responsibility whatsoever for any unfavorable reactions or untoward results due to my refusal to permit the use of blood or its derivatives. It has been clearly explained and I fully understand the possible consequences of such refusal on my part.

Date_____Signed_____

Witness_____Spouse_____

　　　　　　　　　　　　Parents_____

　　　　　　　　　　　　_____

　　　　　　　　　　　　Legal Guardian_____

---

71. RELEASE OF INFORMATION

The physician in charge of an emergency case, and all emergency personnel, should always keep in mind that medical information obtained during the physician-patient relationship is confidential and privileged, and cannot be divulged without proper authorization (Topic 70–8) except by due process of law. Therefore, only factual nonmedical information (name, address, age, how brought in, attending physician, disposition, etc.) can be given to members of the family, friends, attorneys, claim adjustors, investigators, reporters or other interested persons, unless a proper authorization has been signed by the patient or his legal guardian. If an accident requires investigation and report by a law enforcement agency, is covered by the provisions of city, county or state emergency contracts, or concerns a member of the merchant marine or armed services, a brief report, preferably in lay terms, covering the diagnosis, prognosis and disposition may be given to the investigating officer or to the proper law enforcement authorities.

A. Conditions requiring an immediate report to the proper authorities are:

1. Wounds or injuries of any degree, extent or results, self-inflicted with known or suspected suicidal intent.
2. Wounds or injuries inflicted by another person, or other persons, by means of a club, knife, gun, pistol or any other potentially deadly weapon. This includes fists or hands if the assailant is, or has been, a professional pugilist, or has been trained in judo or karate.
3. Injuries or illnesses resulting from conditions which might be dangerous to the general populace.
4. Criminal abortions, proved or suspected.
5. Injuries resulting from violation of any law. This includes minor traffic accidents.
6. Bites, animal, bat, or human.
7. Industrial conditions, i.e., injuries or illnesses covered

by state or federal compensation acts (Topic 76).
8. Conditions or injuries in which objective findings on
   examination are not in accordance with the
   history.

Since the reports completed by law enforcement officers
become public documents, medical information thereon is not
privileged and can be divulged without specific authorization
from the patient or his legal guardian.

  B. Written reports concerning diagnosis, treatment, prog-
      nosis, etc., may be made up at the request of in-
      surance adjustors, attorneys or other interested
      parties, provided a properly witnessed written au-
      thorization (Topic 70–8) signed by the patient (or
      the parent or legal guardian if the patient is a
      minor, or has been legally declared incompetent)
      has been completed and made a part of the file, and
      provided the permission of the emergency physician
      who treated the case (or his superior in a hospital
      or plant emergency department) has been obtained.
  C. Specific authorization is not a requirement for release
      of information concerning an industrial case (Topic
      76). By requesting medical care under the provi-
      sions of any of the several workmen's compensation
      acts the patient waives the physician-patient rela-
      tionship.
  D. The oral or written request or permission of a patient's
      spouse to release medical information is not ade-
      quate if the patient is physically able and mentally
      competent to make the decision regarding release of
      information.

72. RESPONSIBILITIES OF PHYSICIANS EXAMINING AND TREATING EMERGENCY CASES

A. To examine, evaluate and, if possible, establish a diagnosis on all persons with conditions requiring emergency care (Topic 1–1; and B, below) in accordance with the accepted medical standards in the community, and to use diligence, skill and knowledge equivalent to that utilized by other physicians in the same type of practice in the same or a similar community (Topic 69–3).

B. To decide whether or not persons requesting examination and treatment do, in fact, require emergency care. This very important decision is the responsibility solely of the emergency physician. Under no circumstances should it be made by a nurse, orderly, aide or clerk.

C. To be available at all times if assigned to an emergency room, station or ward.

D. To treat patients in order of urgency (Topic 20).

E. To supervise, instruct, direct and assume responsibility for professional assistants, nurses, orderlies, clerks, attendants and other emergency department personnel.

F. To be familiar with the location of, indications for, and adjustment and application of, the various types of mechanical diagnostic and therapeutic equipment available in the emergency department.

G. To be familiar with the application to emergency situations of rites of various religious denominations and sects (Topic 4–8).

H. To be aware of the laws and ordinances relating to emergency situations of the political subdivision in which he is practicing.

I. To be familiar with, and abide by, staff association constitution and by-laws, and by hospital rules, regulations and standing orders, including details of any formally outlined disaster plan, if on duty in an emergency department or ward.

J. To be familiar with accepted actions, doses, side effects and toxicity of commonly used drugs.

K. To arrange for future medical management of all persons with whom he has established a physician-patient relationship through examination, treatment or advice, with full knowledge of his responsibility until another physician takes over active supervision [Topic 65 (*Abandonment*)].

L. To complete and send with any referred or transferred patient a medical résumé giving diagnosis, treatment and recommendations. This résumé should be enclosed in a sealed envelope and a copy made a permanent part of the emergency record.

M. To evaluate the condition of each patient carefully before transfer or referral to be absolutely certain that such transportation or referral will not decrease the patient's chances of recovery or survival. In borderline cases if, in the considered judgement of the emergency physician, transportation is indicated and feasible, supportive measures (oxygen, plasma volume expanders, vasopressor drugs, etc.) should be continued in the ambulance, preferably under the supervision of a physician or registered nurse. In such cases, the attending physician should indicate in the résumé sent with the patient (L, above) his reasons for transfer.

N. To examine and determine the time of death in terminal cases under his supervision and to certify to dead on arrival (DOA) cases (Topic 4–4).

O. To cooperate with the clergy, members of law enforcement agencies, press, photographers and other interested persons within the limits established by the physician-patient relationship, applicable legal restrictions, and staff and hospital regulations.

P. To use courtesy, consideration, tact and kindness in his relations not only with his patients, but also with accompanying members of the family, relatives, friends, neighbors or other interested persons.

> **Q.** To complete a detailed, concise, accurate AND LEGI-
> BLE record on each patient, specifying not only
> WHAT was done but also WHY it was done.

73. SERVICE PERSONNEL AND DEPENDENTS

Only supportive emergency care and measures to prevent
aggravation of a condition should be given to members of any
of the branches of the Armed Services and their dependents—
enough to insure arrival at the closest Armed Services or Government hospital or clinic in satisfactory condition. Obvious or
suspected fractures and dislocations should not be x-rayed unless, in the opinion of the attending emergency physician, such
films are essential for adequate interim care. The injured part
should be splinted with an inexpensive type of splint if possible,
and pain controlled by the usual measures. Transportation, by
government ambulance if necessary, usually can be arranged
by telephonic communication with the proper government facil-
ity in the vicinity.

74. SUBPOENAS

74–1. Appearance in response to subpoena
Any physician can be subpoenaed to appear in person at any
time before any court, any administrative agency or any investigation board by any party to any legal action. Attendance
at the specified time and place is mandatory provided a legal
subpoena has been properly served and accepted. Noncompli-
ance constitutes contempt of court and can be punished ac-
cordingly.

74–2. Relief from unreasonably short notice
If a physician is served with a subpoena which specifies
appearance before an administrative agency or court on un-
reasonably or unusually short notice (for example, service at
6 P.M. to appear the next day at 9:30 A.M.), he or his attorney

usually can obtain relief by informing the clerk of the court of other pressing medical duties, with the request that attendance be continued to a later time so that advance arrangements can be made.

74–3. Duces tecum

A *subpoena duces tecum* is a court or administrative board order which requires production of certain specified documents at a specified place at a given time. This material may include original x-rays and business office records in addition to the medical chart.

74–4. Requirements for a legal subpoena

A. Specification of the date, time and place of appearance.

B. Signature of the proper official of the issuing court or administrative agency.

C. Impress of the official seal of the issuing agency (court or agency) on the original document.

74–5. Proper service

This, as a rule, is considered to mean presentation of the original subpoena (with its impressed official seal) to the subpoenee for inspection, and payment in advance of the appropriate witness fee (Topic 75–5), plus mileage at the established rate per mile from the place at which the subpoena is served to the location of the court or agency at which the subpoenee is ordered by the subpoena to appear.

75. TESTIMONY IN COURT

75–1. Required appearance

Any physician is required by law to appear in court in response to a properly completed and served subpoena (Topic 74). He may be required to appear as a factual (nonmedical), medical or expert medical witness.

75–2. Nonmedical

In this instance the physician may be called upon to testify regarding an incident concerning which he has firsthand (not hearsay) knowledge. He has the same rights, privileges and obligations as any other witness and is entitled to the nominal witness fee (plus mileage). This fee and mileage allowance must be paid in advance when the subpoena is served.

75–3. **Medical**

Any physician may be required to testify regarding findings on medical examination or treatment of any patient under his care, subject to the privileged communication rule. This means that confidential information obtained during examination or treatment, or at any other time when the patient-physician relationship is in effect, cannot be divulged except under certain circumstances. These circumstances vary in details in different localities but in general are:

A. With the permission of the patient (or his legal guardian).

B. In criminal cases.

C. In civil cases where there is a question of the mental competency of a deceased person.

D. In personal injury or wrongful death cases.

E. In certain will contests.

The usual witness fees apply unless prior arrangements have been made with the attorney. However, if the line between factual medical testimony and testimony as an expert witness (75–4, below) is crossed by the request of legal counsel for either side for interpretation of the factual testimony or for a medical opinion of any type, the physician may request that the court award to him an expert witness fee. It is advisable that this request be made to the judge before the physician leaves the witness stand.

75–4. **Expert witness**

Any person who possesses more knowledge than the court about the subject involved may be called upon as an "expert witness." Therefore, in medical matters any physician may be qualified as an expert witness even if he is not particularly trained in a given specialty, and even if he has not actually examined or treated the patient.

An expert medical witness may be required to answer hypothetical questions under oath and to give his opinion concerning diagnosis, disability, further treatment and prognosis. Whenever possible, questions should be answered by "Yes" or "No," but if qualifications are required, they will usually be allowed by the presiding judge. If sufficient facts to permit an accurate and fair answer have not been incorporated in the hypothetical question, the physician may so state and defer his answer until the judge has given his ruling regarding the need for further information.

75–5. **Fees**

Fees for acting as an expert witness vary in different localities, but they are usually based on the time spent in pretrial conferences and in court. Whenever possible, arrangements regarding the fee should be made in advance (75–6, below).

75–6. **Preparation of a court case**

   A. Routine completion of adequate records at the time of examination. In many cases, eventual court appearance can be anticipated at the time of first examination.

   B. Pretrial conferences with the attorney.

   C. Arrangements regarding expert witness fees should be made with the attorney in advance of court appearance. UNDER NO CIRCUMSTANCES should this fee be on a contingent basis. The prearranged fee should cover the pretrial conferences as well as anticipated court appearances and should apply in full regardless of the outcome of the case—won, lost, dismissed, or settled out of court. If court appearance is necessary, the prearranged fee should be in the hands of the expert witness before he goes on the stand.

75–7. **Obligations of a physician as a witness**

   A. To dress and act in a conservative, dignified manner.

   B. To give testimony distinctly with candor, sincerity and truth, avoiding medical terminology as much as possible and explaining those medical terms which are used. Above all, "talking down to" the jury in a condescending manner should be avoided. The original record can be used for reference but if so used may be admissible as evidence.

   C. To avoid taking sides, especially by coloring testimony or in other ways acting as a medical advocate.

   D. To remain calm, even-tempered and alert under cross-examination; and to avoid trying to appear clever in debate or by matching wits with the cross-examiner.

   E. To keep any differences of opinion with other physicians on an impersonal professional level.

   F. To abide scrupulously by any and all rulings made by the trial judge or other presiding officer. Questions regarding the advisability of answering questions concerning privileged or other matters can be asked directly of the judge or hearing officer.

76. WORKMEN'S COMPENSATION (INDUSTRIAL) CASES

76–1. Management on initial visit

Special forms for reporting industrial cases (injuries or illnesses caused by, or arising out of, employment) are used almost universally. ALL MEDICAL INFORMATION ON THESE FORMS MUST BE FILLED OUT IN FULL BY THE EMERGENCY PHYSICIAN AT THE FIRST EXAMINATION. Written permission of the patient is not required; by requesting treatment as an industrial case, he waives all rights to the confidential patient-physician relationship. If, after examination, the physician concludes that the injury or illness of which the patient complained was not caused by, or did not arise out of, employment, he should so inform the patient and write "Nonindustrial" across the face of the industrial form. From this point, any advice or treatment is on a nonindustrial basis.

76–2. Completion of first report of injury

Reports to employers, insurance carriers and governmental agencies must be made up immediately following the first examination. Therefore, for adequate reporting, it is essential that all spaces on the industrial form be filled in. The following is an explanation of the subheadings found on many industrial injury and illness forms.

    A. Diagnosis. This must be specific and descriptive and must indicate the severity of the condition. "Bruised finger" is worthless for industrial reporting purposes; "mild contusion volar surface distal phalanx left index finger" gives a clear picture of the location, type and severity of the injury. If a definite diagnosis cannot be established, a symptom diagnosis should be given. "Diagnosis deferred" is worthless and should never be used under any circumstances.

    Descriptive names for the digits of the hand

should always be given, i.e., thumb, index finger, middle (or long) finger, ring finger and little finger. "First," "second," etc., should never be used. Finger joints should be specified, i.e., "metacarpophalangeal," "proximal interphalangeal" and "distal interphalangeal," not "first," "second" and "third."

Negative findings are of value in diagnosis and prognosis. Examples: "Concussion of the brain— mild. Neurologic examination negative." "Laceration volar surface middle phalanx left ring finger —tendons and nerve supply not injured." "Severe contusion right supra-orbital ridge. No evidence of damage to eye."

B. P.D. (Permanent Disability). On the initial visit, only an estimate regarding ultimate permanent disability can be made. Answer "Yes" or "No." If "Yes" specify:

1. AMPUTATION? Where?
2. LOSS OF FUNCTION from limited motion, weakness or deformity. Specify whether slight, moderate or marked loss of function is anticipated.
3. COSMETIC DISFIGUREMENT sometimes constitutes a ratable permanent disability. For instance, an extensive disfiguring scar on the face might be a handicap in the labor market, while a scar on any portion of the body which is usually covered would not be.

C. Accident Sole Cause? In the majority of cases the answer is "Yes." Certain unusual circumstances, such as syncope causing a fall with resultant injury, do occur. These should be specified under "Contributing."

D. Previous Impairment. Under this heading should be given pre-existent conditions such as arthritis, limited function from old trauma or disease, etc. Aggravation of a pre-existent condition by an industrial injury is a frequent and legitimate cause of disability.

E. Treatment. Include under this heading surgical procedures, splinting, casting, medications, elastic bandages, immunizing injections, administration of anesthetics and antibiotics, and instructions regarding home care. If suturing has been done, the number and type of sutures should be specified.

F. X-Rays. "Yes" or "No." If taken, give impression or working diagnosis, subject to later confirmation by a roentgenologist (Topic 21–1).

G. Hospitalized. Give date of hospitalization, name and location of hospital, and method of transportation (private car, ambulance, etc.).

H. Further Treatment (Length). This is important information for insurance companies or employers because a reserve to meet all expenses of the case usually is set up as soon as the First Report of Injury is received. It is better to overestimate than to underestimate the treatment period.

I. Disability (How Long). If no time loss from work is anticipated, indicate as "N.T.L." (No Time Lost). If in the opinion of the examining physician the patient is unable to do his work, the expected duration of disability should be given in days, weeks or months. As in the case of length of treatment, it is better to overestimate than to underestimate.

J. To Return. The patient should be told to return at a specified time on a specified date, and this date entered on the form. Vague instructions such as "Return if doesn't feel better" or "P.R.N." should never be used.

K. Referred To. If "To Return" (J, above), has been filled out, this space can be left blank. Otherwise, specify the physician or hospital to which the patient has been instructed to report.

APPENDIX

Liquid

0.03 ml.— ½ minim	4 ml.—1 fluidrachm
0.05 ml.— ¾ minim	5 ml.—1¼ fluidrachms
0.06 ml.— 1 minim	8 ml.—2 fluidrachms
0.10 ml.— 1½ minims	10 ml.—2½ fluidrachms
0.20 ml.— 3 minims	15 ml.—4 fluidrachms
0.25 ml.— 4 minims	30 ml.—1 fluidounce
0.30 ml.— 5 minims	50 ml.—1¾ fluidounces
0.50 ml.— 8 minims	100 ml.—3½ fluidounces
0.60 ml.—10 minims	200 ml.—7 fluidounces
0.75 ml.—12 minims	250 ml.—8 fluidounces
1.00 ml.—15 minims	500 ml.—1 pint
2.00 ml.—30 minims	1000 ml.—1 quart
3.00 ml.—45 minims	4000 ml.—1 gallon

Weight

0.10 mg.—1/600 grain	40.00 mg.— ⅔ grain
0.12 mg.—1/500 grain	50.00 mg.— ¾ grain
0.15 mg.—1/400 grain	60.00 mg.— 1 grain
0.20 mg.—1/300 grain	75.00 mg.— 1¼ grains
0.25 mg.—1/250 grain	100.00 mg.— 1½ grains
0.30 mg.—1/200 grain	0.12 gm.— 2 grains
0.40 mg.—1/150 grain	0.15 gm.— 2½ grains
0.50 mg.—1/120 grain	0.20 gm.— 3 grains
0.60 mg.—1/100 grain	0.25 gm.— 4 grains
0.80 mg.—1/80 grain	0.30 gm.— 5 grains
1.00 mg.—1/60 grain	0.40 gm.— 6 grains
1.20 mg.—1/50 grain	0.50 gm.— 7½ grains
1.50 mg.—1/40 grain	0.60 gm.—10 grains
2.00 mg.—1/30 grain	0.75 gm.—12 grains
3.00 mg.—1/20 grain	1.00 gm.—15 grains
4.00 mg.—1/15 grain	1.50 gm.—22 grains
5.00 mg.—1/12 grain	2.00 gm.—30 grains (½ drachm)
6.00 mg.—1/10 grain	3.00 gm.—45 grains
8.00 mg.—⅛ grain	4.00 gm.—60 grains (1 drachm)
10.00 mg.—⅙ grain	5.00 gm.—75 grains
12.00 mg.—⅕ grain	6.00 gm.—90 grains
15.00 mg.—¼ grain	8.00 gm.— 2 drachms
20.00 mg.—⅓ grain	10.00 gm.— 2½ drachms
25.00 mg.—⅜ grain	15.00 gm.— 4 drachms
30.00 mg.—½ grain	30.00 gm.— 1 ounce

APPROXIMATE LIQUID MEASURES
(1 ml. is approximately equal to 1 cc.)

Household Measure	Metric	Apothecary
1 to 2 drops equal (varies with viscosity, specific gravity, type and fullness of container, etc.)	0.06 ml. or	1 minim
1 teaspoonful equals about	4.00 ml. or	1 fluidrachm
1 dessertspoonful equals about	8.00 ml. or	2 fluidrachms
1 tablespoonful equals about	15.00 ml. or	4 fluidrachms
1 teacupful equals about	120.00 ml. or	4 fluidounces
1 glassful equals about	250.00 ml. or	8 fluidounces
1 pint equals about	500.00 ml. or	16 fluidounces
1 quart equals about	1000.00 ml. or	32 fluidounces
1 gallon equals about	4000.00 ml. or	128 fluidounces

APPROXIMATE CONVERSION TABLES—POUNDS AND KILOGRAMS

Kilograms to Pounds		Pounds to Kilograms	
kg.	lb.	lb.	kg.
1 —	2.2	1 —	.45
2 —	4.4	2 —	.9
3 —	6.6	3 —	1.4
4 —	8.8	4 —	1.8
5 —	11.0	5 —	2.3
6 —	13.2	6 —	2.7
7 —	15.4	7 —	3.2
8 —	17.6	8 —	3.6
9 —	19.8	9 —	4.1
10 —	22.0	10 —	4.5
15 —	33.0	15 —	6.8
20 —	44.0	20 —	9.1
25 —	55.0	25 —	11.4
30 —	66.0	30 —	13.6
35 —	77.0	35 —	15.9
40 —	88.0	40 —	18.2
45 —	99.0	45 —	20.5
50 —	110.0	50 —	22.7
55 —	121.0	55 —	25.0
60 —	132.0	60 —	27.3
65 —	143.0	65 —	29.6
70 —	154.0	70 —	31.8
75 —	165.0	75 —	34.1
80 —	176.0	80 —	36.4
85 —	187.0	85 —	38.7
90 —	198.0	90 —	40.9
95 —	209.0	95 —	43.2
100 —	220.0	100 —	45.4
		125 —	56.8
		150 —	68.1
		175 —	79.5
		200 —	90.8

PERCENTAGE SOLUTION TABLE (APPROXIMATE)

Strength of Solution		Solute		Solvent
1–5	(20%)	5.40 gm.	(90.0 gr.)	to 30 ml. (1 oz.)
1–7	(15%)	4.42 gm.	(68.0 gr.)	to 30 ml. (1 oz.)
1–10	(10%)	3.00 gm.	(46.0 gr.)	to 30 ml. (1 oz.)
1–12	(8%)	2.34 gm.	(36.0 gr.)	to 30 ml. (1 oz.)
1–18	(6%)	1.75 gm.	(27.0 gr.)	to 30 ml. (1 oz.)
1–20	(5%)	1.50 gm.	(23.0 gr.)	to 30 ml. (1 oz.)
1–25	(4%)	1.08 gm.	(18.0 gr.)	to 30 ml. (1 oz.)
1–50	(2%)	0.54 gm.	(9.0 gr.)	to 30 ml. (1 oz.)
1–100	(1%)	0.25 gm.	(4.0 gr.)	to 30 ml. (1 oz.)
1–200	(½ of 1%)	0.12 gm.	(2.0 gr.)	to 30 ml. (1 oz.)
1–400	(¼ of 1%)	0.06 gm.	(1.0 gr.)	to 30 ml. (1 oz.)
1–500	—	59.15 mg.	(0.91 gr.)	to 30 ml. (1 oz.)
1–1000	—	32.50 mg.	(0.50 gr.)	to 30 ml. (1 oz.)
1–2000	—	16.00 mg.	(0.25 gr.)	to 30 ml. (1 oz.)
1–3000	—	9.70 mg.	(0.15 gr.)	to 30 ml. (1 oz.)
1–5000	—	7.15 mg.	(0.11 gr.)	to 30 ml. (1 oz.)
1–10000	—	5.8 mg.	(0.09 gr.)	to 30 ml. (1 oz.)
1–15000	—	3.0 mg.	(0.046 gr.)	to 30 ml. (1 oz.)

COMPARATIVE THERMOMETER READINGS

Fahrenheit		Centigrade	Fahrenheit		Centigrade
98.0	—	36.7	102.4	—	39.1
98.2	—	36.8	102.6	—	39.2
98.4	—	36.9	102.8	—	39.3
98.6	—	37.0	103.0	—	39.4
98.8	—	37.1	103.2	—	39.5
99.0	—	37.2	103.4	—	39.6
99.2	—	37.3	103.6	—	39.8
99.4	—	37.4	103.8	—	39.9
99.6	—	37.6	104.0	—	40.0
99.8	—	37.7	104.2	—	40.1
100.0	—	37.8	104.4	—	30.2
100.2	—	37.9	104.6	—	40.3
100.4	—	38.0	104.8	—	40.4
100.6	—	38.1	105.0	—	40.6
100.8	—	38.2	105.2	—	40.7
101.0	—	38.3	105.4	—	40.8
101.2	—	38.4	105.6	—	40.9
101.4	—	38.5	105.8	—	41.0
101.6	—	38.6	106.0	—	41.1
101.8	—	38.7	108.0	—	42.2
102.0	—	38.8	110.0	—	43.3
102.2	—	39.0			

To convert Centigrade into Fahrenheit:

Multiply by 9, divide by 5, and add 32 ($°F = \dfrac{°C \times 9}{5} + 32$)

To convert Fahrenheit into Centigrade

Subtract 32, multiply by 5, divide by 9 ($°C = \dfrac{°F - 32 \times 5}{9}$)

Index